ANESTHESIOLOGY AND THE HEART

DEVELOPMENTS IN CRITICAL CARE MEDICINE AND ANESTHESIOLOGY

Volume 23

For a list of the volumes in this series see final page of the volume.

ANESTHESIOLOGY AND THE HEART

edited by

T. H. STANLEY and R. J. SPERRY

Department of Anesthesiology,
The University of Utah Medical School,
Salt Lake City, Utah, U.S.A.

KLUWER ACADEMIC PUBLISHERS
DORDRECHT / BOSTON / LONDON

ISBN-13: 978-94-010-7379-0 e-ISBN-13: 978-94-009-1966-2
DOI: 10.1007/978-94-009-1966-2

Published by Kluwer Academic Publishers,
P.O. Box 17, 3300 AA Dordrecht, The Netherlands.

Kluwer Academic Publishers incorporates
the publishing programmes of
D. Reidel, Martinus Nijhoff, Dr W. Junk and MTP Press.

Sold and distributed in the U.S.A. and Canada
by Kluwer Academic Publishers,
101 Philip Drive, Norwell, MA 02061, U.S.A.

In all other countries, sold and distributed
by Kluwer Academic Publishers Group,
P.O. Box 322, 3300 AH Dordrecht, The Netherlands.

Printed on acid-free paper

TABLE OF CONTENTS

PREFACE

Theodore H. Stanley, M.D.

Anesthesiology and the Heart contains the Refresher Course manuscripts of the presentations of the 35th Annual Postgraduate Course in Anesthesiology which took place at The Cliff Conference Center in Snowbird, Utah, February 16-20, 1990. The chapters reflect new data and concepts within the general framework of "evaluating myocardial function," "pharmacology and the cardiac patient," "anesthesia for patients with cardiac disease," and "stress, cardiopulmonary bypass, coagulation problems and related issues." The purposes of the textbook are to 1) act as a reference for the anesthesiologists attending the meeting, and 2) serve as a vehicle to bring many of the latest concepts in anesthesiology to others within a short time of the formal presentation. Each chapter is a brief but sharply focused glimpse of the interests in anesthesia expressed at the conference. This book and its chapters should not be considered complete treatises on the subjects addressed but rather attempts to summarize the most salient points. This textbook is the eighth in a continuing series documenting the proceedings of the Postgraduate Course in Salt Lake City. We hope that this and the past and future volumes reflect the rapid and continuing evolution of anesthesiology in the late twentieth century.

LIST OF CONTRIBUTORS

Bailey, P.L.
Department of Anesthesiology, The University of Utah School of Medicine, Salt Lake City, UT 84132, U.S.A.

Barash, P.
Department of Anesthesiology, Yale University School of Medicine, New Haven, CT 06510, U.S.A.

Covino, B.G.
Department of Anesthesia, Brigham and Women's Hospital, Boston, MA 02115, U.S.A.

Foëx, P.
Nuffield Department of Anesthetics, The Radcliffe Infirmary, Oxford OX2 6HE, United Kingdom

Katz, J.
Department of Anesthesiology, University of Texas Health Science Center at Houston, Houston, TX 77030, U.S.A.

Mangano, D.T.
Department of Anesthesia, University of California, San Francisco, CA 94102, U.S.A.

Merin, R.
Department of Anesthesiology, University of Texas Health Science Center at Houston, Houston, TX 77019, U.S.A.

Miller, E.D.
Department of Anesthesiology, College of Physicians and Surgeons, Columbia University, NY 10032, U.S.A.

Muravchick, S.
Department of Anesthesia, Hospital of the University of Pennsylvania, Philadelphia, PA 19104, U.S.A.

Roizen, M.F.
Department of Anesthesiology and Critical Care, University of Chicago Medical Center, Chicago IL 60612, U.S.A.

Schultz, J.R.
Department of Anesthesiology, The University of Utah School of Medicine, Salt Lake City, UT 84132, U.S.A.

Stanley, T.H.
Department of Anesthesiology, The University of Utah School of Medicine, Salt Lake City, UT 84132, U.S.A.

Tinker, J.H.
Department of Anesthesia, University of Iowa College of Medicine, Iowa City, IA 52242, U.S.A.

Williams, J.P.
Department of Anesthesiology, University of Texas at Houston, Houston, TX 77030, U.S.A.

Wong, K.C.
Department of Anesthesiology, The University of Utah School of Medicine, Salt Lake City, UT 84132, U.S.A.

ASSESSMENT OF THE PATIENT WITH ISCHEMIC HEART DISEASE

DENNIS T. MANGANO, PH.D., M.D.

The patient with IHD usually has one of the many symptom complexes associated with varying degrees of ventricular dysfunction. Assessment of a patient with IHD presenting for surgery is usually conducted over a very brief period of time and therefore requires a rather intense assessment of the patient's cardiac status. Other factors add to the difficulties involved in this assessment: 1) The age of the population presenting for surgery is increasing; 2) surgical procedures are becoming more complex; and 3) cost containment procedures will limit the number and type of preoperative tests used to assess risk in patients with IHD, and there will be increasing pressure on us to expedite such an assessment (e.g., come-and-go, come-and-stay surgery). Thus, more than ever, we must know what specific tests are available for assessment of these patients and what information we can obtain from these tests to determine perioperative risk, preoperative therapeutics, intraoperative monitoring, choice of anesthetic, and postoperative care.

IHD is a significant problem and will probably remain so well into the 1990s. This is substantiated by several statistics accumulated in the early 1980s from the United States. It is estimated that 10 million patients have IHD in the United States today, 4 million of whom have had previous myocardial infarctions. In any one year, approximately 1.5 million patients develop a new myocardial infarction and 700,000 deaths are attributed to IHD per year. Surgical procedures performed each year on these patients include approximately 800,000 cardiac catheterizations, with 285,000 coronary artery bypass grafts and an equal number of coronary angioplasties. It is estimated that of the 20 million patients in the United States that undergo surgery each year, approximately 1 to 2 million have IHD or are at high risk for it. Thus, the problem is significant to anesthesiologists. It appears that the prognosis for patients with IHD is related to the development and severity of dysrhythmias, myocardial infarction and ventricular dysfunction. Before proceeding with a discussion of the tests used for IHD, it is important to review the significance of dysrhythmias, infarction and dysfunction in patients with IHD.

T. H. Stanley and R. J. Sperry (eds.), Anesthesiology and the Heart, 1–11.

THE SIGNIFICANCE OF DYSRHYTHMIAS IN IHD

Incidence

In cases of acute myocardial infarction virtually all patients develop premature ventricular contractions within the first five days. Within one to three weeks following infarction, 73-94% of patients develop one or more dysrhythmias. In cases of chronic IHD, the incidence of patients in whom dysrhythmia is the predominant manifestation is unknown. It is known, however, that the most common dysrhythmias with chronic IHD are premature ventricular contractions (PVCs). Also, if chronic PVCs are frequent, multiform, or R-on-T, they are predictive of multivessel disease or significant ventricular dysfunction.

Detection

Detection of dysrhythmias depends on the duration of observation and the degree of stress.

Test	*Incidence of Ventricular Dysrhythmias*
EKG-rest (< 1 minute)	14%
EKG-rest (1 hour observation)	50%
EKG-routine activity (24-hour observation)	88%
EKG-stress testing (< 1 hour)	52-61%

Although 24-hour monitoring detects ventricular tachycardia approximately twice as often as stress testing, in 10% of the patients, serious dysrhythmias (VT, VF) are detected only with stress testing.

Prognosis

The most serious dysrhythmias are ventricular fibrillation and tachycardia, and complex PVCs (R-on-T, multiform, repetitive). These carry the greatest risk of sudden death and are predictive of multivessel disease. Also significant are the conduction disturbances: complete heart block, Mobitz II and bundle branch block (mortality 10 to 70%). Acute atrial dysrhythmias are usually indicative of concurrent disease, and are associated with significant risk if accompanied by acute ischemia or left ventricular failure.

Perioperative Risk

In patients with and without IHD, perioperative dysrhythmias commonly occur (17.9 to 61.7%), and are usually associated with stimulation, CO_2 elevation, hypertension, potassium loss, digitalis therapy and specific anesthetics. Most of these dysrhythmias are supraventricular or PVCs, and few (< 1%) are associated with serious sequelae.

In patients with heart disease (IHD, hypertensive, valvular and congenital) or pre-existing dysrhythmias, the incidence of perioperative dysrhythmias (benign and serious) is increased by as much as threefold. The type of heart disease (IHD vs. valvular) and the severity of the disease (NYHA II vs. IV) appear to be the most critical factors. More informative data are lacking.

It thus seems reasonable to conclude that those patients with IHD who are at highest risk of developing serious perioperative dysrhythmias have: 1) prior infarction complicated by serious dysrhythmias, 2) evidence of ventricular dysfunction, or 3) recurrent or persistent dysrhythmias detected with the rest or exercise EKG.

THE SIGNIFICANCE OF INFARCTION IN IHD

Incidence

Approximately 4 million people in the United States have had one or more myocardial infarctions. Each year, 1.3 million patients develop a new myocardial infarction.

Detection

The hallmarks of the clinical diagnosis are history, EKG and serum enzymes. The classical findings are well known and will not be discussed. But of note are the following:

a. History: Most patients have angina with infarction. However, 20-33% of infarcts are painless, and 35-90% have no prodromal symptoms. Silent extension of MIs has been reported in up to 57% of patients.

b. EKG: With infarction, acute changes in the EKG are characteristic. However, in 20-50% of patients the EKG is non-diagnostic (subendocardial MI, LBBB, WPW, LVH). Furthermore, only 25-50% of old myocardial infarctions can be detected by EKG.

c. Enzymes: In patients with a positive history for acute transmural MI and Q waves on EKG, SGOT, LDH and CPK-MB are elevated virtually all the time (94%, 100%, 100%). However, in patients with a history suggestive of an MI and with persistent ST-T wave changes (> 24 hours), elevation of these enzymes is not as frequent (63%, 71%, 84%).

d. Other Diagnostic Tests: Echocardiography, nuclear radiology and cardiac catheterization are useful for detection of wall-motion abnormalities and evaluation of ventricular function. These are discussed in the last section.

Prognosis

For the past 20 years, the annual mortality following myocardial infarction has been 5-8%. The acute in-hospital mortality is 10-40%. Following infarction, short- and long-term prognoses are most significantly affected by:

a. The degree of ventricular dysfunction following infarction.

Highest risk: CHF symptoms, EF < .40, dyssynergy

b. The site of infarction/extent of disease.
   Highest risk: anterior wall infarct, diffuse 3-vessel, left-main disease
c. The type of post-infarction dysrhythmias and conduction disturbances.
   Highest risk: fascicular block, complete heart block, serious ventricular dysrhythmias

Perioperative Risk

PREVIOUS STUDIES

	1962 (Knapp)	1964 (Tompkins)	1972 (Tarhan)	1978 (Steen)	1978 (Goldman)	TOTAL (Average)
Patients Studied	8,984	12,712	32,877	73,321	1,001	128,895
Previous MI	427	658	422	587	131	2,225
Reinfarction %	6.1%	6.5%	6.5%	6.1%	13.7%	6.8%
Reinfarction Mortality	58%	70%	54%	69%	67%	65%
% Reinfarction:						
0-3 months	100%		37%	27%		
		55%			36%	
3-6 months	100%		16%	11%		

Previous studies have demonstrated that in patients with prior infarction: 1) the overall risk of reinfarction is 6-7% (vs. < 1% without previous MI); 2) with recent infarction (within 6 months), the risk of reinfarction is high (36 to 100%); 3) mortality with reinfarction is high (54 to 70%); and 4) the statistics have not changed over the previous two decades. However, a recent study has found significantly reduced six-month reinfarction rates (5%) and mortality (2%) when aggressive monitoring and therapy are used. These results have significant implication, and certainly warrant independent verification.

Given a patient with a recent infarction, what risk factors place that patient at highest risk?

Preoperative Risk Factors

History:	recent MI (< 6 months), crescendo angina
Physical:	hypertension, CHF
EKG:	Q waves, BBB, CHB, LVH (strain), ventricular dysrhythmia
CXR:	cardiomegaly, CHF
Cath:	2-, 3-vessel disease, left-main disease, EF < .50, valve disease

In addition to these preoperative factors, the intraoperative factors associated with highest risk are: 1) surgery involving the great vessels, thorax, or upper abdomen; 2) emergency surgery; and 3) the degree and duration of intraoperative hypotension.

THE SIGNIFICANCE OF VENTRICULAR DYSFUNCTION IN IHD

Incidence

Approximately 700,000 patients die each year from IHD and its complications. With acute myocardial infarction, death usually results from ventricular dysrhythmias or failure. It appears that the mortality from dysrhythmias has been reduced by EKG monitoring and aggressive therapy. However, mortality from failure remains alarmingly high.

Detection

Quantitated ventriculography, nuclear cardiology and echocardiography provide sensitive measures of ventricular function: ejection fraction, wall motion, and myocardial compliance. The sensitivity of these is summarized by the following.

Measure	*Abnormality first appears with*
Ejection fraction	1-, 2-vessel disease (without MI)
Wall motion (dyssynergy)	3-vessel disease (without MI)
Compliance	MI
Cardiac output	MI + 3-vessel disease
End diastolic pressure	MI + 3-vessel disease

Prognosis

In patients with acute or chronic IHD, the degree of left ventricular dysfunction is of major prognostic importance. Ejection fraction and dyssynergy appear to be the best prognostic indicators of short- and long-term survival. One-year mortality is significantly higher (30%) in patients with ejection fractions < .40. In patients with three-vessel disease and EF < .50, the two-year mortality is 36% (vs. 12% with EF > .50). With single-vessel disease, patients with markedly abnormal wall motion have a five-year mortality of 60% (vs. 10% with normal wall motion). With three-vessel disease, the mortality is 90% (vs. 35% with normal wall motion).

Perioperative Risk

In patients with manifest symptoms and signs of left ventricular failure, the perioperative morbidity and mortality are markedlyincreased. Preoperative assessment is relatively straightforward. However, for the asymptomatic patient with IHD, assessment of the risk of ventricular failure is more difficult. In patients with IHD undergoing non-cardiac surgery, there are no significant data. In patients undergoing myocardial revascularization, the studies indicate that of all the preoperative screening data (routine, EKG, and catheterization), ejection fraction and degree of dyssynergy are the best predictors of left and right ventricular dysfunction during the intraoperative and postoperative periods. Furthermore, studies of short- and long-term survival following cardiac surgery have demonstrated that the preoperative LV ejection fraction is the most useful prognostic guide compared with such measures as cardiac output and end-diastolic pressure.

PREOPERATIVE ASSESSMENT: ADDITIONAL INFORMATION

The preoperative screening data most relevant to the assessment of dysrhythmias, infarction and dysfunction are discussed above. In addition, the following appear to be informative and prognostic.

History

1. Anginal pattern - stable vs. unstable vs. variant
   - stress response, exercise tolerance
2. Dysrhythmia/failure symptoms with stress and effort.
3. Medication compliance (nitrates, beta blockers, Ca^{++} channel blockers)

The history is the focal point of the assessment. However, there does not appear to be a consistent relationship between the historical features of angina (location, duration, precipitation) and the extent of vessel involvement.

Physical Examination

On cardiac exam, the significance of the following four findings is noteworthy.

1. Displaced PMI: Cardiomegaly - usually indicates an EF < .50 and places the patient at increased risk.
2. Precordial systolic bulge: Wall motion abnormality - usually indicates a prior MI or acute ischemia.
3. S_3: Increased LVEDP - usually indicates extensive MI.
4. S_4: Decreased LV compliance - usually indicates a prior MI or ischemia.

Chest X-Ray

In patients with IHD, cardiomegaly (cardiothoracic ratio > .50) is predictive of poor ventricular function (EF < .50) in approximately 70% of patients. Other changes (increased LV volume, increased total heart volume) are equally predictive.

EKG (resting)

Positive Findings: The EKG is a reliable predictor of IHD only when: 1) significant Q waves are present, or 2) ST changes occur with spontaneous angina (stable, unstable or variant). Other findings on the EKG (ST-T wave changes, LBBB, LVH) are non-specific.

Negative Findings: A normal EKG does not preclude IHD. In 25-50% of patients with IHD the resting EKG is normal. However, it is rarely normal in the patient with significant left ventricular dyssynergy.

EKG (vector)

Vectorcardiography is useful in depicting infarction patterns where the scalar EKG is equivocal. There is also evidence that selected abnormal vector patterns are indicative of severe abnormality of left ventricular function.

EKG (ambulatory-Holter)

Compared with other methods of EKG monitoring, ambulatory monitoring significantly increases the yield of dysrhythmias. However, stress-response dysrhythmias may be missed. The yield of ST-segment changes is also increased, and a good correlation exists between ST depression occurring during normal activity and angiographic findings. However, the artifact problem is significant, and affects the reliability of ST interpretation.

EKG (stress-testing)

For dysrhythmia detection, the "exercise EKG (EEKG)" increases the yield of PVCs threefold (over the rest EKG) and eightfold for repetitive forms of ventricular dysrhythmias. Approximately 52% of patients with IHD exhibit PVCs on EEKG. The dysrhythmias usually occur not only at peak exercise, but also during the initial 3 minutes of recovery. In fact, ventricular fibrillation is most likely to occur during recovery.

For ischemia detection, the EEKG is informative if 1) the ST change is significant (> 2 mm); 2) symptoms or hypotension occur with the ST change; or 3) the changes occur during the early testing period. Without these changes, it appears that exercise stress testing does not significantly improve diagnostic capability.

Echocardiography

One dimensional (M-mode) and two-dimensional (2D) echocardiography are safe and non-invasive techniques used in IHD primarily for assessing left ventricular wall motion and function (LV volumes, ejection fraction). They have also been used for detection of left-main stenosis, LV aneurysms, septal rupture, papillary muscle abnormality and mural thrombus formation.

Wall Motion

1. M-mode echocardiography is not satisfactory. Although 1-2 mm sensitivity can be achieved, the beam is narrow (one dimensional) and only the basal LV is viewed.

2. 2D echocardiography is useful and reasonably accurate in 80-90% of patients with IHD. 2D wall-motion abnormalities correlate well with the location and extent of acute MI scarring (post-mortem studies in dogs). Comparison with angiography demonstrates good correlation (84-97%), specificity (84%), and sensitivity (95%). Limitations include: 1) the technique varies from laboratory to laboratory; 2) technical difficulties (COPD, anatomic abnormalities) limit use; 3) multiple cross-sectional views are necessary; and 4) inferior-posterior dyssynergy is more difficult to detect (vs. anterior).

Left Ventricular Function

1. M-mode echocardiography is inaccurate when dyssynergy is present. LV function is assessed by measuring the internal diameter of the LV along the beam at end-diastole ($LVID_d$) and end-systole ($LVID_s$). $LVID_d$ is accurate with or without dyssynergy. $LVID_s$, in the presence of dyssynergy, is inaccurate. Thus, estimates of ESV, SV, CO and EF may be inaccurate.

2. 2D echocardiography provides useful information if multiple cross-sections (> 2) are used. 2D ejection fraction correlates well with angiographic ejection fraction (.78 to .94). However, 2D left ventricular volumes consistently underestimate angiographic volumes by 30%, especially when less than 4 cross-sections are used. Thus, stroke volumes and cardiac outputs are underestimated. Estimates of ejection fraction are more accurate because of cancellation of errors. However, 3 or more cross-sections should be used for accurate estimation of ejection fraction.

Nuclear Cardiology

Radioisotope imaging for detection of myocardial infarction and quantitation of ventricular function is safe and relatively non-invasive.

Myocardial Infarction

Use of radioisotope imaging for detection of myocardial infarction is useful when conventional methods (symptoms, EKG, enzymes) are equivocal or untimely (LBBB, WPW, < 6 hours or > 48 hours post-MI). Two different techniques are used: "hot spot" and "cold spot" imaging.

	"Hot spot" Imaging	*"Cold spot" Imaging*
Radionuclide	Technetium ^{99}m-pyrophosphate	Thallium-201
Uptake by	Infarcted tissue	Normal tissue (normal perfusion and metabolism)
Positive with	Acute MI (> 5 gm infarct)	Acute MI (> 5 gm infarct) Old MI Ischemia
Timing:		
Earliest positive test	12-16 hours (post MI)	immediately
Most sensitive	48-72 hours	< 24 hours
Other uses	RV MI Subendocardial MI Infarct size (+/-)	Chamber size LVH, RVH, ASH Stress testing

Left Ventricular Function

Two techniques are used: first pass radionuclide angiography and gated cardiac blood pool.

	First-Pass	*Gated-Pool*
Radionuclide	Any technetium (99m) labeled pharmaceutical	Technetium (99m) labeled albumin or RBC
Type of technique	Transient (30 seconds) Multiple injections/hour	Steady state (6 hours) Single injection/hours
EF correlation with angiography	>.90	>.90
Uses	LVEF Exercise testing Dyskinesis RVEF Intracardiac shunt	LVEF Exercise Testing Dyskinesis
Geometric Assumptions	None	Several

Cardiac Catheterization

Coronary angiography and ventriculography are the "gold standards" for definition of coronary anatomy and quantitation of ventricular function. In these regards, no other techniques are as accurate or informative.

Procedure

1. The catheter is advanced retrograde: peripheral artery to left ventricle.
2. Pressure measurements (systemic, ventricular, atrial) are made.
3. Ventriculography (single-plane or bi-plane) is performed using a highly osmotic contrast dye (10-18 ml/sec over 3-4 seconds).
4. Left ventricular volumes are measured (area-length method)
5. Segmental wall motion is quantitated (using hemiaxial shortening, segmental ejection fraction or percent asynergic segments)
6. Pressure measurements are repeated.
7. Selective coronary angiography is performed.

Information

Ventricular Function Data:
1) Ejection fraction (most important)
2) Dyssynergy
3) Stroke work
4) End-systolic volume
5) End-diastolic volume
6) Change in end-diastolic pressure (dye)
7) Cardiac output
8) End-diastolic pressure

Angiographic Data:
1) Number and degree of vessel involvement
2) Presence of left main (equivalent) disease - especially with a high grade right coronary lesion or a left-dominant circulation.

REFERENCES

Background

1. Kannel WB, McGee D, Gorden T: A general cardiovascular risk profile: The Framingham Study. Am J Cardiol 38:46, 1976
2. Gorleri R: Coronary Artery Disease. WB Saunders, Philadelphia, 1976
3. Cohn PF: Diagnosis and Therapy of Coronary Artery Disease. Little, Brown and Co, Boston, 1979

Dysrhythmia

1. Ruberman LD, Weinblatt E, Goldberg JE et al: Ventricular premature beats and mortality after myocardial infarction. N Engl J Med 279:759, 1977

2. Jelinek MV and Lown B: Exercise stress testing for exposure of cardiac arrhythmia. Prog Cardiovasc Dis 26:497, 1974

3. Angelini P, Feldman MI, Lufschanowski R et al: Cardiac arrhythmias during and after heart surgery. Prog Cardiovasc Dis 16:469, 1974

Myocardial Infarction

1. Tarhan S, Moffitt EA, Taylor WF et al: Myocardial infarction after general anesthesia. JAMA 220:1451, 1972

2. Goldman L, Caldera DL, Nussbaum SB et al: Multifactorial index of cardiac risk in noncardiac surgical procedures. N Engl J Med 297:845, 1977

3. Rao TLK, El-Etra A: Myocardial reinfarction following anesthesia in patients with recent infarctions. Anesth Analg 60:271, 1981

Ventricular Dysfunction

1. Moraski RE, Russell RO, Smith M et al: Left ventricular function in patients with and without myocardial infarction and one, two or three vessel coronary artery disease. Am J Cardiol 35:1, 1975

2. Cohn PF, Gorlin R, Cohn LH et al: Left ventricular ejection fraction as a prognostic guide in surgical treatment of coronary and valvular heart disease. Am J Cardiol 34:136, 1979

3. Mangano DT, Van Dyke DC, Ellis RJ: The effect of increasing preload on ventricular output and ejection in man: Limitations of the Frank-Starling mechanism. Circulation 62:535, 1980

Assessment

1. Proudfit WL, Shirey EK, Sones FM: Selective cine coronary arteriography: Correlation with clinical findings in 1,000 patients. Circulation 33:901, 1966

2. Borer JS, Brensike JF, Redwood DR et al: Limitations of the electrocardiographic response to exercise in predicting coronary artery disease. NEJM 293:367, 1975

3. Reeder GS, Seward JB, Tajik AJ: The role of two-dimensional echocardiography in coronary artery disease. Mayo Clin Proc 57:247, 1982

4. Folland ED, Hamilton GW, Larson SM et al: The radionuclide ejection fraction: A comparison of three radionuclide techniques with contrast angiography. J Nucl Med 18:1159, 1977

5. Mangano DT: Preoperative assessment of cardiac catheterization data: Which parameters are most important? Anesthesiology 53:S106, 1980

EVALUATING THE RIGHT VENTRICLE

P.Foëx

Introduction

Experimental evidence in which extensive destruction of the free wall of the right ventricule did not cause a significant increase in central venous pressure (1) or a marked reduction in cardiac output (2), has led to the view that right ventricular contraction may not be essential for the maintenance of adequate circulatory function. This may be true when the pulmonary circulation offers a low resistance to right ventricular ejection, but is untrue when pulmonary vascular resistance is high, or in the presence of an extensive myocardial infarction.

Relatively recently, Laver recognized that acute right ventricular dysfunction occurs in critically ill patients and is an important determinant of the overall effect of acute illnesses, especially respiratory failure, on the circulation (3). Indeed, marked abnormalities of their cardiovascular function have been identified in patients with respiratory failure. These include pulmonary arterial hypertension, elevated pulmonary vascular resistance, and depressed ventricular performance. Intermittent positive pressure ventilation, especially when associated with positive end-expiratory pressure improves arterial oxygenation but may exert adverse effects on the cardiovascular system, because it increases pulmonary vascular resistance.

Similarly, it is only relatively recently that the clinical significance of right ventricular infarction has been recognized (4). As right ventricular infarction occurs in about 25% of patients suffering from posterior left ventricular infarction, it is far from being an uncommon condition.

T. H. Stanley and R. J. Sperry (eds.), Anesthesiology and the Heart, 13–24.

In order to understand the clinical features and special modalities of treatment of right ventricular failure, it is important to consider the functional anatomy of the right ventricle.

Functional anatomy of the right ventricle

The right ventricle is a crescent shaped, thin walled cavity bordered by a concave free wall and the convex interventricular septum. The right ventricle extends from the right atrioventricular (tricuspid) valve nearly to the cardiac apex and then continues upwards and to the left forming the infundibulum that reaches the pulmonary orifice. The right ventricle possesses an inflow orifice (tricuspid valve), an inflow tract leading at an obtuse angle to an outflow tract (infundibulum), and an outflow orifice (pulmonary valve). The infundibulum provides support for the pulmonary valve cusps as it remains contracted during early diastole.

The myocardium of the right ventricle consists of fibres within a network of supportive connective tissue. The direction of imbrication of fibres reverses at the equator in a figure of eight. The attachment of the right ventricular free wall to the left ventricular and septal myocardium contributes to the inter-dependence between the ventricles and facilitates right ventricular emptying (5,6). Because of this attachment of the free wall, ventricular output may be maintained provided the wall offers sufficient elastance so that traction by adjacent muscle fibres displaces it towards the septum.

Patterns of right ventricular contraction

Contraction begins with the downward motion of the tricuspid valve, followed by the inward motion of the free wall (Figure 1). Finally, an inward motion of the septum completes ejection. Further complexity results from the relative asynchrony of contraction of the free wall. Contraction starts in the inflow tract and progresses toward the outflow tract in a peristalsis-like fashion. Outflow tract contraction lags behind inflow tract contraction by at least 25 milliseconds (7), so that in the early phase of contraction the inflow tract contracts while the outflow tract dilates (Figure 2). During early diastole, shortening in the outflow tract persists and it has been postulated that the outflow tract supports the pulmonary valve.

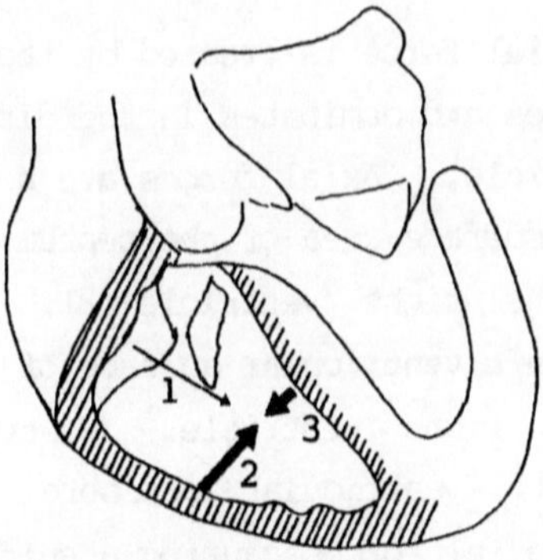

Figure 1. Diagrammatic representation of the three phases of right ventricular contraction

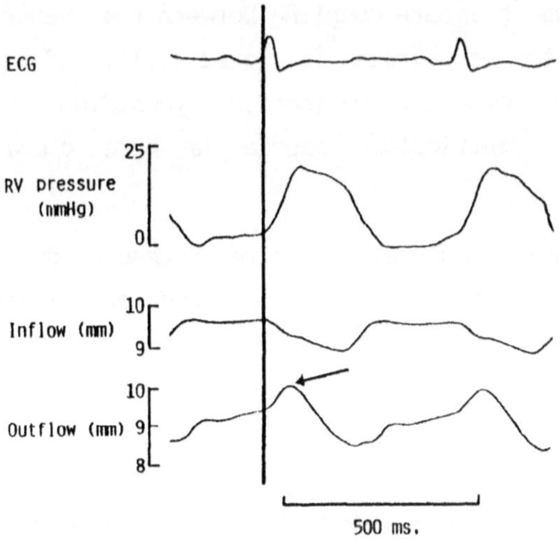

Figure 2. Differences in the time of onset of shortening are observed in the right ventricle. The arrow shows that the outflow tract dilates as the inflow tract contracts.

Interactions between right and left ventricles

a) Muscle: As some fibre pathways run continuously from the free wall of the right ventricle to the septum and the anterior wall of the left ventricle there is mechanical linkage. Thus, changes in the dimensions and performance of one ventricle influence the geometry and dynamics of the other.

b) Septum: A radial force is created by the tethering action of the muscle fibres and dominates in the direction of the free wall of the left ventricle. Axial forces are a function of the chamber pressure and the surface area of the septum and tend to bow the septum toward the right ventricle (8). Normally, axial forces dominate on the left ventricular surface of the septum so that it bowes into the right ventricle. However, acute or chronic increases in right ventricular pressure or volume, alter the distribution of axial forces causing a shift of the septum towards the left ventricle (3,8). Thus, the geometry and distensibility of the left ventricle are modified by changes in right ventricular dynamics and vice-versa.

c) Pericardium: pressure coupling between the ventricles is very close when the pericardiun is closed (9,10) and the heart is best viewed as a composite pericardium-myocardium shell. In this shell, the ventricular muscle is more compliant than the pericardium.

d) Intrathoracic pressure: negative pressure during inspiration increases the pressure gradient between extra- and intrathoracic veins; this facilitates the filling of the right heart. However, venous return to the left ventricle is impeded during inspiration because of an increase of the capacitance of the pulmonary vascular bed (11). With intermittent positive pressure ventilation, mean intrathoracic pressure increases and this augments the resistance to right ventricular ejection; an increase in the radius of curvature of the septum may be observed (8).

Determinants of right ventricular performance

Right ventricular performance, depends on at least four major determinants: afterload, preload, contractility and compliance. Furthermore, interactions with left ventricular function must be taken into consideration.

a) Afterload. The marked influence of afterload on the right ventricular stroke volume has been demonstrated by Ghignone, Girling and Previtt (12). Increases in pulmonary vascular resistance by embolisation cause marked reductions of stroke volume. As the wall of the right ventricle is thin, it is more sensitive to an increase in afterload than the left ventricle.

b) Preload. Weber and his colleagues (13) have shown that and increase in end-diastolic volume causes a shift to the right of the pump function curve of the right ventricle.

c) Contractility. Dobutamine, at constant end-diastolic volume, causes a shift to the right of the ventricular pump function curve, demonstrating that right ventricular function responds to positive inotropic interventions (13).

d) Compliance. As the wall of the right ventricle is thin, its compliance is high. However, the pericardium and interventricular mechanical linkages reduce it. Because of the linkages, increases in left ventricular end-diastolic pressure reduce, while reductions in left ventricular end-diastolic pressure increase right ventricular compliance. Similarly, increases in right ventricular end-diastolic presure decrease left ventricular compliance. In many patients suffering from the adult respiratory distress syndrome, the pulmonary capillary wedge pressure is elevated even though the end-diastolic volume of the left ventricle is not increased. This indicates that right ventricular dilatation (due to pulmonary hypertension) decreases left ventricular compliance (6). Pharmacologically mediated reductions in pulmonary vascular resistance unload the right ventricle and by this mechanism increase left ventricular compliance, presumably by reducing the degree of leftward shift of the septum.

Coronary circulation

Coronary blood flow to the right ventricle occurs during both systole and diastole. This is not surprising since the "coronary driving pressure" (the difference between aortic pressure and right ventricular pressure) is high throughout the cardiac cycle (14). However, in the presence of pulmonary hypertension, right ventricular pressure increases and systolic coronary flow is maintained only as long as aortic pressure is high (15). It is now recognised that an adequate aortic pressure is essential if right ventricular function is to be maintained in the face of pulmonary hypertension.

Evaluation of RV function.

a) Radionuclides

The marked variability in the anatomy of the right ventricle makes it difficult to use geometric assumptions to calculate ventricular volumes and ejection fractions. However, as scintigraphic techniques are independent from geometric assumptions, they are theoretically more accurate.

With first pass radionuclide angiography, high count rates from a multicrystal scintillation counter after injection of a technetium-labelled radiopharmaceutical, can be obtained. Analysis of the right and left ventricular time curves allows ventricular ejection fractions to be calculated. With gated first pass radionuclide angiography, data acquisition is gated to the "R" wave of the electrocardiogram and 14 to 16 frames are obtained for each cardiac cycle. From the sums of end-diastolic and end-systolic counts, RV ejection fraction may be calculated.

Gated cardiac blood pool imaging allows the entire equilibrium blood pool to be imaged at various phases during the cardiac cycle, the "R" wave being used to determine the onset of data acquisition. A large number of frames (14 to 32) per cardiac cycle are usually obtained. Technetium-labelled albumin or red blood cells are used because they remain within the intravascular space. From equilibrium studies, regional wall motion may be evaluated, as well as global ejection fraction.

Radionuclides may be used to determine the presence of right ventricular infarction. Technetium pyrophosphate is taken up by infarcted myocardial tissue, so that infarction is detectable as early as 12 to 16 hours after onset of symptoms. The extent of right ventricular infarction, assessed by scintigraphy is a predictor of right ventricular failure (16).

b. Thermodilution techniques

The development of fast response thermistors has made it possible to measure right ventricular ejection by the thermodilution technique (17). This technique relies on the conservation of heat energy during successive cardiac cycles. The plateaus of blood temperature at the end of the first three cardiac cycles during the recovery of temperature after a bolus of cold saline are used to calculate two mean residual fractions, and from them the mean ejection fraction. This method correlates well with the first pass radionuclear technique (18). Difficulties arise when patients are in atrial fibrillation, suffer from tricuspid regurgitation or intracardiac shunts. However, this method is simple, inexpensive, and is particularly useful for the serial monitoring of right ventricular performance, especially in respiratory failure.

c. Echocardiography

Two-dimensional echocardiography provides accurate measurements of right ventricular size. This is important in order to detect non-invasively right ventricular overload and its effect on the septum and hence on left ventricular dynamics. In pulmonary hypertension, and during ventilation with high levels of PEEP, right ventricular pressure overload can be demonstrated by echocardiography.

Right ventricular infarction

Right ventricular infarction occurs in about 25% of patients suffering from posterior left ventricular infarction, usually in association with a severe stenosis of the coronary artery responsible for perfusing the posterior wall. The association of transmural infarction of the ventricular septum is a critial factor in the development of the characteristic haemodynamic profile of right ventricular infarction.

Depending on the extent of right ventricular damage, right atrial presure may be elevated, being equal or greater that the pulmonary capillary wedge pressure. If right ventricular output is impaired, a picture of hypotension, low cardiac index, elevated central venous pressure associated with clear lung fields and relatively low pulmonary capillary wedge pressure will develop. Typically the right ventricle is distended and extensive wall motion abnormalities are observed, together with a greatly reduced ventricular ejection fraction. ST-segement elevation in the more rightward-placed chest leads (V_3R, V_4R) is a reliable sign of right ventricular infarction (19).

The therapeutic implications of right ventricular infarction are: 1) the need to maintain adequate biventricular filling; 2) the need to preserve or restore an appropriately timed atrial contraction (this may require cardioversion in patients with atrial fibrillation, or sequential atrial and ventricular pacing in those with heart blocks); 3) caution in the use of morphine or glyceryltrinitrate because they may acutely decrease right ventricular filling.

Afterload mismatch

In patients suffering from acute, or acute on chronic pulmonary hypertension, acute right ventricular failure may develop. This failure may be due to the increase in right ventricular afterload alone. However, besides the purely mechanical effect of increased afterload, relative myocardial ischaemia may play an important role. This is suggested by the results of experimental studies involving acute pulmonary hypertension. In such studies, the administration of phenylephrine, given to increase systemic arterial pressure, and therefore the coronary perfusion pressure of the right ventricle, has been shown to increase coronary blood flow and to improve stroke volume (Figure 3;20). As right ventricular afterload

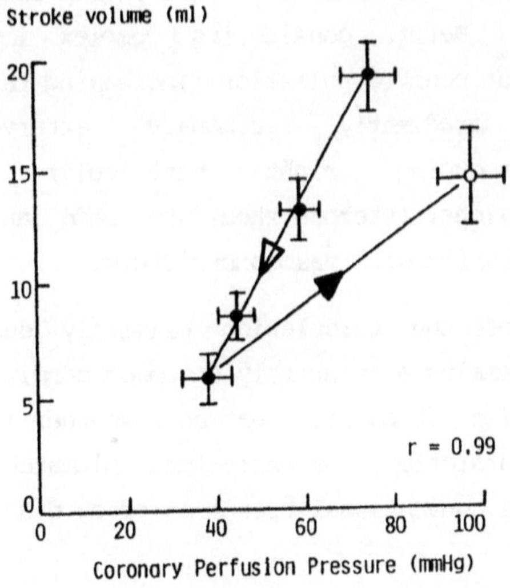

Figure 3. Gradual pulmonary hypertension (▷) causes a marked reduction in stroke volume. Phenylephrine increases stroke volume (▶)

remained unchanged, the improvement in right ventricular function must be ascribed to better myocardial perfusion. Several studies have shown that relative hypoperfusion of the right ventricular myocardium occurs when acute, or acute on chronic pulmonary hypertension develops (21). An imbalance of oxygen supply and demand occurs even though the coronary arteries are normal. A syndrome of relative coronary ischaemia leading to right ventricular failure is now recognized in patients suffering from pulmonary arterial hypertension. In such patients, peripheral vasoconstriction using phenyelephrine or noradrenaline may cause a dramatic improvement in right ventricular function because it restores an adequate right ventricular coronary perfusion pressure gradient. In these patients, it may be tempting to use vasodilators to decrease right ventricular afterload. However, most vasodilators exert their effects on both the systemic and the pulmonary circulation; their administration may be associated with the worsening of right ventricular perfusion if aortic pressure is reduced. Indeed, attempts at reducing pulomnary pressure by the use of prostacyclin have been successful only when systemic arterial pressure was maintained by the simultaneous administration of vasopressors (22). Before considering complex interventions such as aortic balloon counter pulsation (increasing the diastolic coronary perfusion gradient), pulmonary artery balloon counterpulsation (reducing right ventricular afterload), ventricular assist devices, attempts should be made at improving right ventricular perfusion with vasoconstrictors.

While failure of the circulation primarily due to right ventricular failure remains a relatively uncommon condition, it is important to recognize it as its treatment, whether it is due to right ventricular infarction, or afterload mismatch, differs substantially from the conventional treatment of cardiac failure.

References

1 Starr I, Jeffers WA, Meade JR. Am Heart J, 1943; **26**: 291-301.

2 Brooks H, Kirk ES, Vokonas PS, Urschel CW, Sonnenblick EH. J Clin Invest, 1971; **50**: 2176-2183.

3 Laver MB, Strauss HW, Pohost GM. Crit Care Med, 1979; **7**: 509-519.

4 Cohn JN, Guiha NH, Broder MI, Limas CJ. Am J Cardiol, 1974; **33**, 209-214.

5 Streeter DD jr, Vaishnav RV, Patel DJ, Spotniz HM, Ross J jr, Sonnenblick EH. Biophys J, 1970; **10**: 345-363.

6 McCallum JB. On the muscular architecture and growth of the ventricles of the heart. Welch Festschrift. Johns Hopkins Hosp Reports, 1900; **9**: 307-335.

7 Raines RA, LeWinter MM, Covell JW. Am J Physiol, 1976, **231**: 1395-1400.

8 Weber KT, Janicki JS, Shroff SG, Likoff MJ. Clin Chest Med, 1983; **4,(2)**: 101-110.

9 Laks MM, Garner D, Swan HJC. Circulation Res, 1967; **20**, 565-569.

10 Elzinga G, von Grondelle R, Westerof N, van den Bos GC. Am J Physiol, 1974; **226**: 941-947.

11 Weber KT, Janicki JS, Shroff SG, Likoff MJ, St.John Sutton MG. Crit Care Med, 1983; **11**: 323-328.

12 Ghignone M, Girling L, Prewitt RM. Am J Physiol, 1984; **246**: H339-H343.

13 Weber KT, Janicki JS, Shroff SG, Likoff MJ. Clin Chest Med, 1983; **4,(2)**: 101-110.

14 Kolin A, Ross G, Gaal P, Austin S. Nature (Lond), 1964; **203**, 148-150.

15 Vlahakes GJ, Turley K, Hoffman JIE. Circulation, 1981; **63**: 87-95.

16 Brown KA, DeSanctis RW, DiCola V, Boucher CA, Pohost GM, Okada Rd. Am Heart J, 1986; **112**: 1321-1322.

17 Vincent JL, Thirion M, Brimioulle S, Lejeune P, Kahn RJ. Intens Care Med, 1986; **12**: 33-38.

18 Dhainaut JF, Brunet F, Villemant D. Evaluation of right ventricular function by thermodilution techniques. In:Cardiopulmonary Interactions in Acute Respiratory Failure, JL Vincent and PM Suter eds. Springer-Verlag,Berlin, 1987, pp 95-106.

19 Andersen HR, Nielsen D, Falk E. Right ventricular infarction: diagnostic value of ST elevation in lead III exceeding that of lead II during inferior/posterior infarction and comparison with right-

chest leads V_3R to V_7R. Am Heart J, 1989; **117**: 82-86.

20 Foëx P. Right ventricular function. In: Update in Intensive Care and Emergency Medicine, J.L.Vincent ed. Springer-Verlag, Berlin, 1986, pp 181-185.

21 D'Ambra MN, LaRaia PJ, Philbin DM, Watkins WD, Hilgenberg AD, Buckley MJ. J Thorac Cardiovasc Surg, 1985; **89**: 567-572.

22 Pennington DG, Merjavy JP, Swartz MT, Codd JE, Barner HB, Lagunoff D, Bashiti H, Kaiser GC, Willman VL. Ann Thor Surg, 1985; **39**: 16-24.

CARDIOVASCULAR PHYSIOLOGY OF CONGENITAL HEART DISEASE

Alan Jay Schwartz, M.D., M.S.Ed.

Classification of Congenital Heart Disease

Congenital heart disease (CHD) is comprised of a vast array of anatomic variations producing specific alterations of physiology which are manifest in a limited number of clinical presentations. The number of anatomic combinations in CHD are so numerous that they defy memorization. A simple and logical classification of CHD can be based primarily upon pathophysiology. This type of classification attempts to distill the myriad of congenital heart lesions into categories from which the answers to several basic questions are provided.

1. Is there an abnormal pathway for blood flow (shunting) through an intracardiac, extracardiac, or combined defect?
2. Is there obstruction to and reduction of blood flow due to a supravalvular, subvalvular, or primary valvular abnormality?
3. What are the consequences of abnormal cardiovascular (CV) pressures or volume which result from shunting of or obstruction to blood flow?
4. What are the consequences on the pulmonary and systemic vasculatures, and pulmonary and systemic blood flows?

The pathophysiological classification separates the congenital heart lesions into three groups. In two of the groups the primary problem is shunting of blood through abnormal

T. H. Stanley and R. J. Sperry (eds.), Anesthesiology and the Heart, 25–35.

circulatory pathways. Alteration of pulmonary blood flow (PBF) is the major consequence of shunt lesions. PBF will either be increased, resulting in a volume and/or pressure overload to the pulmonary circulation (e.g., ventricular or atrial septal defect, patent ductus arteriosus), or decreased, resulting in a relative inability to oxygenate blood (e.g., tetralogy of Fallot). Also included in these groups are complex congenital heart lesions in which there is a functional shunt (e.g., common ventricle, transposition of the great arteries, truncus arteriosus) which may or may not be associated with an anatomic obstruction to pulmonary and/or systemic blood flow. These more complex congenital heart malformations have the same effect of either ↑ or ↓ the effective PBF. A functional ↓ in PBF occurs, for example, when desaturated venous blood is shunted to the systemic circulation rather than to the pulmonary circulation because of the presence of a common mixing chamber such as a single ventricle.

There is no shunting of blood in the third group of congenital heart lesions (e.g., aortic or pulmonic stenosis, coarctation of the aorta). The primary problem in this group is obstruction to blood flow. The major consequences of obstruction to blood flow include the increased ventricular workload(s) necessary to overcome the obstruction(s) and the relatively reduced circulation distal to the obstruction(s).

Cyanosis or CHF are the two major clinical states which result from the abnormal anatomy. Cyanosis occurs most commonly in lesions where (1) PBF is ↓ or (2) mixing of systemic and pulmonary venous return occurs (e.g., transposition of the great arteries). CHF occurs most commonly in shunt lesions with ↑ PBF. Excessive pulmonary venous return to the left heart results in pulmonary vascular congestion. Less commonly, pulmonary venous congestion may occur when obstructive lesions or myocardial dysfunction impair forward cardiac output (CO).

Pathophysiology of Congenital Heart Disease - The "Plumbing" Principle

The pathophysiology of shunting of and/or obstruction to blood flow is explained by considering two fundamental principles of physics; Ohm's Law and the Hagen-Poiseuille relationship. While neither of these are used quantitatively, in a qualitative sense they are very helpful in describing blood flow.

When applied to CV physiology, Ohm's Law relates blood flow to the pressure generating it and the resistance impeding it.

Ohm's Law (Cardiovascular Equivalent)

$$Q \propto \frac{P}{R}$$

where:

Q = Shunt blood flow

R = Resistance(s) to blood flow

P = Pressure gradient(s)

The Hagen-Poiseuille relationship describes the laminar flow of a homogeneous fluid through a rigid tube of constant caliber and length. When applied to CV physiology it is "assumed" that blood is a homogeneous fluid and the blood vessels are relatively constant size conducting tubes.

Hagen-Poiseuille Relationship

$$Q = \frac{DP\pi r^4}{8L\eta}$$

where:

Q = Blood flow

DP = Pressure drop in fluid as it flows through a vascular channel

r = Radius of the vascular conduit

L = Length of the vascular conduit

η = Viscosity of fluid (assumed to remain constant)

In this relationship, $\pi r^4/L$ represents the cross-sectional area of the vascular conduit over its length. This is a more specifically defined resistance factor than that used in Ohm's Law.

Combination and modification of Ohm's Law and the Hagen-Poiseuille relationship yields a versatile learning tool which can be used to understand the pathophysiology of CHD. The reaggregation of these expressions results in a CV "plumbing" principle (Figure 1) expressed as:

$$Q \alpha \frac{P \times D^4}{R}$$

where:

Q = Blood flow (cardiac output and/or shunt flow)

P = Pressure gradient(s) (across valve(s), outflow tract(s), and/or intracardiac or extracardiac communication(s))

D = Diameter(s) (of valves, and/or intracardiac or extracardiac communication(s))

R = Resistance(s) (to blood flow (ventricular outflow tract(s), cross-sectional area(s) of a vascular bed(s), and/or length(s) of vascular channel(s))

FIGURE 1

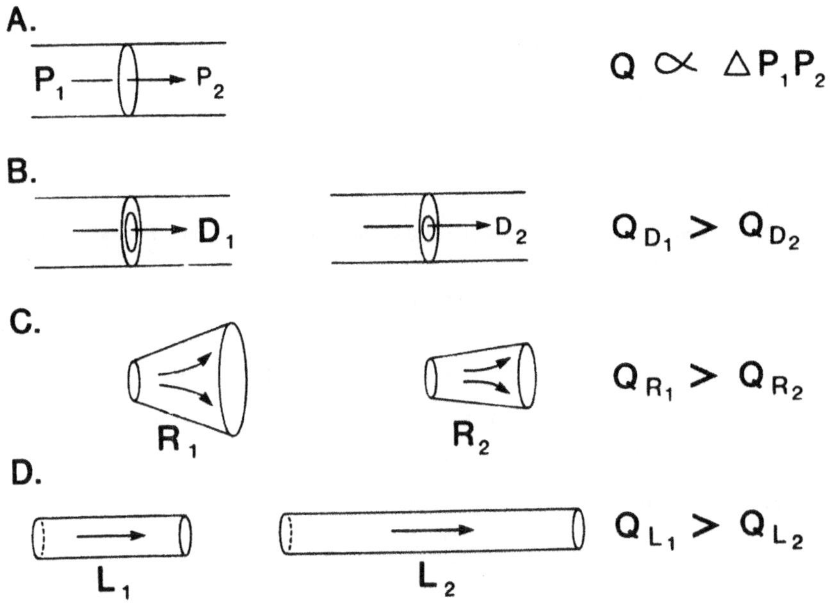

Figure 1: Schematic representation of the individual factors which influence the flow of blood through vascular channels. The quantity of flow is determined by pressure gradients in vascular channels, the diameter of the vascular channel, the resistance offered by the circuit into which the vascular channel empties, and the length of the vascular channel. Q=difference between; P=pressure; D=diameter; R=resistance; L=length. A. Q is proportional to D P_1 and P_2. In the diagram, P_1 is > than P_2, therefore, Q is in the direction of P_2. B. Two vascular channels of different diameters are shown. Q through the channel with the larger diameter, D_1, is > Q through the channel with the smaller diameter, D_2. C. Two vascular channels of equal initial diameter (the opening of each on the left) are shown emptying into circuits offering different resistance. Q through the channel offering less resistance, R_1, is > Q through the channel offering more resistance, R_2. D. Two vascular channels of equal diameter and different length are shown. Q through the shorter channel, L_1, is > Q through the longer channel, L_2.

Applied Pathophysiology of Congenital Heart Disease

Ventricular septal defect (VSD) is an example of an ↑ PBF lesion (Figure 2). Blood is shunted into the lungs because left ventricular (LV) pressure is higher than right ventricular (RV) pressure, and right ventricular outflow tract (RVOT) resistance (including that contributed by the pulmonary vasculature) offers less impedance to flow than that of the systemic circulation. The existence of any shunted blood, and its total quantity is dependent upon the resistance to flow offered by the VSD itself. The larger the diameter of the VSD, the less resistance it offers, and the greater the flow across it from the higher pressure LV to the lower pressure RV and ultimately to the pulmonary circuit. This information can be conceptualized in the relationship.

$$\text{VSD Q(pulmonary shunt)} \propto \frac{\text{P(LV>RV)} \times D^4\text{(VSD)}}{\text{R(PVR<SVR)}}$$

where:

LV = left ventricle   PVR = pulmonary vascular resistance

RV = right ventricle   SVR = systemic vascular resistance

Tetralogy of Fallot (TOF) is an example of a ↓ PBF flow lesion (Figure 2). Blood is shunted away from the lungs because the muscular portion of the RVOT is obstructed (infundibular pulmonic stenosis) and offers more resistance to blood flow than the intraventricular communication, i.e., the VSD, which is present. The VSD actually serves as a "pop off valve" that decompresses the RV which can not empty normally due to its obstructed outflow tract. The pressure in the RV, which commonly equals or exceeds the pressure in the LV, is elevated in response to the resistance of the normal pathway for RV emptying. As long as the SVR is relatively low in comparison to the resistance offered by the obstructed RVOT, the LV empties in a normal fashion and an additional quantity of blood will flow from the RV through the VSD to the LV and ultimately to the systemic circuit. This information can be conceptualized in the relationship:

$$\text{TOF Q(systemic shunt)} \propto \frac{\text{P(RV>LV)} \times D^4\text{(VSD)}}{\text{R(RVOT>SVR)}}$$

where:

RVOT = Right ventricular outflow tract

Aortic stenosis (AS) is an example of a non-shunt obstructive lesion. The normal quantity of blood flows through the normal pathway. To satisfy the flow-pressure-resistance relationship, LV pressure must be markedly increased in order to overcome the resistance offered by the reduced diameter of the aortic orifice. This information can be conceptualized in the relationship:

$$\text{AS Q(systemic flow)} \propto \frac{\text{P(LV>Aorta)} \times D^4\text{ (Aortic valve)}}{\text{R(LVOT)}}$$

where:

LVOT = Left ventricular outflow tract

FIGURE 2

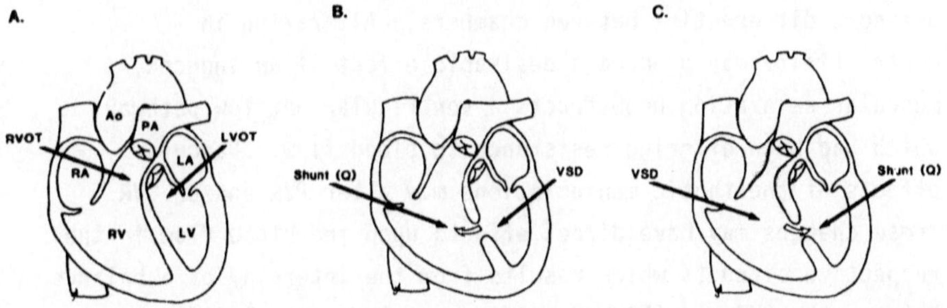

Figure 2: Diagrammatic representation of a normal heart and congenital heart lesions in which there are pathophysiological alterations in PBF. Ao=aorta; LA=left atrium; LV=left ventricle; LVOT=left ventricular outflow tract; P=pressure; PA=pulmonary artery; Q=shunt blood flow; R=resistance to blood flow; RA=right atrium; RV= right ventricle; RVOT=right ventricular outflow tract; VSD=ventricular septal defect. A. A normal heart showing the anatomic relationships between the cardiac chambers and the outflow tracts of the ventricles. B. An ↑ PBF lesion is exemplified by a VSD. When 1) the VSD is large diameter offering low R, and 2) RVOT and PA offer low R, then 3) $P_{LV}>P_{RV}$, and Q, indicated by the open arrow, is left-to-right. C. A ↓ PBF lesion is exemplified by tetralogy of Fallot. When 1) the VSD is large diameter offering low R, 2) RVOT is obstructed (subpulmonic muscular hypertrophy indicated by the shaded areas), 3) RVOT R> LVOT R, then 4) $P_{RV}\geq P_{LV}$, and Q, indicated by the open arrow, is right-to-left.

Anesthetic Application of the Pathophysiological Principles of CHD

Anesthetic manipulations alter the pathophysiological expression of CHD and have the potential to affect several components of the flow-pressure-resistance relationship. Cardiac depressant effects of anesthesia may limit the ability of each ventricle to produce flow (CO). If the ventricles' ability to generate pressure is affected, there may be a change in the pressure differential between chambers. Alteration in contractility may produce a desirable effect if an induced muscular relaxation unobstructs a ventricular outflow pathway which had been offering resistance to blood flow. Vascular effects of anesthetic manipulations may alter PVR and/or SVR. These changes may have direct effects upon the blood flow in their respective circuits which results from the interplay of a balance between the PVR and SVR. Specific examples will clarify these effects.

In children with lesions that ↑ PBF, anesthetic manipulations are designed to reduce the shunt and increase systemic perfusion by increasing the ratio of right heart pressures to left heart pressures. While it not clinically feasible to independently regulate the right and left heart filling pressures (preload), chamber compliance, or inotropic state, right and left heart pressures may be altered by manipulation of the impedance to outflow of the respective ventricles. Less blood may be shunted into the lungs by ↑ the ratio PVR/SVR. Increasing PVR promotes shunting of blood away from the lungs. Hypoxia, hypercarbia, acidosis, high mean airway pressure, sympathetic stimulation, and hypervolemia predispose to ↑ PVR. In the absence of clinically useful pulmonary vasoconstrictors, the avoidance of hypocarbia and the use of high mean airway pressures during ventilation (including positive end-expiratory pressure) may be used to maintain PVR. The use of vasodilators to reduce SVR, thereby increasing PVR/SVR, is of uncertain benefit. Vasodilators, including anesthetics, often exert similar actions on the pulmonary and systemic vasculatures resulting in no net change in PVR/SVR. Generalized vasoconstriction resulting from a high sympathetic tone due to light anesthesia, or from vasopressor administration, similarly may not alter the ratio of PBF to systemic blood flow.

In children with ↓ PBF, anesthetic manipulations are designed to avoid further ↑ in right-to-left shunting. PBF may be promoted and right-to-left shunting ↓ by decreasing the ratio of right heart pressure to left heart pressure. This favorable alteration in the pressure gradient across the VSD may be accomplished by ameliorating the degree of right heart obstruction where possible, and by maintaining or elevating SVR. Manipulation of SVR in the presence of an elevated and relatively fixed impedance to right heart outflow will produce observable alterations in shunt flow. Increasing SVR generally promotes shunting of blood into the lungs. Light levels of anesthesia and the administration of α-adrenergic agonists predispose to maintenance or elevation of SVR. Infusion of phenylephrine into children with TOF produces ↓ in intracardiac shunting and ↑ in systemic O_2 tension. In this instance, the vasopressor ↑ SVR and impedance to left heart outflow relative to right heart outflow. This results in a decrease in the right-to-left interventricular pressure gradient that reduces RV to LV shunting. Decreasing SVR, on the other hand, promotes shunting of blood away from the lungs and could intensify the shunt and create cyanosis. Vasodilators and deep levels of anesthesia can predispose to ↓ SVR. If hypovolemia and systemic ↓ BP are superimposed on a congenital heart lesion with obstruction to PBF, both the right-to-left shunt and cyanosis are intensified. This physiologic sequence leads to shock and cardiac arrest if unreversed. Reduction in PVR may also help in promoting PBF. This is accomplished by hyperventilation with a high inspired O_2 concentration and avoiding high mean airway pressure.

The flow-pressure-resistance relationship can also be applied to the non-shunt obstructive lesions. Reducing ventricular function limits the heart's ability to generate a pressure gradient and produce CO in a setting in which obstruction to blood flow is present. The ability of the heart to eject stroke volume depends on the adequacy of ventricular filling and inotropic state. Excessive myocardial depression, hypovolemia, and loss of properly timed atrial systole are to be avoided. Adequate regulation of SVR is essential to provide important coronary perfusion pressure. Control of impedance to LV outflow is equally important, however, and excessive increases in this resistance to flow are to be avoided in non-shunt obstructive lesions.

Anesthetic depression of cardiac contractility is not always detrimental. In contrast to adults with valvular stenosis, AS and PS in children is often subvalvular (i.e., infundibular) in location. Forward blood flow and myocardial O_2 balance may be altered by modifying the degree of infundibular obstruction in these lesions. In TOF, for example, the RVOT is obstructed by a subvalvular muscular stenosis. Infundibular RVOT obstruction can be exacerbated by tachycardia and hypovolemia, which reduce ventricular size, and by excessive contractility. This can increase the degree of muscular contraction and obstruction intensifying the abnormal shunt. Systemic vasodilation may also impair RV infundibular outflow by causing a reflex increase in heart rate and contractility. Avoidance of excessive sympathetic tone, provision of adequate venous return, and control of SVR are desirable in this setting. The negative chronotropic and inotropic actions of anesthetics and β-adrenergic antagonists can be used to advantage to reduce an obstructing degree of muscular RVOT obstruction.

SUMMARY

Application of the flow-pressure-resistance relationship, i.e., the "plumbing" principle enables one to understand the pathophysiology of CHD and selection of an anesthetic technique for children with these lesions.

Suggested Reading

1. Fink BW: Congenital Heart Disease: A Deductive Approach to its Diagnosis, 2nd ed. Chicago: Year Book Medical, 1985
2. Kawabori I: Pediatr Clin North Am 25:759-795, 1978
3. Moore RA: Anesthesiol Rev 8(no. 12):23-29, 1981
4. Schwartz AJ, Campbell FW: In Pediatric Cardiac Anesthesia, Edited by CL Lake, Norwalk, Appleton & Lange, 1988, pp 7-25
5. Schwartz AJ, Jobes DR: Congenital heart disease-special anesthetic considerations. In Cardiac Anesthesia, Edited by TJ Conahan, Menlo Park, Addison-Wesley, 1982, pp 62-91
6. Stevenson JG: Pediatr Clin North Am 25:725-158, 1978
7. Young D: Int Anesthesiol Clin 18:5-26, 1980

MYOCARDIAL LYMPHATICS AND CARDIAC FUNCTION

JOHN P. WILLIAMS, M.D.

Discussions of myocardial edema frequently focus on manipulation of the coronary arteries; lesser attention is given to the rich plexus of lymphatics within the myocardium, although this is the normal avenue of exit for all interstitial edema fluid. To understand the variety of effects and problems encompassed with any manipulation of the interstitium and lymphatics, one must have some knowledge of the anatomy and physiology of the microvascular exchange area and its drainage. This paper will delineate the microvascular exchange area, describe the physiology of microvascular fluid exchange, detail the anatomy of the lymphatic network and discuss the clinical relevancy of alterations in lymphatic and interstitial function with particular attention to myocardial edema.

ANATOMY

The lymphatics originate in the subendocardium and extend through the myocardium into the subepicardium where they join the major draining trunks leading by the innominate vein and ultimately draining into the superior vena cava (Figure 1) (1). The lymphatic capillary walls have anchoring or tethering filaments attached to them (Figure 2) (1) which may serve to maintain the lymphatic lumen during grossly edematous states (2). Lymphatic capillaries can generally be identified by their thin and irregular endothelial walls, protruding mucleus and a luminal content of slightly acidophilic material (3). These

T. H. Stanley and R. J. Sperry (eds.), Anesthesiology and the Heart, 37–51.

endothelial cells are joined by three types of intercellular junctions: end to end, overlapping and interdigitation. Occasional scattered "open" junction (intercellular spaces of > 50 nm) also occur; however, their incidence is < 1% of all junctions. Tight junctions account for 80-95% of all identifiable cellular contacts (3). The difficulty in obtaining reliable serial sections of a given intercellular contact accounts for this wide range.

<u>Figure 1</u>

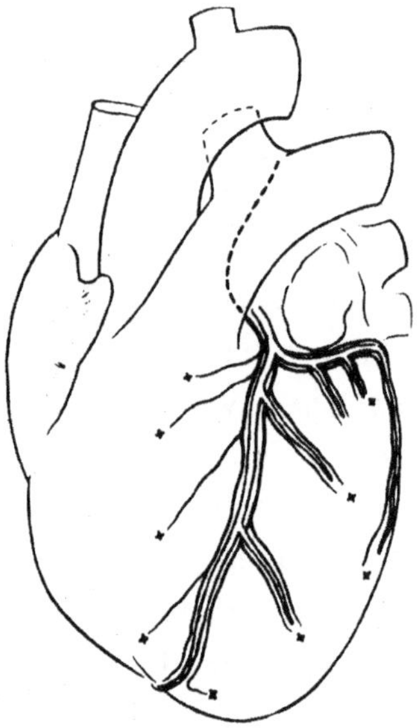

Fig. 1. Typical representation of the arrangement of lymphatic draining trunks. The cardiac node would be located posteriorly to the aorta near the superior vena cava and would lead to the thoracic duct.

Figure 2

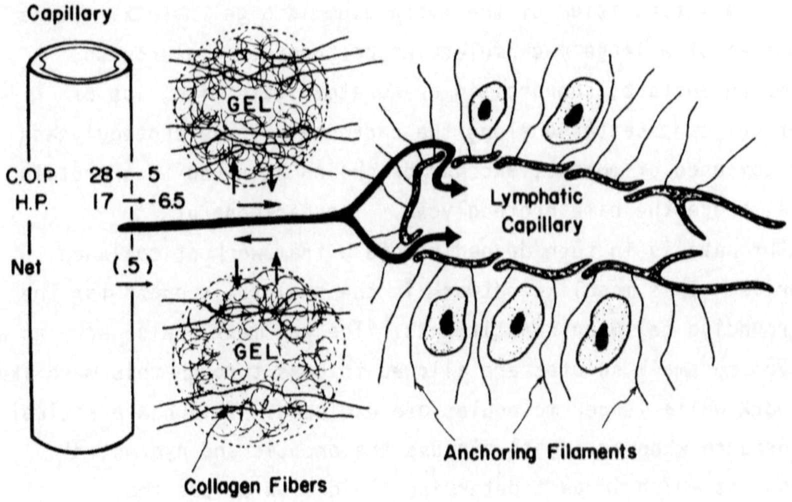

Fig. 2. Artist's rendering of the tethering fibrils which are attached to the endothelial walls of the lymphatic capillaries. (By permission R. Drake).

The physiologic significance of the type of junctions noted in the myocardial lymphatic vessels is uncertain. Some authors feel that open junctions are the entrance point for lymph under normal conditions (4). The junctions would be "open" during the diastolic portion of the cardiac cycle and would "close" during the systolic phase. This phasic opening and closing would also correlate with peak flow in the coronary microvasculature and presumably the period of peak microvascular fluid flux.

The ground substance or connective tissue matrix surrounding and supporting the lymphatic capillaries is principally composed of collagen fibers; although, elastic fibers and fibroblasts are also present (3). This region is the interstitial matrix and serves as both a sponge and molecular sieve between the lymphatics and the microvascular exchange region. It is this region which undergoes remodeling following a prolonged edematous stimulus (5).

INTERSTITIAL MATRIX

The interstitium of the myocardium is a gel matrix. It is composed of a large macromolecular backbone of hyaluronate, dermatan sulfate, chondroitin or keratosulfate with ribs of proteoglycan scattered along the backbone. These proteoglycans are composed of mucopolysaccharide chains attached to a protein core, hence the name proteoglycan. The backbone of hyaluronate is in turn draped around a framework of collagen fibrils. This meshlike network is the skeletal support for the surrounding cellular constituents. The gel matrix also acts as a sieve; so small solutes are allowed to pass through this meshlike network while larger molecules are excluded. This has practical importance when trying to discuss the oncotic and hydrostatic pressures which in part determine fluid flux across the interstitium. The gel matrix composition of the interstitium also has practical significance because of the steric (molecular charge) and elastic forces. These forces become more important as the hydration state of the matrix is acutely altered. The sum of these many forces (elastic, steric, hydrostatic and oncotic) will ultimately seek equilibrium and a net matrix pressure can be measured. The mechanical deformation of the myocardium contracting around a given volume of fluid also contributes to the matrix pressure. The net matrix pressure is the interstitial pressure which we will be discussing later in the chapter.

MICROVASCULAR EXCHANGE

The microvasculature of the myocardium is similar anatomically to that found in all other organs. However, the transmicrovascular fluid and protein fluxes are an order of magnitude higher in the myocardium on a per weight basis (2). This is probably secondary to the higher capillary density and large exchange surface area available in the myocardium (6). The control of flow to various capillary beds within regions in the myocardium is directed by a series of precapillary sphincters. These are in turn regulated by a variety of physiologic mediators such as: nitric oxide (EDRF), ADP, ATP, hydrogen ion and CO_2 to name a few. These factors govern flow and available surface area, which control capillary pressure, which ultimately determine the driving pressure for fluid transudation. There are also post capillary venous sphincters but these are less important than the total number or size of venous channels available for drainage. In the myocardium approximately 75% of total myocardial outflow occurs through the coronary sinus (7). The remaining 25% exits primarily through the anterior cardiac and thebesian system.

Although the microvascular exchange area in the myocardium exchanges both solvent and solutes, we will discuss primarily the solvent portion of the equation here. None of the interventions I will discuss disturb microvascular permeability but do alter the rate of fluid filtration. This is not meant to imply that the normal myocardial exchange area does not filter large amounts of protein, which it does. Rather for simplicities sake I will deal only with fluid flow through the lymphatics for now.

Those forces within the myocardium which normally govern the flow of fluid into the interstitium and subsequently the lymphatics are similar to the Starling forces anywhere in the body. The Starling equation (1) describes fluid flux across any biological membrane.

$$Jv = Lp \cdot A\,[(P_{cap} - P_{int}) - \sigma(\pi cap - \pi int)] \quad (1)$$

where LpA is the microvascular hydraulic conductivity - surface area product, commonly known as Kf the filtration coefficient, Jv is the rate of fluid filtration, Pcap and π cap are the hydrostatic and oncotic pressures respectively within the capillaries and Pint and π int the identical pressures within the interstitium. The normal interstitial pressure in the myocardium is about 15 mmHg and the oncotic difference is about 6 mmHg (2). The positive interstitial pressure is interesting as in many tissues (skin, cornea, skeletal muscle, subcutis and lung) the interstitial matrix pressure is negative or subatmospheric. The brain and heart are the only two organs which are supplied by continuous capillaries and maintain positive interstitial pressures; interestingly they are also the only two organs which create a fluid filled cavity.

The normal amount of lymph production in the canine myocardium is approximately 6-7 ml/hr with a protein concentration of approximately 0.8 of the plasma concentration. This protein concentration difference translates into the 6 mmHg oncotic pressure drop we and others have measured (1, 8).

As the interstitial fluid moves toward the initial lymphatics it is imperative to recognize that in the normal myocardium the cellular mass is only 1/3000th as permeable to the movement of water as the endothelial barrier the fluid and solutes have just crossed (9). Thus the majority of fluid and solute should rapidly be removed by the lymphatics. Once into the initial lymphatics the lymph is slowly propulsed up into the collecting lymphatics and eventually into the cardiac node. This rests behind the aorta and either on the trachea or superior vena cava. From here the lymphatics empty into the thoracic duct or into the innominate vein on the left (commonly) or the right subclavian (rarely).

The rate of myocardial lymphatic drainage is then dependent upon changes in superior vena caval pressure. As superior vena caval pressure is elevated the outflow pressure for the lymphatics is elevated and hence the drainage of the myocardial interstitium is impaired. This impairment of interstitial drainage does not seem to cause acute alterations in interstitial water content (10). However, this is a very special circumstance where only superior vena caval pressure is elevated but not right atrial pressure. Once right atrial pressure or more importantly coronary sinus pressure is elevated, any elevation in superior vena caval pressure will lead to a rapid gain in myocardial water content (10). The secondary increase in capillary pressure with the increase in coronary sinus pressure leads to an increase in transudation across the microvascular exchange barrier. Following an intervention to elevate capillary pressure and to impede myocardial lymph flow, we have noted increases in the net weight of the left ventricle of 28% over a four hour period (10).

Although it is tempting to relate Jv in equation 1 to total lymph outflow this is not accurate until the steady state is reached. The time required for the attainment of steady state is dependent upon the magnitude of the fluid flux, the compliance of the system and the resistance and height of the cannula used to measure lymph flow. Thus one cannot describe the total lymphatic conduit system without knowing the resistance of the lymphatic system which is replaced by the cannula used to measure lymph flow. We are presently engaged in work to delineate this quantity for the myocardium. We have however, previously shown that in the lung and liver the segments of lymphatic replaced by the cannula demonstrate greater resistance to flow than the cannula (22).

Cannula height above the heart can be utilized as a measure of relative changes in interstitial pressure (Figure 3). That is the higher the position at which flow from a cannulated lymph vessel ceases, the greater the interstitial pressure.

Figure 3

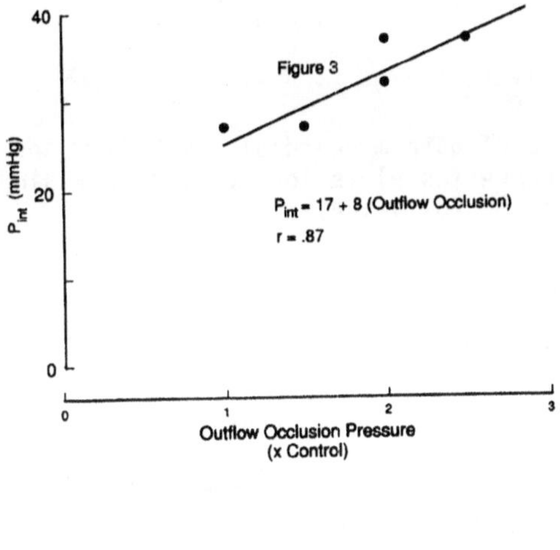

Fig. 3. Relationship between myocardial lymphatic outflow occlusion pressure (cannula height above the heart required to stop lymphatic flow) and myocardial interstitial pressure (P_{int}) in mmHg.

Unfortunately this relationship is fairly steep but it is helpful to relate changes in interstitial pressure. The positive relationship with interstitial pressure also includes both the coronary sinus pressure and lymph flow (Figure 4). That is the higher the coronary sinus pressure (up to a maximum of 45-50 mmHg) the greater the lymph flow and similarly the higher the interstitial pressure (1).

Figure 4

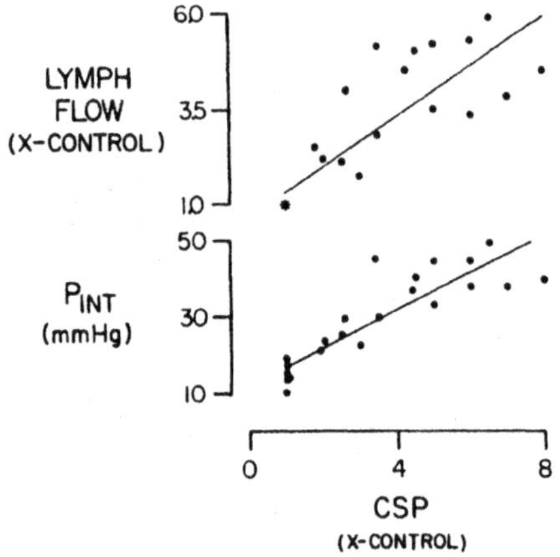

Fig. 4. Relationship of both myocardial lymph flow and interstitial pressure versus elevations of coronary sinus pressure (CSP in multiples of control value).

CLINICAL IMPLICATIONS

Ischemia and infarction - Ischemia generally produces an increase in lymph flow and extracellular water depending upon the model for ischemia examined and the method of estimating myocardial water content (12, 13). Changes in permeability are more difficult to quantitate because of the high concentration of most proteins in the myocardial lymph. We have shown that one of the larger proteins, β-lipoprotein, can be utilized as a measure of alterations in myocardial permeability (2, 14). The same may be said of $(dP/dt)_{max}$ but only under non-ischemic conditions, thus making the application of $(dP/dt)_{max}$ less useful in the setting of ischemic disease.

What is more interesting perhaps is the aggravation of an ischemic insult if carried out under the setting of lymphatic obstruction (15, 16). This may be indicative of the limited ability of the myocardium to augment contractility in the face of an edematous myocardial interstitium. It is also tempting to speculate that a portion of the beneficial effect noted with nitroglycerin is related to either venous capillary or lymphatic dilatation. In the former case the venous capillary dilation will lead to a reduction in capillary hydrostatic pressure (17) while in the latter, the rate of lymph egress would be increased. In either case interstitial pressure would decrease.

HYPERTENSION

Chronic arterial hypertension elevates interstitial pressure in the myocardium, alters microvascular permeability and increases lymph flow (Figure 5) (18). Some hypertensive patients have angina with angiographically normal coronary arteries. One of the possible causes of this angina has been described as microvascular angina (19, 20). This description appears to be independent of our observations of the effect of chronic hypertension upon interstitial pressure.

Microscopic myocardial sections from patients with hypertension who died from accidental causes demonstrate not only the expected myocardial cellular hypertrophy but interstitial fibrosis as well (21, 22). We have previously demonstrated that chronic myocardial edema results in the rapid proliferation of collagen within the myocardium (4). The chronic elevation of interstial pressure with hypertension may gradually reduce the coronary vascular reserve and lengthening diffusion distances for O_2 by increasing the volume of the interstitial matrix. These changes of supply characteristics in combination with the increase in oxygen demand by the hypertrophied muscle may contribute to this "microvascular angina". Those same factors may also contribute to the development of ischemia in the periumbral area following infarction in the hypertensive patient (23-25).

Figure 5

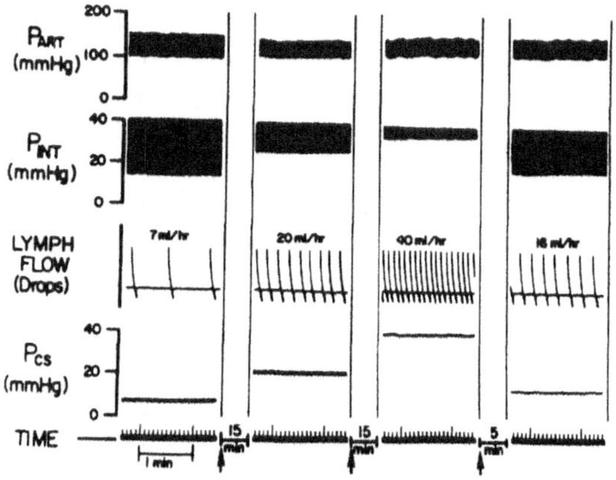

Fig. 5. Typical recording of interstitial pressure, lymph flow, coronary sinus pressure (CSP) and arterial pressure in normal and hypertensive dogs before and after an elevation in CSP.

CARDIOPULMONARY BYPASS

The drainage of canine cardiac lymph is not effected by cardiopulmonary bypass (CPB) per se but rather by the subsequent interventions which follow. Perfusing the heart through an extracorporeal circuit has little effect (26); however, once the heart has been filbrillated or excluded from aortic perfusion, lymph flow changes rapidly.

Lymph flow rates following fibrillation drop by 50% but rise steeply following restoration of sinus rhythm, generally exceeding the baseline state. Not unexpectedly cessation of coronary perfusion results in a rapid decline in the rate of lymph egress which rapidly returns and exceeds baseline once perfusion is restored. The restoration of lymph flow in the latter condition is often accompanied by blood tinging of the lymphatic flow; presumably indicative of permeability changes

(26). Others have noted increases in the myocardial water content (27, 28), extracellular space (27) and a coincident decrease in the diastolic compliance (27, 29) of the canine left ventricle following CPB. Many of these changes relate to the administration of cardioplegia as well as the ischemic hypothermia arrest (28, 30).

The effect of a hypothermia ischemic arrest without cardioplegia also increases myocardial water content while concomitantly causing decreases in left ventircular function (max dP/dt, peak LVP, LVEDP, LVSWI) and coronary blood flow following restoration of flow (31). This prompted our group to examine the acute effects of myocardial edema upon cardiac function (4, 14).

Using the elevated coronary sinus pressure model of myocardial edema, we rendered canine myocardium edematous for two hours and then constructed cardiac function curves. These curves were then compared to the same animal prior to the edematous challenge. In addition, changes in max dP/dt were plotted as a function of time. Both measures of global left ventricular function revealed marked alterations with the edematous challenge (see Figure 6).

<u>Figure 6</u>

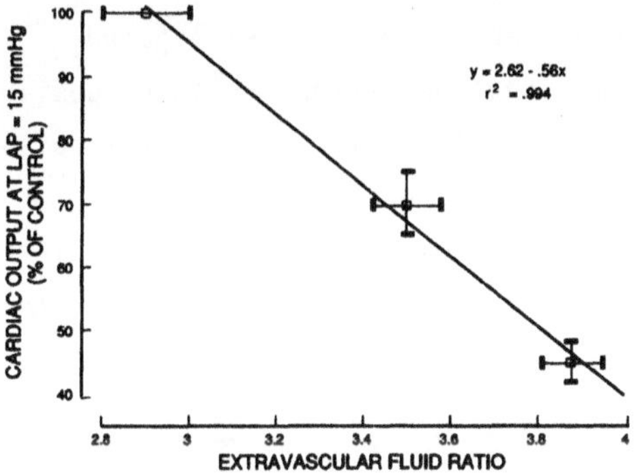

Fig. 6. Cardiac output and left ventricular (dP/dt) max expressed as percentage changes following an acute edemagenic insult.

VENOUS AND LYMPHATIC OBSTRUCTION

Chronic lymphatic obstruction studies are difficult to interpret. The lymphatic vessels regenerate very rapidly (32). This makes it very difficult to attain complete lymphatic obstruction for any prolonged period. The studies which examine this issue in the canine rarely demonstrate complete lymphatic interruption, but often obtain partial obstruction and note a wide variety of changes. The most common anomaly is thickening and opacification of the mitral valve leaflets (33). Commonly dilatation of the interstitial space and lymphatic capillaries are noted early (within 3 weeks) after obstruction. Generally thickening of the valve cusps only becomes apparent after four or more weeks of obstruction. Stain injected into the valve leaflets after obstruction reveal an extensive lymphatic network which is not present in control dogs (34). Other less frequent changes are thickening of the endocardium (33, 35), increased elastic and fibrous tissue (33, 35) and subendocardial hemorrhaging (33, 35). In man dilated and tortuous lymphatic channels have been associated with fibroelastosis (36).

Chronic isolated venous or coronary sinus obstruction does not occur in man. However, early in the second half of this century Beck described an operation which created an arteriovenous fistula from the coronary sinus to the aorta (37).

In animals this procedure conferred a protective effect when their coronary arteries were later (weeks) ligated. Unfortunately in humans this operation caused congestive heart failure and a more rapid demise. In all of these patients their hearts were described as edematous.

In canines this retrograde connection results in an increase in coronary sinus pressure and flow for a period of four to five weeks after which time the flow is lost and antegrade flow returns. Pathologic venous changes in these animals reveal greater density of collagen around the veins, increased thickness of the adventitia, proliferation of intimal connective tissue and occasionally replacement of the veins by connective tissue. All of the canine hearts with the Beck procedure were heavier although no measurements of interstitial size or wet weights were made (38).

At present the only clinical application of the impairment of venous drainage is in patients with elevated right atrial pressures. Lymphatic obstruction is very similar but also includes patients with high levels of positive end-expiratory pressure and mediastinal tumor involvement which results in superior vena caval obstruction.

As mentioned in the first section of this paper chronic elevation of right-sided myocardial pressures (i.e. conpulmonale, pulmonary hypertension, etc.) can accelerate the formation of lymph by elevating coronary sinus pressure and decrease the rate of elimination of lymph by elevating superior vena caval pressures (10). These alterations in microvascular fluid flux can and do lead to deterioration in the function of not only the right but also the pressure spared left ventricle (39).

Although the relative protein concentration in the lymph is initially depressed, total protein excretion is elevated secondary to the enhancement of surface area made available by the elevation of coronary sinus pressure (40). It is presumably this increase in capillary exchange area which accounts for the brief improvement in contractility we and others have noted when obstructing the coronary sinus (14, 38, 40).

CONCLUSION

The myocardium has a rich and well-developed lymphatic system to assist in the drainage of microvascular fluid and solutes. The interactions between the interstitium, microvascular endothelial filtration barrier, and lymphatics are complex and only partially explored. The rate of egress of lymphatic fluid is not linearly related to the microvascular filtration rate once the lymphatic is cannulated. In the steady state however microvascular fluid flux can be assessed by measuring lymphatic outflow.

The myocardial interstitium is relatively non-compliant although the lymphatic interstitial border is more compliant than other similar beds in the body (skeletal and hepatic). This means that relatively small changes in Jv will bring about large changes in interstitial pressure but these changes are not met with similarly large changes in lymph flow. This has the practical effect of increasing interstitial pressure to oppose further transudation across the microvascular exchange barrier. Clinical implications of these changes are discussed in detail with regards to ischemia, infarction, cardiopulmonary bypass, hypertension and venous and lymphatic obstruction. The validation of a technique for exploring the effects of various interventions upon myocardial microvascular permeability is described. A variety of unexplored areas remain to be examined with this technique including the effect of vasodilation on permeability, alterations in solute excretion following permeability changes, assessment of interstitial function following permeability alterations and many others. Hopefully this chapter has served to assist in the exploration of interstitial fluid dynamics in the myocardium.

REFERENCES

1. Leak LV, Schannahan A, Scully H, Daggett WM: Anat Rec 191:183-202, 1978.
2. Laine GA, Granger HJ: Am J Physiol 249:H834-H842, 1985.
3. Bouchor Y, Roberge S, Paul-Emile R: Microvasc Res 29:305-319, 1985.
4. Casley-Smith JR: Lymphology 12:177-183, 1980.
5. Laine GA: Circ Res (In Press), 1989.
6. Wean JT: J Exp Med 47:273-291, 1928.
7. Scharf SM, Bromberger-Barnea B, Permutt S: J Appl Physiol 20:657-622, 1971.
8. Drinker CK, Warren MF, Maurer FW, McCarrell JD: Am J Physiol 130:43-55, 1940.
9. Landis EM: Annals New York Academy of Science:713-731, 1948.
10. Williams JP, Drake RE, Allen SJ, Gabel JC, Laine GA: Fed Proc 46:1545, 1987.
11. Elk JR, Drake RE, Williams JP, Gabel JC, Laine GA: Am J Physiol 254:G748-G752, 1988.
12. Sunnengren and Poveto: J Mol Cell Cardiol 12:1011-1031, 1980.
13. Feola M and Glick G: Am J Physiol 229:44-48, 1975.
14. Laine GA: Circ Res 61:203-208, 1987.
15. Kline IK, Miller AJ, Pick R and Katz LN: Am Heart J 68:515-523, 1964.

16. Pick R, Miller AJ, and Glick G: Am Heart J 87:627-632, 1974.
17. Endrich B, Franke N, Peter K, Messmer K: Anesthesiology 66:605-613, 1987.
18. Laine GA: Circ Res 62:953-960, 1988.
19. Cannon RO, Epstein SE: Am J Cardiol 61:1338-1343, 1988.
20. Brush JE, Cannon AO, Schenke WH, Bonow RO, Leon MB, Maron BJ, Epstein SE: NEJM 319:1302-1307, 1988.
21. Losse B, Kuhn H, Rafflenbeul D, Kronert H, Hort W, Feinendegen LE, Loogen F: Z Kardiol 69:523-530, 1980.
22. Opherk D, Zebe H, Weihe E, Mall G, Durr C, Gravert B, Mehmel HC, Schwarz F, Kubler W: Circulation 63:817-825, 1981.
23. Rabkin SW, Mathewson FAL, Tate RB: Am J Cardiol 40:604-610, 1977.
24. Koyanagi S, Eastham CL, Harrison DG, Marcus ML: Circ Res 50:55-62, 1982.
25. Raison J, Achimastos A, Asmar R, Simon A, Safar M: Am J Cardiol 57:223-226, 1986.
26. Ullal SR: Ann Roy Coll Surg Engl 51:282-298, 1972.
27. Pogatsa G, Dubeez E and Gabor G: Basic Res Cardiol 73:551-558, 1978.
28. Laks H, Standeven J, Blair D, Hohn J, Jellineck M and Williams VL: J Thorac Cardiovasc Surg 73:129-138, 1977.
29. Allen WB, Blackstone EH, Kouchoukes NT: Circulation 49/50 (Suppl):III-19, 1974.
30. Foglia RP, Steed DL, Follete DM, DeLona E and Buckburg GD: J Thorac Cardiovasc Surg 78:217-222, 1979.
31. Amano J, Sunamori M, Kameda T, Okamura T, Suzuki A: Adv Myocardial 4:465-471, 1983.
32. Reichert FL: Arch Surg 13:871-881, 1926.
33. Miller AJ, Pick R, Katz LN: Circ Res 8:941-947, 1960.
34. Ullal SR, Kluge TH, Gerbode F: Surgery 71:328-334, 1972.
35. Miller AJ, Pick R, Katz LN: Br Heart J 25:182-190, 1963.
36. Kline IK, Miller AJ, Pick R, Katz LN: Circulation 30:728-735, 1964.
37. Beck CS, Hahn RS, Leighninger D, McAllister FF: JAMA 147:1726-1731, 1951.
38. Eckstein RW and Leighninger DS: Circ Res 11:60-72, 1954.
39. Kelly DT, Spotnitz HM, Beiser D, Pierce JE, Epstein SE: Circulation 44:403-412, 1971.
40. Scharf SM and Bromberger-Barnea B: Am J Physiol 224:918-925, 1973.

PATHOPHYSIOLOGY OF THE CORONARY CIRCULATION

P.Foëx

The heart receives its blood supply via the right and left coronary arteries. The latter divides into the left anterior descending coronary artery (LAD) and the left circumflex artery (LC). The former (LAD) supplies blood to most of the ventricular septum, the anterior, lateral and apical wall of the left ventricle and the anterolateral papillary muscle. The latter (LC) supplies the left atrial wall, the posterolateral left ventricular wall, the posteromedial papillary muscle and in 40-50% of patients the sinus node. The right coronary artery supplies blood to the sinus node (50-60% of patients), the right ventricular wall, the crista supraventricularis and the right atrium.

Blood flow to the human myocardium is approximately 70 ml/min/100g (1). As oxygen extraction is high, increases in oxygen demand must be matched by increases in coronary blood flow. Thus, the major control of the coronary blood flow occurs at the cellular level and is determined by metabolic needs. Even during exercise, increases in oxygen extraction are limited and coronary sinus oxygen content remains relatively constant (2).

A variety of substances may be utilized by the heart for energy production. These include glucose, free fatty acids, lactate and pyruvate. Under aerobic conditions, 20-30% of arterial lactate is extracted and metabolized (3). High energy phosphates (ATP, creatine phosphate) and their degradation products (ADP, AMP, inorganic phosphates) serve to regulate cellular metabolism.

The matching of oxygen supply and demand, i.e. the local regulation of coronary blood flow, is not fully understood. Many

T. H. Stanley and R. J. Sperry (eds.), Anesthesiology and the Heart, 53–64.

substances have been implicated as mediators for this regulation. These include reduced cellular oxygen tension, carbon dioxide, hydrogen ions, lactic acid, potassium ions, osmolarity, polypeptides, histamine, prostaglandins and adenine nucleotides; the latter are currently favoured (4).

Blood flow in the coronary arteries depends on coronary arterial tone and aortic perfusion pressure (5). Coronary arterial resistance has three components: (i) basal viscous resistance; (ii) autoregulatory resistance secondary to metabolic needs; (iii) compressive resistance. The latter is particularly important in the left ventricle, as the coronary circulation must supply oxygenated blood at an adequate pressure to a constantly exercising muscle with high metabolic demand. For the thick walled left ventricle, tissue pressure exerted by the contracting myocardium exceeds the driving pressure at the origins of the coronary arteries so that systolic flow cannot penetrate the myocardium. Thus, left ventricular coronary flow is mainly diastolic, particularly for the subendocardial myocardium. The major haemodynamic determinant of myocardial blood flow is the diastolic pressure-time index, which depends upon the gradient between aortic and left ventricular pressures, and the duration of diastole (6). By contrast, myocardial oxygen demand is approximated by the systolic pressure-tissue index. Even in the presence of normal coronary arteries, the combination of high left ventricular diastolic pressure, low aortic diastolic pressure and tachycardia may cause myocardial ischaemia.

Coronary pressure-flow data suggest that coronary flow stops at an inflow pressure (P_{zf}) that is substantially greater than left ventricular end-diastolic pressure (Figure 1). The closing pressure appears to depend upon vascular tone. Thus, under conditions of maximal coronary vasodilatation, the critical closing pressure is of the order of 12 to 18 mmHg, while under resting conditions it may be in the region of 40 to 50 mmHg (7).

In the presence of coronary artery stenoses, coronary flow is limited and becomes exquisitely sensitive to changes in perfusion pressure and duration of diastole. Increased myocardial oxygen demand cannot be met because of the inadequacy of the flow reserve. Moroever, hydraulic factors tend to worsen the effect of fixed stenoses. As demand increases, the pressure drop across stenoses increases, and a substantial part of the pressure energy is converted into kinetic energy and then to turbulent energy; this is associated with a redistribution of coronary flow towards the epicardial layers.

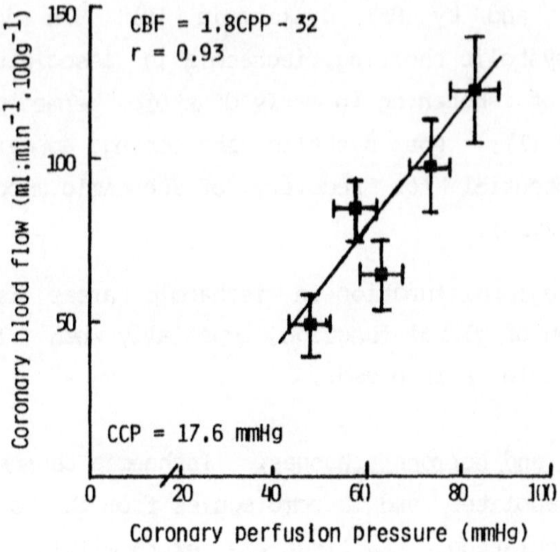

Figure 1. Coronary closing pressure (CCP), also called zero flow pressure (P_{zf}) obtained by extrapolation of pressure/flow relation.

Effects of myocardial ischaemia

a. Electrophysiological changes. An immediate effect of ischaemia is to cause positively and negatively charged ions (K^+, Cl^-) to leak across the cell membrane. This causes an imbalance of electrical potentials at the boundaries between ischaemic and non-ischaemic myocardium. Such differences in electrical potentials create a current of injury that flows from injured to normal tissue during electrical diastole and is seen on the surface electrocardiogram as ST segment changes. Another consequence of ischaemia is the development of re-entry circuits at the boundaries of ischaemic segments, leading to ventricular dysrhythmias, including ventricular fibrillation (8).

b. Mechanical effects. The left ventricular myocardium shortens by 15-20% of its resting length during systole and the wall thickens in the same proportion. Regional ischaemia causes hypokinesia (reduced shortening and thickening), akinesia (absence of shortening and thickening), and dyskinesia (systolic lengthening and systolic thinning). In case of coronary artery constriction, a reduction of coronary blood flow by 10-20% causes hypokinesia, by 80% akinesia, and by 95% dyskinesia (9). In addition to the reduction in systolic shorting, ischaemia is associated with the continuation of shotening in early diastole, termed post-systolic shortening (10,11). Post-systolic shortening appears to be a marker of potential for recovery of ischaemic myocardium after reperfusion (12,13).

Altered regional function in ischaemic areas is associated with depression of global function, especially when a large area of the left ventricle is involved.

c. Biochemical and hormonal changes. Ischaemia causes the leakage of ions, metabolites and macromolecules from the ischaemic cells into the circulation. Earliest is extracellular leakage of potassium ions, caused by impaired activity of energy-requiring ion pumps (14). In prolonged ischaemia, raised catecholamine levels drive potassium ions back into the cells and hypokalaemia may develop. Inadequate energy supply causes lactate production, leakage of adenosine and macromolecules, associated with an increase in the isoenzyme of creatine-kinase, CK-MB.

d. Cellular damage advances as a wavefront from the endocardium to the epicardium giving the completed infarct the shape of a truncated pyramid with its base on the subendocardium.

Collateral circulation

Collateral channels link the coronary arteries in humans. These native collaterals are small in diameter and number. In response to myocardial ischaemia, there is widening and disruption of the architecture of collateral vessels followed by perivascular inflammation. This subsides in a later phase and the vessels become thinner and larger. A massive increase in diameter (up to eight-fold) is associated with cellular proliferation and wall thickening. Angiographically visible collateral channels may provide enough blood flow to maintain structure and function in areas supplied by occluded coronary arteries.

In patients with coronary artery disease, several types of anatomical patterns of lesion have emerged (15). In approximately 23% of patients, a steal prone anatomy is present. This associates the complete occlusion of one artery, a stenosis of another, and the presence of demonstrable collaterals between both territories (Figure 2). In 51% of patients, one or more stenoses

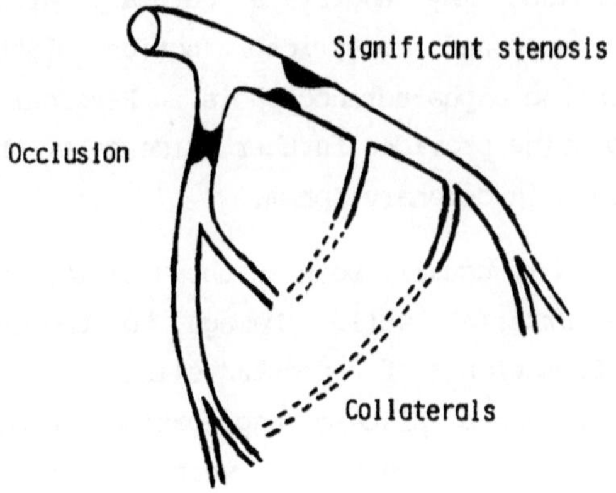

Figure 2. Diagrammatic representation of a steal-prone coronary anatomy as described by Buffington et al (1988).

are present but no vessel is occluded; in 10% of patients, a total occlusion is observed, but no collaterals can be identified; and in 16% a total occlusion is noted, collaterals are visible, but without stenosis in the territory which supplies the collaterals.

Coronary spasm

Coronary spasm is a well recognized feature of Prinzmetal angina. Coronary spasm may be a critical factor in effort angina and occasionally of myocardial infarction. Transmural defects in uptake of radionuclide tracers have been observed in areas of myocardium supplied by a vessel in spasm, and found to be associated with ST-segment elevation. Humoral factors may play an important role in coronary spasm. Indeed, alpha and beta-adrenoceptors are present in coronary arteries. Alpha-adrenoceptor stimulation increases the cell membrane permeability to calcium ions, thus increasing smooth muscle tone. Conversely, beta-adrenoceptor stimulation causes hyperpolarization of the cell membrane and increases the production of cyclic AMP. This reduces calcium ion concentration and decreases vascular smooth muscle tone. When vascular tone is normal, adrenergic stimulation causes vasodilatation because beta-adrenoceptors predominate. Beta-adrenoceptor blockade may aggravate coronary artery spasm by permitting the unopposed constrictor action of the sympathetic nervous system on the alpha-adrenoceptors. Reversal of coronary spasm by phentolamine provides further evidence of the role of the alpha-adrenoceptors in coronary spasm.

Coronary spasm is usually seen in the vicinity of morphologic changes of the arterial wall. Damage to the endothelium may preclude the formation of prostacyclins. If too little prostacyclin is released, platelet aggregation can occur and cause the release of vasoactive substances which in turn will cause vasoconstriction. This is another possible mechanism for coronary artery spasm. While most episodes of ischemia occuring during anesthesia relate to an imbalance between oxygen supply and demand caused by large haemodynamic changes, some may be due to coronary spasm. Indeed, coronary spasm has been shown to occur during anesthesia in response to interventions that increase sympathetic activity. Before tachycardia and hypertension can be detected, substantial reductions in coronary blood flow have been documented.

Effects of anaesthesia on the coronary circulation.

a. Normal myocardium. Most of the experimental and human studies of the effects of inhalational and intravenous anaesthetic agents on the normal coronary circulation have shown that coronary blood flow changes as an almost direct function of myocardial oxygen requirement. This indicates that local regulation of coronary blood flow is maintained, and thus the global effects of the anaesthetic agent on the circulation cause appropriate changes in coronary vascular tone. Inhalational agents decrease contractility and systolic pressure in a dose-dependent fashion, so that oxygen demand is substantially reduced. Local regulation of coronary blood flow operates and coronary blood flow decreases. With enflurane, the reduction of coronary flow is slightly less than that of oxygen demand, suggesting modest vasodilatation (16). Isoflurane, however, interferes with the regulation of coronary flow, because it is a powerful vasodilator (17,18). Thus, during isoflurane anaesthesia coronary blood flow exceeds the oxygen requirements and oxygen extraction is reduced. The profound coronary vasodilatation induced by isoflurane is of no consequence in the normal heart. However, it may promote coronary steal in the compromised heart (17).

Nitrous oxide does not appear to alter the coronary flow regulation in experimental animals with normal coronary arteries (19). However, nitrous oxide appears to constrict epicardial coronary arteries (20), and may cause dysfunction in compromised myocardium (21).

The intravenous anaesthetics used for induction of anaesthesia tend to increase coronary blood flow, mainly because they elicit tachycardia and, therefore, increase myocardial oxygen consumption. Etomidate differs from thiopentone, and methohexitone, in that it causes an increase in coronary blood flow without increasing myocardial oxygen consumption. This indicates coronary vasodilation (22). Morphine may increase coronary vascular resistance (23) whilst fentanyl exerts little effect on coronary blood flow and resistance (24).

Irrespective of the anaesthetic agents used for maintenance of anaesthesia, alterations of the coronary blood flow regulation may occur because of changes in carbon dioxide tension (25). Hypercapnia causes coronary vasodilatation associated with reduced oxygen extraction, while hypocapnia causes vasoconstriction associated with increased oxygen extraction.

b. Compromised myocardium. Early studies of the effects of anaesthesia on ischaemic myocardium have used models of acute, complete occlusion. With such models halogenated anaesthetics and opioids appear, in most studies, to minimize the extent of ischaemic damage (26,27). However, in models of critical coronary artery stenosis, selective depression of the compromised myocardium associated with regional dysfunction has been reported (10,28). These adverse effects are due mostly to the dose-dependent reduction in coronary perfusion pressure that attends the administration of inhalational anaesthetics (Figure 3). In such

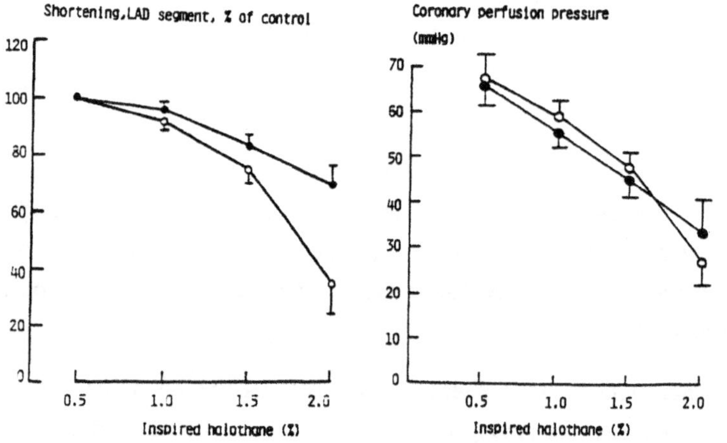

Figure 3. Before (●—●) and after critical constriction of the left anterior descending coronary artery (o—o) halothane reduces the coronary perfusion pressure. Selec--tive depression of function is noted in the compromised territory (after Lowenstein et al, 1981).

models, opioids do not cause selective depression and dysfunction of compromised myocardium because they do not reduce the coronary perfusion pressure (21). However, the addition of nitrous oxide to opioids may cause myocardial dysfunction (21,29). A specific question is that of drug induced coronary steal. Poweful vasodilators such as dipyridamole and isoflurane may induce sufficient dilation of resistance coronary vessels to reduce blood supply in territories that rely exclusively on collateral flow to maintain function and cell integrity. Experimental and clinical studies (17,30,31) suggest that changes in regional function, electrocardiographic alterations, and modifications of lactate metabolism indicative of ischaemia may develop during isoflurane anaesthesia, especially when relatively high concentrations are administered, and the patient has a steal-prone anatomy of the coronary circulation.

It must be borne in mind that cardiovascular drugs play an important role in the anaesthetic management of patients with coronary heart disease, and may modify the responses of the circulation to anaesthesia and surgery. Experimentally, beta-adrenoceptor blockade appears to protect the function of compromised territories (32), while calcium antagonists exaggerate the adverse effects of anaesthesia on ischaemic territories (33). Clinical studies have shown that beta-adrenoceptor blockers are effective in preventing the development of mycoardial ischaemia (34,35,36), while calcium antagonists are not (36,37).

It is well established that increases in heart rate, through an increase in oxygen demand and a reduction of blood supply (because of the shorter duration of diastole) facilitates the development of myocardial ischaemia in patients with coronary artery disease. Similarly, increases in arterial pressure compromise the oxygen balance of the ischaemic myocardium because the coronary reserve is limited and thus coronary blood flow may not increase in the same proportion as oxygen demand. Finally, hypotension compromises the ischaemic myocardium because the reduction of diastolic pressure decreases the effective perfusion pressure of the coronary circulation (the gradient between diastolic pressure and critical closing pressure), thus causing inordinate reductions of coronary flow. All of these changes have been shown to be associated with myocardial ischaemia and myocardial infarction in patients with ischaemic heart disease; it is imperative to try to prevent these changes and to treat them rapidly should they develop during anaesthesia, surgery, or recovey.

References:

1 Klocke FJ, Bunnell Il, Greene DG, Wittenberg SM, Wisco JP. Circulation, 1974; **50**: 547-559.

2 Stone HL. Ann Rev Physiol, 1983; **45**: 213-217.

3 Gertz EW, Wisneski JA, Neese R, Bristow JD, Searle GL, Hanlon JT. Circulation, 1981; **63**: 1273-1279.

4 Olsson RA, Bunger R. Prog Cardiovasc Res, 1987; **29**: 369-387.

5 Epstein SE, Canenn RO III, Talbot TL. Am J Cardiol, 1985; **56**: 4E-10E.

6 Buckberg GD, Fixler DE, Archie JP, Hoffman JIE. Circ Res, 1972; **30**: 67-81.

7 Bellamy RF Circ Res, 1987; **43**: 92-100.

8 Janse MJ, Kleber AG. Circ Res, 1981; **49**: 1069-1081.

9 Vatner SF. Circ Res, 1980; **50**: 547-559.

10 Lowenstein E, Foëx P, Francis CM, Davies WL, Yusuf S, Ryder WA. Anesthesiology, 1981; **55**: 349-359.

11 Doyle RL, Foëx P, Ryder WA, Jones LA. Cardiovasc Res, 1987; **21**: 507-514.

12 Brown MA, Norris RM, Takayama M, White MD. Cardiovasc Res, 1987; **21**: 702-716.

13 Takayama M, Norris RM, Brown MA, Armiger L, White HD. Circulation, 1988; **78**: 994-1007.

14 Hearse DJ, Crome R, Yellon DM, Wyse RKH. Cardiovasc Res, 1983; **17**: 452-458.

15 Buffington C, Davis K, Gillipsie S, Pettinger M. Anesthesiology, 1987; **66**: 293-300.

16 Merin R. Anesthesiology, 1981; **55**: 398:408.

17 Reiz S, Balfors E, Sorensen MB, Ariola S, Friedman A, Truedsson H. Anesthsiology, 1983; **59**, 91-97.

18 Cutfield GR, Francis CM, Foëx P, Jones LA, Ryder WA. Br J Anaesth, 1988; **60**: 784-790.

19 Thorburn J, Smith G, Vance JP, Brown DM. Br J Anaesth, 1979; **51**: 937-942.

20 Wilkowski DAW, Sill JC, Bonta W, Owen R, Bove AA. Anesthesiology, 1987; **66**: 659-665.

21 Philbin DM, Foëx P, Drummond G, Lowenstein E, Ryder WA, Jones LA. Anesthesiology, 1985; **62**: 166-174.

22 Kettler D, Sonntag H. Acta Anaesth Belg, 1974; **3**: 384-401.

23 Vatner S, Marsh JD, Swain JA. J Clin Invest, 1975; **55**: 207-217.

24 Sonntag H, Hellberg K, Schenk H-D, Donath U, Regensburger D, Kettler D, Duchanova H, Larsen R. Acta Anaesth Scand, 1975; **19**: 69-78.

25 Foëx P, Ryder WA. (1979). Bull Europ Physiopath Resp, **15**: 625-638.

26 Bland JHL, Lowenstein E. Anesthesiology, 1976; **45**: 287-293.

27 Theroux P, Ross J, Franklin D, Kemper WS, Sasayama S. Circulation, 1976; **53**: 302-314.

28 Priebe H-J, Foëx P. Anesthesiology, 1987; **66**: 293-300.

29 Leone BJ, Philbin DM, Lehot J-J, Foëx P, Ryder WA. (1988). Anesth Analg, **67**: 814-822.

30 Reiz S, Ostman M. Anesth Analg, 1985; **64**: 570-576.

31 Moffitt EA, Barker RA, Glenn JJ, Imrie DD, DelCampo C, Landymore RW, Kinley E, Murphy DA. Anesth Analg, 1986; **65**: 53-61.

32 Leone BJ, Lehot J-J, Francis CM, Cutfield GR, Foëx P. (1987) Anesth Anal, **66**: 607-614.

33 Leone BJ, Philbin DM, Lehot J-J, Wilkins M, Foëx P, Ryder WA. (1988). Anesth Analg, **67**: 205-210.

34 Stone JG, Foëx P, Sear JW, Johnson LL, Khambatta HJ, Triner L. (1988). Br J Anaesth, **61**: 675-679.

35 Slogoff S, Keats AS. Anesthesiology, 1988; **68**: 676-680.

36 Chung F, Houston PL, Cheng DCH, Lavelle PA, McDonald N, Burns J, David TE. Anesthesiology, 1988; **69**: 343-347.

THE AGING HEART

S. MURAVCHICK

The most important advance in our understanding of the physiology of aging has been the recognition of the need to distinguish clearly between processes of aging and age-related disease. Only those manifestations of altered tissue and organ system function and structure which are universally present in all elderly individuals, and which increase in severity or magnitude with increasing age, represent aging. Changes in function or structure which are not universally present or which do not demonstrate a direct relationship between severity and chronologic age reflect age-related disease. Sixty-five percent of the geriatric population has definable cardiovascular disease; therefore, it is futile to attempt to assess the intrinsic effects of aging on cardiovascular function using large-scale epidemiologic investigations alone. Even for patients in the seventh decade of life free of cardiac symptoms, there is a 12% incidence of coronary artery disease, a figure which does not include those individuals with other forms of cardiovascular pathology such as valvular dysfunction or hypertension.

The major anatomic and histologic cardiac changes in the aging human heart include an increase in ventricular wall thickness, diffuse myocardial fibrosis, and valvular fibro-calcification. Intramyocardial lipofuscin deposition may result in "brown atrophy of the heart". The mechanical consequences of increased myocardial thickness and stiffness are predictable: ventricular compliance decreases, making relatively small changes in intravascular volume, venous capacitance or loss of the

T. H. Stanley and R. J. Sperry (eds.), Anesthesiology and the Heart, 65–68.

synchrony between atrial and ventricular systoles important determinants of cardiac function in the aged patient. There is also a loss of elasticity in the aorta and other branches of the arterial tree. As a consequence, there is increased impedance to ejection of stroke volume, a rise in systolic pressure and widened pulse pressure, and generalized hypertrophy of the left ventricular wall. These age-related reductions in arterial elasticity are seen even in populations in which pathologic arteriosclerosis is virtually unknown. Hypertension and arteriosclerotic disease, with or without myocardial ischemia, is the most common presentation of age-related pathology in the geriatric population. Half of all elderly patients evidence this type of age-related disease, and it may be the major factor in perioperative death for 10% of this group.

Overall, however, age changes cardiac function less that it changes its structure. The classic data suggest a relentless decline in cardiac index with advancing age[1]. More recent studies indicate, however, that normally active, adequately-conditioned elderly individuals maintain cardiac output at resting levels indistinguishable from their younger counterparts[2]. They also appear to be capable of increasing cardiac output appropriately to meet metabolic demand, not by increasing heart rate alone as seen in younger individuals, but by a unique ability to increase left ventricular diastolic volume in response to augmented preload[3]. Stroke volume and cardiac output are thus increased through the Frank-Starling mechanism, instead of by augmentation of ejection fraction[4]. Homeostatic cardiac mechanisms requiring increased rate or velocity of myocardial contraction also diminish in importance with advancing age. Both human and animal studies demonstrate an age-related prolongation of the time required for myocardial contraction as well as myocardial relaxation[5]. Maximum heart rate decreases at a rate of approximately 5% per decade after the fifth decade of life[6].

More than 40 years ago, one report indicated that only 39% of patients over 70 years of age without known heart disease had normal EKG tracings[7]. Thirty-one percent had minor changes such as low voltage or occasional premature contractions, and the remaining 31% had definite and consistent abnormalities. More recently, when patients were screened by treadmill tests and thalium scans to exclude those with ischemic heart disease, 89% of patients studied nevertheless had ventricular, and 87% atrial, ectopic complexes during 24-hour monitoring[8]. The nonpathological, truly age-related changes in EKG configuration appear to be decreased S- and T-wave amplitudes, some left shift of axis, increased P-R interval, and a shortened duration of the QRS complex[9]. Some of these changes may reflect the loss of fascicles within the His bundle and a decreased SA-node pacemaker cell population. There is also progressive age-related reduction of resting heart rate seen in the elderly.

The chronotropic and inotropic effects of all beta-agonist drugs are significantly less in elderly than in young individuals, supporting the general concept that aging, at least on an adrenergic level, can be thought of as progressive beta-blockade. Although the maximal contractile response to calcium infusion is the same in elderly as in young subjects, isoproterenol responses are diminished. However, a similar reduction of response is seen with dibuteryl cyclic AMP, an agent with actions independent of the cyclic AMP receptors. It would appear therefore, that biochemical differences in cardiac muscle due to aging may exist in the sequence of events needed for excitation-contraction coupling after the process of adrenergic receptor activation, but before calcium is released from the sarcoplasmic reticulum. In fact, the maximal contractile responses to paired atrioventricular pacing is age-independent, an observation which suggests that the final intracellular steps required for cardiac muscle contraction remain intact.

REFERENCES

1. Brandfonbrener, M., Landowne, M., Shock, N.W. Circulation 12:557-566, 1955.

2. Gerstenblith, G., Fredericksen, J., Yin, F.C.P., Fortuin, N.J., Lakatta, E.G. Circulation 56:273-278, 1977.

3. Port, S., Cobb, F.R., Coleman, R.E., Jones, R.H. N. Engl. J. Med. 303:1133-1137, 1980.

4. Grawath, A., Jansson, B., Strandell, T. Acta. Med. Scand. 176:425-446, 1964.

5. Lakatta, E.G. Fed. Proc. 38:163-167, 1979.

6. Astrand, I., Astrand, P.O., Rodahl, K. J. Appl. Physiol. 14:562-566, 1959.

7. McNamara, R.J. Geriatrics 4:150-160, 1944.

8. Fleg, J.L., Kennedy, H.L. Chest 81:302-307, 1982.

9. Bachman, S., Spanow, D., Smith, L.K. Am. J. Cardiol. 48:513-516, 1981.

HYPERTENSION: IS IT REALLY IMPORTANT

EDWARD D. MILLER, JR., M.D.

The anesthesiologist frequently encounters patients with hypertension. The difficult decision for the anesthesiologist is - is it really important or should we proceed without further information. Elevation in blood pressure results in a dose-dependent increase in morbidity and mortality. This elevation in blood pressure has broad implications for the anesthesiologist because it denotes potential underlying structural and functional changes in various organs of the body. Those alterations result in a diminished "margin of safety" for that organ. The main organs affected by hypertension are the heart, the brain and the kidney. (1) Since the perioperative period results in significant changes induced by anesthesia and surgery, it is not surprising that dysfunction of one of these organs occurs more frequently in the hypertensive patient than in the normotensive patient. Systemic arterial hypertension by definition is a blood pressure greater than 160/95. More recently, studies have examined the consequences of borderline hypertension (140/90 - 160/95) and have found these patients will also develop complications of high blood pressure. It is now established that the severity of the hypertension and the length of time hypertension is present without drug therapy result in an increased incidence of myocardial infarction, stroke or renal dysfunction. This discussion will examine some of the factors involved in hypertension, some of the therapies aimed at the treatment of

T. H. Stanley and R. J. Sperry (eds.), Anesthesiology and the Heart, 69–78.

hypertension and recommendations for the anesthetic management of these patients.

Systemic hypertension may be divided into two broad categories: primary or essential hypertension and secondary hypertension. Secondary hypertension includes hypertension due to identifiable factors such as primary aldosteronism, stenosis of the renal artery resulting in renovascular disease, parenchymal disease such as nephrosclerosis, and pheochromocytoma.

Secondary Hypertension

Secondary hypertension comprises about 10% of all hypertension. Specific treatment of the underlying condition results in a complete cure of the hypertension in most cases. While these patients represent only a small percentage of all hypertensives, an understanding of their basic pathophysiology may be helpful in the diagnosis and treatment of patients with essential hypertension.

Primary Aldosteronism

Primary aldosteronism is a condition in which an adenoma in the adrenal gland produces excess amounts of aldosterone. Aldosterone is a potent steroid which results in sodium retention and subsequent potassium excretion by the kidney. With increased sodium retention, effective blood volume is increased and blood pressure becomes elevated. The patient presents with hypertension, hypokalemia, low plasma renin activity and metabolic alkalosis. Removal of the adenoma results in a cure of the hypertension.

Renal Artery Stenosis

If one or both renal arteries become stenotic, hypertension may result. In younger individuals, the stenosis is due to fibromuscular thickening of the renal artery, while in older patients, it is due to atherosclerosis. The stenosis causes a decrease in pressure within the kidney. This decrease in pressure is sensed, and renin, a protolytic enzyme, is released from the kidney. Renin acts on a plasma protein to form angiotensin I which is converted to angiotensin II in passage through the pulmonary circulation. Angiotensin II is a potent vasoconstrictor, as well as a stimulus to aldosterone secretion. These two factors work in concert to raise arterial blood pressure. With correction of the stenosis, arterial pressure falls toward control levels if the hypertension has not been too long-standing.

Renal Parenchymal Disease

Renal parenchymal disease often results in patients with an increased arterial blood pressure. It appears that about 80% of these patients have increased arterial pressure secondary to increased extracellular volume. This increased volume is due to the patient's inability to excrete solutes because of his renal dysfunction. If renal dialysis is employed, blood pressure can be controlled with this therapeutic modality alone. The other 20% of these patients appear to have a renin-dependent hypertension and are greatly helped by inhibition of the renin-angiotensin system.

Pheochromocytoma

Pheochromocytoma still remains one of the anesthetic challenges of today. In the past, operative mortality for removal of this tumor was high. Because of better understanding of the underlying pathophysiology and improvement in drug therapy, this is no longer true.

Successful anesthetic and surgical management is often assured with good preoperative management. Because of persistent catecholamine excess, blood volume and plasma volume may be decreased. With preoperative treatment with phenoxybenzamine, not only is blood pressure decreased but also blood volume is restored toward normal. Blood transfusion because of anemia may be instituted at this time as well if it is indicated. Metyrosine (alpha methyl tyrosine), an inhibitor of tyrosine hydroxylase, has also been used as a preoperative drug instead of phenoxybenzamine. Many believe that beta blockade is also helpful in these patients especially if ventricular arrhythmias are present or if heart rate is greater than 100 beats/minute.

Arterial catheter for monitoring blood pressure and either a CVP or Swan-Ganz catheter prior to anesthesia are helpful for the induction of anesthesia. While a variety of anesthetic techniques have been used with success, forane or enflurane offer theoretical advantages. (2) Increases in blood pressure are treated with sodium nitroprusside; and ventricular arrhythmias, with propranolol or esmolol. Labatol is also effective. Fluid replacement is vigorous prior to tumor removal.

With tumor removal, blood pressure may decrease markedly; but if volume replacement is adequate, this if often not a problem anymore. Persistent hypotension should be treated with a vasopressor to "buy time" until appropriate measurements can be made to determine the underlying cause. Postoperatively, blood pressure tends to return toward more normal levels. However, patients with long-standing hypertension may remain elevated for some time before baroreceptor resetting begins. While only 0.1-0.2% of all hypertensive patients have a pheochromocytoma, it is one of the few surgically treatable forms of hypertension.

Primary Hypertension

While the secondary causes of hypertension are well understood, the common variety of hypertension--essential hypertension--still remains without a specific etiology. Page and McCubbin proposed the mosaic theory of hypertension which linked several factors together. These included heredity, salt intake, psychological influences, and the sympathetic nervous system.

Presently, investigators have begun to look more closely at amounts of catecholamines on target organs, the sodium-potassium transport systems of a variety of cells, and the search for a putative hormone that might initiate or maintain the hypertensive state. Investigators have also sought the nature of a substance called naturetic factor and have tried to implicate it in hypertension. None of these studies is conclusive. Whether one factor or a combination of factors will prove to be crucial for the development of hypertension remains to be proven.

Whatever the cause of hypertension, certain hemodynamic findings are similar. First, cardiac output is normal and the hypertension is due to an increased peripheral vascular resistance. Second, any stimuli which causes constriction of vascular smooth muscle will have more pronounced effect in the hypertensive patient as compared to the normotensive patient. This means that the blood pressure response will be greater in the hypertensive patient at intubation, for example. These exaggerated responses may be modified by appropriate drug therapy. (3,4)

<u>Drug Therapy</u>

In the classic pharmacological study of the importance of drug therapy of hypertension by Freis and coworkers, it was well established that the morbidity and mortality of severe hypertension could be greatly decreased if blood pressure was lowered. It appears that the manner in which blood pressure is lowered is not as important as the fact that the blood pressure remains in the normal range. Patients' lack of compliance with drug therapy has been one major reason for the development of new drugs with fewer side effects.

Mild hypertension has been shown to be effectively treated with diuretics. How diuretics lower blood pressure is not known. Patients with essential hypertension have been shown to have a decreased plasma volume. Perhaps diuretics cause the loss of sodium from cells important in blood pressure control.

Beta blockers have been added to the list of drugs which are now used to treat hypertension. Because the antihypertensive effect of such drugs requires weeks for onset, the blockade of B-receptors alone does not adequately explain their mode of action. Beta blockers are known to inhibit renin release, and part of their antihypertensive action may be due to this mechanism.

Much of the drug therapy of moderate to severe hypertension has been directed at agents which act directly on the sympathetic nervous system. Guanethidine, reserpine, and prazosin have a predominant effect on the peripheral sympathetic nervous system while agents such as clonidine and methyldopa work centrally.

Drug therapy aimed at inhibition of the renin-angiotensin system with enalapril and captopril has now been shown to be extremely effective in patients with renovascular hypertension and also, surprisingly, in patients with essential hypertension. Currently, calcium channel blockers such as diltiazem, which cause relaxation of peripheral vascular smooth muscle, has shown to be an effective antihypertensive agent. The newer agents (beta blockers, converting enzyme inhibitors and calcium channel blockers) have grown in popularity because of the decreased incidence of side effects and the need of therapy only once or twice a day. Such improvements have resulted in better patient acceptance and therefore compliance.

Data and experience have now shown that when a hypertensive patient comes to a surgical operation, antihypertensive agents should be continued up to, and after, the surgical procedure. Concern that the sympathetic nervous system dysfunction caused by the antihypertensive agents would result in severe hypotension intraoperatively has not been verified.

Anesthetic Considerations

The most important consideration in the care of the hypertensive patient is to recognize that the patient is hypertensive. Initial blood pressure recordings may be high and subsequently are in the normotensive range. These patients are the labile hypertensive patients and often have the largest changes in blood pressure in the perioperative period. While severe intraoperative hypertension may be effectively treated, a better course of treatment would be the prevention of such episodes. If the patient is diagnosed as being hypertensive, then appropriate lab work would include BUN, creatinine, serum K^+, EKG and chest x-ray. If history or physical findings suggest cardiac dysfunction, other tests may be indicated. It is now well appreciated that patients with hypertension often have left ventricular wall thickening as detected by echocardiography. EKG and chest x-ray is often normal in such patients. In such patients, history of angina should be carefully sought and evaluation of the coronary system may be indicated prior to major surgery.

The type of surgery may also be an important factor in determining if the patient is ready for surgery. It is known that cerebral autoregulation is altered in hypertensive states. Recent data suggest that antihypertensive therapy will partially restore cerebral autoregulation. (5) Therefore, the decision whether to use either controlled hypotension or allow blood pressure to decrease significantly for a particular procedure will partially be based on the adequacy of antihypertensive therapy prior to surgery.

Since much of the knowledge concerning morbidity and mortality is based on arbitrary limits of blood pressure, so also are the recommendations concerning when a patient should be cancelled for elective surgery. A guideline which may be useful is a diastolic pressure greater than 110 mm Hg. Then, surgery should be cancelled and appropriate drug therapy instituted. Since these pressures are seen only in a small minority of patients, surgery need not often be postponed. The majority of patients who are found to have hypertension prior to surgery or who are inadequately controlled have diastolic pressures less than 110 mm Hg and can be managed safely intraoperatively. (6)

Preoperative Medication

As has been stated, oral antihypertensive agents should be continued up to the time of surgery and begun postoperatively as soon as possible. Other premedicants include the use of benzodiazepines or barbiturates to lessen the anxiety of the patient prior to surgery. Often intravenous sedation prior to anesthesia gives some indication of the degree of lability of blood pressure. Such information portends the anesthetic agents that will be most useful.

Recent data would suggest that inhibition of the sympathetic nervous system prior to induction may be very beneficial in the patient at risk. Stone and colleagues demonstrated that a single small oral dose of beta adrenergic blocking agent decreased myocardial ischemia in the perioperative period in patients with moderate hypertension. (7) While the number of patients studied was small and outcome studies were not done, the implications of such a study are great. Similarly, the use of clonidine preoperatively clearly demonstrated that intraoperative lability of blood pressure was decreased and that requirements for inhalational agents and narcotics was diminished. In another study in which clonidine was given, the incidence of postoperative shivering was decreased. The implications from such studies are that preoperative blunting of the sympathetic nervous system is important for the perioperative management of the hypertensive patient. (8,9)

Intraoperative Management

The main aim of intraoperative management of the hypertensive patient should be to diminish large increases in blood pressure seen at times of intubation, incision and at completion of surgery. This is often best accomplished by the use of generous doses of short acting narcotics, increased amounts of barbiturates at induction and skillful intubation. Attention to decreasing heart rate at this time by narcotics or beta blockers is important. Regional anesthesia is also an acceptable form of anesthesia but shows no distinct advantage over general anesthesia except for the stress of intubation. If intraoperative hypertension should occur, treatment with increased anesthesia and/or vasodilating agents is indicated.

Postoperative Management

Most authors would now agree that hypertension and tachycardia at the end of the procedure or in the recovery room are probably responsible for the morbidity and mortality that attends a hypertensive patient. It must be emphasized that the patient who has hypertension may have increased left ventricular wall mass, may have coronary artery disease and if allowed to be stressed by pain, shivering, increased carbon dioxide or hypoxia, go on to have myocardial ischemia and infarction. Vigorous treatment of tachycardia first and hypertension second can be accomplished in many ways. Labetalol has been shown to be very effective in such situations. (10)

Conclusions

A well-controlled, hypertensive patient presents minimal anesthetic problems. With the excellent pharmacological agents available for effectively decreasing the patient's blood pressure preoperatively, the goal of the anesthesiologist should be to identify patients with undiagnosed hypertension and have therapy begun. When this is not possible, the anesthetic and surgical experience may result in significant morbidity and mortality if appropriate modes of therapy are not instituted.

References

1. Strandgaard S, Olesen J, Skinghof E, Lassen NA: Br Med J 1:507-509, 1973
2. Suzukawa M, Michaels I, Ruzbarsky J, Kopriva C, Kitahata L: Anesth Analg 62:100-103, 1983
3. Prys-Roberts C: Anesthesiology 50:281-284, 1979
4. Prys-Roberts C: Int Anesthesiol Clin 4:18, 1980
5. Hoffman WE, Miletich DJ, Albrecht RF: Anesthesiology 58:326-332, 1983
6. Goldman L, Caldera DL: Anesthesiology 50:285-292, 1979
7. Stone JG, Foex P, Sear JW, et al: Anesthesiology 68:495-500, 1988
8. Longnecker DE: Anesthesiology 67:1-2, 1987
9. Roizen M: Anesthesiology 68:482-484, 1988
10. Leslie JB, Kalayjian RW, Sirgo MA, et al: Anesthesiology 67:413-416, 1987

PERIOPERATIVE MYOCARDIAL ISCHEMIA: DIAGNOSIS AND TREATMENT

DENNIS T. MANGANO, PH.D., M.D.

Ischemic heart disease continues to be prevalent in the United States and throughout the world. There are approximately 10 million patients in the United States with ischemic heart disease. This incidence will continue to be high because of the growth of our aging population. To anesthesiologists the impact is significant. Approximately 1 million patients with ischemic heart disease undergo noncardiac surgery in the United States every year. This population represents a significant challenge to the anesthesiologist because of the associated perioperative morbidity. Previous studies have addressed the question of perioperative myocardial reinfarction. They found a 7% incidence of perioperative reinfarction with a mortality of 40 to 70%. These alarmingly high statistics precipitated more recent studies in an effort to control the morbidity associated with ischemic heart disease. One such study suggested that morbidity may be reduced by aggressive intraoperative and postoperative monitoring and therapy, in addition to meticulous preoperative preparation. Using these techniques, reinfarction rates were 2 to 6%, versus the previously reported rates of 6 to 37%. Additional studies focused on a variety of techniques, including routine electrocardiograms, multiple lead electrocardiograms, Holter monitors, echocardiograms, and pulmonary artery catheters. It was demonstrated that the incidence of intraoperative ischemia is high, occurring in 20 to 69% of patients. In addition, three of these studies demonstrated an increased rate of perioperative myocardial infarction in patients who became ischemic when compared to those who did not. Finally, a limited number of studies have considered the role of therapeutic intervention. However, reduction in morbidity remains to be proved conclusively.

Because of the results of these studies and the influx of more sophisticated monitoring equipment into the operating room, there is an increasing emphasis on the detection of intraoperative ischemia. In this chapter, we will address this by reviewing: 1) The pathophysiology of myocardial ischemia; 2) The detection of the ischemic response.

T. H. Stanley and R. J. Sperry (eds.), Anesthesiology and the Heart, 79–90.

THE PATHOPHYSIOLOGY OF MYOCARDIAL ISCHEMIA

Myocardial ischemia occurs when the metabolic demands of the myocardium are not adequately met. Specifically, ischemia represents an imbalance between myocardial oxygen supply and demand. Treatment attempts to restore this balance.

Myocardial Oxygen Demand

High-energy phosphates generated through aerobic metabolism are the principal source of myocardial energy. Unlike skeletal muscle, the accumulation of significant oxygen debt during strenuous activity is not well tolerated. A high degree of oxygen extraction (at least 75%) is necessary to maintain normal myocardial function even during minimal activity. Myocardial oxygen consumption (MVO_2) is determined by six factors. The three major factors are myocardial wall tension, contractility and heart rate. The three minor factors are basal metabolism, energy of activation and fiber shortening. *Myocardial wall tension* is directly proportional to the radius of the ventricle and the developed pressure; it is inversely proportional to the thickness of the left ventricular wall. Increases in intraventricular pressure and volume, and in vascular afterload, increase intramyocardial wall tension and systolic wall stress. *Myocardial contractility* is classically defined using isolated muscle strip preparations. Unfortunately, clinical measurements of the velocity of fiber shortening are difficult to obtain. *Heart rate*, the third major determinant, has both direct and indirect effects on oxygen consumption. As heart rate increases, so does contractility and, therefore, oxygen consumption; in contrast, as heart rate increases, diastolic filling may decrease and, therefore, intramyocardial wall tension. The degree to which these factors offset one another depends on individual pathophysiology. *Basal metabolism* of the heart accounts for approximately 15 to 20% of the total oxygen requirements and is necessary for maintenance of intracellular metabolism. *Activation energy* accounts for approximately 1% of oxygen consumption and is necessary for maintenance of electrical activity and transmission. *Fiber shortening* is determined during the ejection of a volume of blood from the left ventricle to the aorta under constant pressure conditions. The oxygen consumption associated with volume work is significantly less than that of pressure work. Eighty percent of the total oxygen consumed by the heart occurs prior to aortic valve opening during isovolemic contraction. Only 20% of the work occurs during volume transmission from the left ventricle to the aorta.

Myocardial Oxygen Supply

Myocardial oxygen supply is dependent on two factors: arterial oxygen content and coronary blood flow. In normal patients breathing room air, the arterial oxygen content is approximately 20 ml per 100 ml of blood. Under resting conditions, the heart extracts approximately 15 ml per 100 ml of blood.

Thus, the effects of content on oxygen supply become manifest when oxygen saturations approach 75% or when hemoglobin decreases below 10 grams/100 ml. Even under increased oxygen requirements, arterial oxygen content does not appear to be a major factor affecting supply since both anemia and pulmonary shunt can be effectively managed clinically.

However, coronary blood flow is a major factor affecting myocardial oxygen supply. Either acute decreases in flow or failure to increase flow as metabolism increases are the usual causes of acute myocardial ischemia. Coronary blood flow is inversely proportional to the coronary vascular resistance (CVR) and directly proportional to the perfusion pressure and the duration of diastole (for the LV).

Coronary Vascular Resistance

CVR is affected by changes which occur in both the larger epicardial conductance vessels and the smaller intramyocardial arteriolar vessels. The epicardial vessels contribute to the CVR when significant atherosclerosis is present or when coronary spasm occurs. With respect to the epicardial vessels, fixed lesions can occur concentrically or excentrically, with varying degrees of stenosis. Stenoses of 50% or less (luminal diameter) do not affect coronary flow at rest or during maximal arteriolar vasodilation. With 60 to 80% occlusion, resting flow is maintained by compensatory arteriolar dilation. Critical stenoses of 80% or greater cause decreases in resting flow. Resistance is also affected by the length of the stenosis, the number of stenotic segments, and the anatomy of the stenosis (concentric, excentric or crescent-shaped).

With respect to the arteriolar vessels, both intrinsic and extrinsic factors affect vasomotor tone. Intrinsic factors directly affect the smooth muscle of the vessel wall and include autoregulation, metabolic factors, neural factors, and the effects of pharmacologic agents. Extrinsic factors consist mainly of mechanical compression of the vessel wall, usually occurring during active myocardial contraction.

In response to local metabolic factors, the coronary vessels have the ability to autoregulate, i.e., maintain flow over large ranges of pressure. Adenosine, a product of ATP metabolism, appears to be the most significant mediator. Autoregulation confers a degree of vascular reserve on the coronary bed such that when flow is impeded in one portion of the vessel, the remaining portion can dilate to compensate. For example, with significant stenosis in a proximal epicardial vessel, maximal coronary vasodilation of the distal arteriolar vessel occurs, using coronary vascular reserve with flow becoming entirely pressure dependent. As perfusion pressure decreases, so does coronary flow, until flow ceases (at approximately 35 mm Hg). Thus, coronary autoregulation plays a critical role in the maintenance of coronary flow, especially when proximal atherosclerosis or spasm exists. In addition to coronary autoregulation, a second "compensatory" mechanism exists. Upon relief of obstruction or spasm of a vessel, flow can increase by two- to threefold to compensate for the degree and duration of the occlusion. The absence of this reactive hyperemia implies that coronary vasodilation is maximal and no coronary reserve exists. Any increase in the metabolic requirements would be accompanied by myocardial ischemia.

Coronary Perfusion Pressure

Coronary perfusion pressure is generally regarded as diastolic aortic pressure minus the left ventricular end-diastolic pressure (LVEDP). Although this is a useful clinical definition, several comments are necessary. During systole, left ventricular intercavitary pressure increases, markedly as does subendocardial intramyocardial pressure. Subendocardial flow effectively ceases and can even reverse during systolic contraction. The intramyocardial tension in the subepicardial region is less, and flow during systole is diverted to the subepicardial layer. The total left ventricular flow during systole represents only approximately 15% of total flow. The majority of flow in the left ventricle occurs during diastole. (In contrast, the right ventricle receives 50% or more of its flow during systole because of the lower intercavitary pressures.)

Approximately 85% of the left ventricular flow occurs during diastole because of the lower intercavitary pressure during this period. Although the left ventricular mean diastolic and end-diastolic pressures represent the intercavitary pressures, they do not necessarily reflect the true back pressure on the coronary artery. Studies in animals demonstrate that the pressure at which zero flow (P_{ZF}) occurs in the left coronary system can be significantly higher than the intercavitary LVEDP and may represent a truer back pressure. However, for clinical purposes, it is reasonable to assume that the LVEDP is a correlate of back pressure, and that increases in LVEDP may cause significant decreases in coronary flow.

Duration of Diastole

Since 85% of left ventricular coronary flow occurs during diastole, the total duration of diastole is an important determinant of total coronary flow. As heart rate increases, the duration of both systole and diastole decreases, but the diastolic decrease is proportionately greater. This response is nonlinear, however, with the most significant effects occurring at the lowest heart rates. As heart rate increases from 50 to 70, the relative percent of time spent in diastole decreases by 20%; whereas, as heart rate increases from 90 to 110, the percent of diastole decreases by only 5%. Thus, increases in heart rate, particularly over the lower ranges, can significantly decrease coronary flow to the left ventricle.

THE DETECTION OF THE ISCHEMIC RESPONSE

Methods for detection of intraoperative myocardial ischemia are rapidly evolving. Four principal methods are either in clinical use or under study: 1) single lead, multiple lead, and computerized electrocardiographic detection; 2) echocardiographic detection of wall motion abnormalities; 3) pulmonary wedge pressure measurement for detection of alterations in myocardial compliance; and

4) lactate measurement for detection of alterations in myocardial metabolism. These techniques have the potential of providing sensitive measurement of the electrical, mechanical and metabolic components of the ischemic response. Over the coming decade, these and other methods (such as magnetic resonance imaging) will be introduced to the intraoperative setting via clinical studies. Adaptation to the intraoperative environment will depend not only on the accuracy and sensitivity of these methods, but also on the demonstrated effectiveness of these techniques in decreasing perioperative morbidity and mortality. Each of these will be discussed individually, with a focus on background physiology.

Electrical Conduction Effects and the EKG

The surface electrocardiogram, in particular the QRS complex, is a reflection of the total electrical potential of the left and right ventricles. The ST segment represents the period between ventricular depolarization (QRS complex) and repolarization (T wave). In the normal heart, no potential difference exists following depolarization, and the ST segment is isoelectric. With ischemia, the membrane permeability of the myocardial cells is affected and results in intracellular acidosis, sodium and water accumulation, and extracelluar hyperkalemia. Resultant changes in action potential alter ventricular depolarization and repolarization. Characteristic changes in the ST segment occur as well. The most sensitive layer, the subendocardium, produces electrical changes which are opposite in direction from the QRS vector. Thus, precordial measurement of the ST segment will reveal ST depression, and intracavitary measurement will reveal ST elevation. Location of the ST depression correlates well with the anatomic location of injury. However, Blackburn has demonstrated that approximately 89% of the ST changes which occur during exercise tests can be detected with a bipolar lead system with the negative electrode near the V_5 position. It has been demonstrated that even using multiple lead systems, ischemia can occur without detection using the precordial EKG. Thus, a generalized and significant change in subepicardial flow is necessary to produce electrically detectable ischemia. ST segment elevation occurs with acute myocardial infarction, Prinzmetal's variant angina, and ventricular wall motion abnormalities, principally aneurysms. With acute transmural infarction, ST segment elevation is associated with subepicardial ischemia and can vary in amplitude from less than 1 mm to more than 10 mm. With Prinzmetal's angina, the characteristic at-rest ST segment elevations return to baseline following the ischemic episode, without further evolution of Q or T wave changes. Cardiac enzymes are usually negative. These transient ST segment elevations reflect reversible transmural ischemia and are attributed to coronary vasospasm. Persistent ST segment elevation is seen after acute myocardial infarction and usually reflects ventricular dyssynergy, with or without associated aneurysm.

The intraoperative monitoring of the electrocardiographic signs of myocardial ischemia has undergone a marked change over the last decade. Clinical practice has evolved from the use of single lead EKG systems to selective leads to multiple and simultaneous lead monitoring. Recently, automatic detection of ST segment deviation has been introduced using computerized signal processing. Although this process is both timely and interesting, the accuracy and usefulness of such systems must be substantiated before being placed into widespread clinical use.

For those patients at significant risk of developing intraoperative ischemia, older patients undergoing major and prolonged surgery, five electrode electrocardiograhic systems are in common use. The lead systems consist of either a bipolar arrangement, measuring the potential between two electrodes, or a unipolar electrode, measuring the potential between an electrode and a combination of the remaining electrodes. The standard limb leads (I, II, III) are bipolar, whereas the precordial leads (V_1-V_6) and the augmented limb leads (AVR, AVL, AVF) are unipolar. For ischemia detection, in awake man undergoing exercise stress testing, lead V_5 is associated with the largest number of ST segment abnormalities. Furthermore, the diagnostic mode, which filters frequencies below 0.14 Hz, is more useful than the monitor mode (high pass at 4 Hz) for the detection of these ST segment changes. As well, electrical calibration of all signals must be performed if the desired accuracy is to be achieved. What are the criteria for ST ischemia? Based on studies performed in coronary care units and exercise stress testing laboratories, the criteria for ischemic ST changes are a horizontal or downsloping depression of 1 mm or more occurring 80 msec beyond the J point. This depression can be either new or additive and is associated with a greater incidence of complications. Other changes such as isolated J point depression, with an upsloping ST segment are usually rate related and can be a normal response. The depth of depression of the ST segment has been related to subsequent coronary events. Certainly, a 2 mm or more depression carries the most significant prognosis. Recently, the comparative height of the R wave, used as a normalizing factor, has been shown to give greater validity to the standard ST change. Clinical application of this technique will be forthcoming.

Nonspecific ST T wave changes, including less than 1 mm deviation of the ST segment, T wave flattening and inversion, may be associated with myocardial ischemia or other nonischemic causes. For example, these can be normal variants, or can be associated with hyperventilation, strain patterns, or drug effects (digitalis, hypokalemia).

Intraoperative studies using standard, multiple lead and Holter systems have demonstrated a 20 to 69% incidence of intraoperative ischemia in patients with coronary disease undergoing surgery. This rather high incidence has been reported even with intermittent EKG monitoring. Thus, the incidence of intraoperative ischemia may be even higher. The relationship of intraoperative ischemia to supply and demand factors has been addressed in several studies. Initially, it was felt that the double or triple product best correlated with ischemia; however, most recent data implicate heart rate increases as being particularly detrimental. Other studies have demonstrated that there may be no relationship between supply and demand factors, and ischemia occurs spontaneously. The relationship of intraoperative ischemia to postoperative outcome is presently under study. Recently, it has been demonstrated that, in patients who develop intraoperative ischemia, the risk of postoperative infarction is increased two- to threefold. These data imply that intraoperative ischemia should be agressively monitored and treated. With respect to treatment, the usual correction of supply and demand imbalances in combination with the agents which enhance coronary flow to ischemic areas (the nitrates) is the standard of therapy. However, prophylactic use of nitrates, beta blockers or other pharmacologic agents has not been demonstrated to consistently reduce the incidence of intraoperative ischemia.

Wall Motion, Wall Thickening and the Echocardiogram

Studies in animals have demonstrated that soon after coronary occlusion, the ischemic myocardium develops wall motion and wall thickening abnormalities. Both systolic shortening and thickening of the myocardial fibers become impaired. The regional effects on contractility produce abnormal contractions of the wall known as dyssynergy, which passes through the phases of hypokinesis, akinesis and, finally, dyskinesis or aneurysmal-type bulging. These local segmental effects often occur before reductions in local ATP, possibly suggesting the early role of calcium. With depletion of ATP, impairment of contraction becomes complete.

The effects of ischemia on wall thickening are important as well. In fact, wall thickening may be a more specific index of ischemia than wall motion. In the area of acute myocardial infarction, segmental lengths of the involved tissue are increased; paradoxical bulging is noted, and systolic thinning of the wall occurs. Transition regions between the area of infarction and normal tissue show similar abnormalities, but to a lesser degree. Normal regions of the myocardium compensate for these changes with shortened fiber length and increased wall thickening during systolic contraction.

The effects of ischemia on global contractility are complex and depend on a number of factors: the degree of ischemia, the type of wall motion abnormality (akinetic vs dyskinetic), and the amount and performance of the remaining normally functioning myocardial fibers. During the early phases of ischemia, when dyssynergy occurs, energy is lost via the paradoxical dilation of the dyssynergic segment. With time, an akinetic myocardial scar develops at that site and may improve the general contractile state. Thus, the early acute stages of myocardial ischemia can be more critical than the actual infarction-scar formation phase.

Significant advances in echocardiography have enabled this technique to be used in patients with ischemic heart disease. Both M-mode and two-dimensional echocardiography are noninvasive and relatively inexpensive and may offer advantages over the standard electrocardiographic techniques. With the development of wall motion abnormalities, systolic thinning may occur before abnormalities of the ST segment or increases in intracavitary left ventricular pressure. Intraoperatively, transesophageal echocardiography is a relatively straightforward technique which can provide an improved quality of echo signal over the conventional precordial technique. The device consists of a single element transducer (3.5 or 5 MHz) or a multi-element phased array transducer (3.5 MHz) attached to the tip of a commercially available gastroscope. This 9 mm-in-diameter device is readily advanced into the esophagus of the anesthetized patient. It enables views of the aortic valve, the four cardiac chambers, the LV short axis, and the apex. For the detection of regional wall motion abnormality, the LV short axis view at the level of the papillary muscles (at approximately 45 cm) is recommended. Regional wall motion abnormalities can be detected and time-sequenced during the operative period. There are several major disadvantages to transesophageal echocardiography. First, it requires considerable attention to detail to diagnose wall motion abnormalities. It therefore has the potential of focusing attention away from the patient and on the monitoring device. Second, quantitative measurements are difficult to perform on a real-time basis by the clinician. Until software is developed to provide real-time digitized information to the clinician, its use for quantitation of ejection fraction and intracardiac planar dimensions is limited to off-line research applications. Third, the cost of echocardiography is substantial ($50,000-$100,000). In summary, transesophageal echocardiography does indeed play a role in patient monitoring and provides sensitive and specific information useful for the diagnosis of myocardial ischemia and infarction. It may have even greater sensitivity than electrocardiographic monitoring. The widespread clinical applicability of this device is yet to be determined, but with resolution of cost and quantitation problems, there will be increasing demand for its use in patients with coronary disease undergoing major surgery.

Diastolic Relaxation and LVEDP

Ischemia affects diastolic relaxation of the ventricular muscle and results in incomplete relaxation between systolic contractions. Inadequate ventricular filling and impaired ventricular contraction result. The net effect is an increase in the LVEDP, producing increased wall tension and myocardial oxygen consumption. Thus, the increases in LVEDP seen with myocardial ischemia not only reflect impaired systolic function, but also incomplete diastolic relaxation. The rise in LVEDP is further exacerbated by the effect of left atrial systole, causing a sudden deposition of blood into a stiffer ischemic left ventricle. The increases in LVEDP with ischemia tend to be greater in the presence of previous myocardial infarctions, hypertrophied ventricles, and during tachycardic and afterload stresses. Some observers have reported, particularly during exercise studies, that the rises in LVEDP begin almost immediately with the onset of exercise, peak before the onset of ST depression, and return to normal before ST segment recovery. Both the LVEDP changes and the ST changes occur before the onset of angina. Rises in the pulmonary capillary wedge pressure (PCWP) often do not reflect the increases in LVEDP because end-atrial systole occurs over such a short period of time that the LVEDP spike is not reflected in the mean diastolic pressure or in the PCWP.

The intraoperative use of the PCWP as a monitor of myocardial ischemia has yet to be rigorously studied. There is evidence that increases in the PCWP may precede changes in the ST segment during episodes of intraoperative ischemia. However, the sensitivity and specificity of the PCWP in relationship to the ST segment or echocardiographic wall motion changes has yet to be determined. The most significant problem with relying on the PCWP as an ischemia monitor has been outlined above. With ischemia, acute rises in LVEDP may occur and not be reflected in the PCWP. Thus, PCWP may be a relatively insensitive marker for myocardial ischemia. With respect to its specificity, sudden rises in the PCWP in patients with coronary artery disease may reflect either impaired diastolic relaxation or impaired systolic contraction. It is difficult to determine which of these occurs first. Therapy should address the reduction of PCWP by altering preload, afterload or contractility, and sudden increases in the PCWP should be aggressively treated in patients with coronary artery disease.

Myocardial Metabolism and Lactate Determination

The principal substrates for myocardial metabolism are fatty acids and glucose. Fatty acids taken into the myocardial cell are converted to acetyl CoA in the mitochondria. Acetyl CoA, via the Krebs cycle, provides the necessary hydrogen for the cytochrome system, enabling oxidative phosphorylation to occur. Thirty-six ATP's are produced via oxidative phosphorylation. Other sources of acetyl CoA are ketones and pyruvate which enter the mitochondria and enhance oxidative phosphorylation. The second major substrate, glucose, enables the production of 2 ATP's via glycolysis. Thus, 36 of the 38 of the high energy phosphates are produced by oxidative metabolism within the mitochondria, and only 2 of the 38 phosphates are produced via anaerobic metabolism in the cytoplasm.

During myocardial ischemia, the flow of blood to myocardial cells is diminished and results in inadequate delivery of oxygen. The transition of metabolic pathways from aerobic to anaerobic metabolism occurs with an increased use of extracellular glucose and intracelluar glycogen stores. Lactate metabolism is also altered. Under normal conditions, extracellular lactate is used as a substrate, being converted to pyruvate and thence to acetyl CoA in the mitochondria for aerobic metabolism. With myocardial ischemia, this conversion does not take place, and lactate as a substrate is no longer used. Furthermore, anaerobic metabolism produces lactate as an end-product, and since this form of metabolism is much less efficient than aerobic metabolism, significant amounts of lactate are produced in the cytoplasm of the cell when ischemia occurs. Lactic acid production has been used as a marker for myocardial ischemia, and measurements in man have been made using coronary sinus lactate assays. Limitations to this method exist, however, since 1) cytoplasmic lactate may not be effectively removed by the venous effluent because of decreased coronary flow, and 2) smaller regional areas of lactate production may be masked when combined with the effluents from larger areas of normally functioning myocardium.

The result of myocardial metabolism is the production of ATP, which enables cellular function, i.e., it effects contractility of fibers. The myocardium of the ventricle consists of a series of interlocking cells which are cross-banded to serve as functional units. Each cell is surrounded by a sarcolemma through which ion exchange occurs and action potentials are generated. Within the sarcolemma are fibrils which embody the contractile proteins actin and myosin, structurally arranged in units called sarcomeres. Other regulating proteins, such as troponin and tropomyosin are also embodied in the sarcomere. Active contraction of the cell is produced by generation of the action potential at the sarcomere. Conversion of this electrical energy to mechanical contraction is accomplished by an increase in the intracellular concentration of calcium ion from extracellular influx, as well as intracellular release from the sarcoplasmic reticulum of the cytoplasm. The increase in intracellular calcium, in association with ATP and magnesium ion, effects the actin and myosin interaction via regulating proteins and produces shortening of the fiber. Relaxation of the fibers is thought to be effected by a re-entry of the calcium ion into the sarcoplasmic reticulum. Myocardial ischemia affects cellular function in a number of ways. Ischemia not only depletes the major energy source of the cell, ATP, but also inhibits sarcolemma ion exchange, action potential generation and possibly calcium release from the sarcoplasmic reticulum. Calcium dynamics probably play a key role in the depression of the myocardial contractility associated with ischemia. With acute ischemia, calcium entry into the cell is inhibited, thereby shortening the duration of the action potential and depressing myocardial contractility. With continuation of the ischemia, intracellular acidosis produces increased binding of calcium to the sarcoplasmic reticulum and impairment of calcium release necessary for the actin-myosin interaction. Ischemia also affects relaxation of the myocardial fibers by prolonging the relaxation phase which becomes incomplete during the next systolic contraction. This incomplete or impaired relaxation is energy inefficient and does not allow adequate ventricular filling to fully effect the Frank-Starling mechanism.

The intraoperative use of metabolic markers of ischemia is currently limited to the research setting and includes coronary sinus lactate and radiolabeled lactate determinations, free fatty acid and carbohydrate assays, and magnetic resonance spectroscopy. Coronary sinus catheterization has been performed in a number of studies which have principally addressed the comparative effects of anesthetics on the ischemic state. For clinical purposes, routine catheterization is neither practical nor warranted at present. In the future, several of these techniques, in particular, magnetic resonance spectroscopy, will find clinical application. The comparative benefits of any of these techniques must be fully evaluated first and related to those benefits of more standard techniques, such as electrocardiographic and echocardiographic monitoring.

In conclusion, the detection of intraoperative myocardial ischemia is relatively new and still rapidly evolving. There is no doubt that we will be besieged by a number of invasive and noninvasive monitors which will allow more sensitive and specific detection. However, regardless of any significant improvements, we must address whether the use of these monitors really affects morbidity before we consider widespread clinical acceptance.

References

1. Kannel WB, McGee D, Gordon T: A general cardiovascular risk profile: The Framingham Study. Am J Cardiol 38:46, 1976
2. Roy WL, Edelist G, Gilbert B: Myocardial ischemia during non-cardiac surgical procedures in patients with coronary-artery disease. Anesthesiology 51:393-397, 1979
3. Coriat P, Harari A, Daloz M: Clinical predictors of intraoperative myocardial ischemia in patients with coronary artery disease undergoing non-cardiac surgery. Acta Anaesth Scand 26:287-290, 1982
4. Goldman L, Caldera DL, Nussbaum SB et al.: Multifactorial index of cardiac risk in noncardiac surgical procedures. N Engl J Med 297:845, 1977
5. Rao TLK, Jacobs KH, El-Etr AA: Reinfarction following anesthesia in patients with myocardial infarction. Anesthesiology 59:499-505, 1983
6. Steen PA, Tinker JH, Tarhan S: Myocardial reinfarction after anesthesia and surgery. JAMA 239:2566, 1978
7. Kaplan JA, King SB: The precordial electrocardiographic lead (V_5) in patients who have coronary-artery disease. Anesthesiology 45:570-574, 1976
8. Sonntag H, Merin RG, Donath U, Radke J, Schenk HD: Myocardial metabolism and oxygenation in man awake and during halothane anesthesia. Anesthesiology 51:204-210, 1979
9. Blackburn H, Taylor HL, Okamoto N: Standardization of the exercise electrocardiogram: A systematic comparison of chest lead configurations employed for monitoring during exercise. In: Maroven M, Barry AJ, eds., Physical Activity and the Heart. Springfield: Charles C Thomas, pp 101-133, 1966
10. Fuchs RM, Achuff SC, Grunwald L, Yin FCP, Griffith LSC: Electrocardiographic localization of coronary artery narrowings: Studies during myocardial ischemia and infarction in patients with one-vessel disease. Circulation 66:1168-1176, 1982
11. Fox AM, Hakki A, Iskandrian AS: Relation between electrocardiographic and scintigraphic location of myocardial ischemia during exercise in one-vessel coronary artery disease. Am J Cardiol 53:1529-1531, 1984
12. Tubau JF, Chaitman BR, Bourassa MG, Watters DD: Detection of multivessel coronary artery disease after myocardial infarction using exercise stress testing and multiple ECG lead systems. Circulation 61:44-52, 1980
13. Hollenberg M, Budge WR, Wisneski JA, Gertz EW: Treadmill score quantifies electrocardiographic response to exercise and improves test accuracy and reproducibility. Circulation 61:276, 1980
14. Kotrly KJ, Kotter GS, Mortara D, Kampine JP: Intraoperative detection of myocardial ischemia with an ST segment trend monitoring system. Anesth Analg 63:343-345, 1984

15. Schlüter M, Langenstein BA, Polster J, Kremer P, Souquet J, Engel S, Hanrath P: Transesophageal cross-sectional echocardiography with a phased array transducer system: Technique and initial clinical results. Br Heart J 48:67-72, 1982

16. Souquet J, Hanrath P, Zitelli L, Kremer P, Langenstein BA, Schlüter M: Transesophageal phased array for imaging the heart. IEEE Trans Biomed Eng 29:707-712, 1982

17. Reeder GS, Seward JB, Tajik AJ: The role of two-dimensional echocardiography in coronary artery disease. Mayo Clin Proc 57:247, 1982

BETA-ADRENERGIC BLOCKING DRUGS: NEW DEVELOPMENTS

R. MERIN

INTRODUCTION

Although beta-adrenergic blocking drugs can no longer be classified as "new drugs", and although for many uses other drugs have surpassed the beta blockers in popularity (calcium blockers, ACE inhibitors, etc.), the drugs are still an important component of the management of both ischemic and hypertensive cardiovascular disease. In addition, they still play a unique role in anesthesia and critical care medicine as far as control of tachycardia is concerned. This review will concentrate on new developments in beta-adrenergic pharmacology with the emphasis on beta blockers rather than beta agonists.

Physiology and Pathophysiology

The original classification of Lands et al of beta-1 and beta-2 receptor specificity (1) where the beta-1 receptor mediated the cardiac actions of sympathetic nervous system activation and beta-2 receptor mediated the smooth muscle effects has now become much more complicated. For instance, it is now apparent that beta-1 receptors mediate the release of renin from the kidneys and increase lipolysis in fat tissue. On the other hand, besides their smooth muscle relaxing effect, beta-2 receptors also mediate some cardiac effects as well as controlling liver and skeletal muscle glycogenolysis and increasing potassium influx in the latter, and even affecting the function of the heart. Under normal circumstances, the beta-1 receptor is still the maximal mediator for the cardiac effects of beta agonism. However, in the failing heart, where classically

T. H. Stanley and R. J. Sperry (eds.), Anesthesiology and the Heart, 91–99.

sympathetic stimulation has proved ineffective, it has become apparent that the predominance of beta-1 receptors (90%) may shift so that now in terminal heart failure 50% of the beta receptors are of the beta-2 category (2). Obviously, this has led to the use of beta-2 agonists for treating terminal heart failure. This discovery also suggests that perhaps in the failing heart where it would be preferable to uncouple the effect of beta agonism on heart rate from contractility the use of a beta-1 selective antagonist might be advantageous. The hypokalemic effect of epinephrine is predominantly mediated through beta-2 agonism, so that if this is a desirable effect, beta-2 blockade would not be advantageous.

Uses

In one recent interview, 51 different clinical syndromes were reported as having been treated with beta-adrenergic blocking drugs (3)! However, the predominant indications for beta-adrenergic blockade have not changed appreciably over the last 10 years. By far, the most widespread use is for cardiovascular diseases. Although the initial indication, supraventricular arrhythmias, is still current, the two most widely treated disease syndromes are certainly myocardial ischemia and hypertensive cardiovascular diseases. Although the calcium blocking drugs have become very popular for the treatment of both of these syndromes, beta blockers still form a cornerstone for therapy, particularly for ischemic heart disease. In fact, the widespread substitution of calcium blocking drugs for beta blocking drugs to treat ischemic heart diseases has resulted in problems for the anesthesiologist taking care of these patients. Calcium blocking drugs do not effectively prevent the tachycardia and hypertension that may occur during induction of anesthesia and perioperatively (4,5). The availability of a new ultra-short acting beta blocking drug may be very advantageous for this indication (see below). As a rule, the beta-adrenergic blocking drugs are used in combination to treat hypertension, unless the etiology is excess renin secretion from the kidney. Another syndrome where the calcium blocking and beta blocking drugs have a common use is hypertrophic cardiomyopathies, both of the left (asymmetric septal hypertrophy) and the right ventricle (pulmonary infundibular stenosis and tetralogy of Fallot). Beta blocking drugs have also proved to be useful for preventing migraine headaches, treating congenital tremor states, calming at least the sympathetic nervous response to anxiety, modifying the sympathetic nervous hyperactivity that accompanies withdrawal from abused drugs (alcohol and narcotics), the treatment of thyrotoxicosis, especially surgical preparation, and, of course, treatment of glaucoma. Obviously, the anesthesiologist is likely to see a significant number of patients presenting for anesthesia and surgery who are still being treated with beta-adrenergic blocking drugs. In addition, the drugs may be useful in the perioperative period as well (see below).

The Drugs

The major difference between the eight beta-adrenergic blocking drugs available for chronic administration today is in the so-called associated side effects and in pharmacokinetics (6). In fact, the most important differentiation is probably the kinetics, for the side effects are probably of minimal importance. Certainly, the membrane stabilizing activity (MSA) or local anesthetic effect has essentially no importance as far as clinical usefulness is concerned. In some circumstances, a beta-1 selective drug may be useful when beta-2 blockade is harmful, particularly in patients with vaso- or bronchospastic disease. As to whether partial agonist activity (PAA) is important or not is very controversial. In any event, Table 1 lists the comparison of these drugs in terms of potency, associated side effects and kinetics. Propranolol, timolol, metoprolol, pindolol and acebutolol are all drugs of moderate to high lipid solubility which are predominantly biotransformed in the liver and the metabolities excreted in the kidney and bile. Consequently, the drugs have a relatively limited and unpredictable bioavailability when given by mouth because of the high hepatic extraction. In addition, they are approximately the same duration of action with elimination half-lives of ±4 hours. Nadalol, atenolol and the new penbutolol are different pharmacokinetically. They are barely lipid soluble and are metabolized very little by the liver. As a result, their bioavailability is more predictable when taken by mouth and they are predominantly excreted unchanged by the kidneys with their elimination half-life being considerably longer. However, with these drugs, the level of renal function markedly affects their elimination and dosage.

Associated Side Effects

As I mentioned, the only important associated side effect is beta-1 selectivity. Of the available drugs, only metoprolol, atenolol and esmolol have appreciable beta-1 selectivity. Consequently, they can be used more safely in patients with broncho- and vasospastic diseases. However, this selectivity is only that and in higher doses these drugs all produce beta-2 blockade. Often these dose levels are necessary for effective therapy. In addition, there are some circumstances where beta-1 selectivity may not be desirable. For instance, in patients with acute myocardial infarction who are treated with diuretics and become hypokalemic, there may be a higher incidence of cardiovascular collapse in patients treated with selective compared with non-selective beta blockers. On the other hand, as suggested above, it is possible that beta-1 selective blockers may be more effective in treating ischemic heart patients with failing ventricles if the evidence that beta-2 receptors predominant in the failing ventricle is confirmed.

The New Drugs

One of the new drugs is not really new. Labetalol has been approved for more than five years now, but is only now receiving attention in the critical care and anesthesia literature. Labetalol has the unique property of possessing alpha-adrenergic blocking activity as well as beta blocking activity. It is nonspecific as far as the beta blocking is concerned with no associated side effects. The alpha blocking activity is between 1/5th and 1/10th as potent as the beta blocking activity and, hence, labetalol should be considered basically to be a beta blocker. However, this alpha blocking activity has made the drug of considerable use in treating perioperative hypertension. Although it is marketed for use as intravenous infusion, in fact, the drug is not a rapid-onset, rapid-offset drug like esmolol, but has a kinetic profile that is similar to propranolol. Consequently, considerable caution should be used when infusing the drug as significant accumulation can occur.

The newest of the beta blockers is one that is unlikely to be useful in anesthesia. Penbutolol (Levatol) joins nadalol and atenolol as relatively lipid insoluble, renal excreted, long duration drugs. From the information available, it is unclear as to what advantage penbutolol has over nadalol. They appear to be essentially identical drugs. The major consideration for the anesthesiologist is the realization that these are long half-life drugs and that if a patient is being treated with one of these drugs, maintenance of normal oral dosing on the morning of surgery will probably allow for reasonable beta block through the perioperative period.

Acebutolol is the only beta blocker that possesses all three associated pharmacologic properties. It is beta-1 selective and has partial agonist and membrane stabilizing activity. However, all are relatively weak and the major difference of acebutolol from the other beta blockers is the fact that it is metabolized to an active metabolite, diacetol, which then confers a much longer duration of action on the compound. Acebutolol itself has an elimination half-life of only three to four hours, but in combination with diacetol, the beta-adrenergic blocking half-life is of similar duration to the longer acting atenolol (Table 1).

Certainly, the most useful of the new beta blockers to the anesthesiologist is esmolol. I believe that esmolol is a very important drug for anesthesia and critical care. The basic reason is that this drug with its rapid onset (less than 1 minute) and short duration (less than 10 minutes) allows the anesthesiologist to try beta blockade as a treatment especially for resistant tachycardia in patients where there may be relative contraindications. For instance, in the patient with bronchospastic disease, especially since esmolol is a beta-1 selective blocker, a trial of this drug for treatment of tachycardia, hypertension, myocardial ischemia, etc., is unlikely to result in serious consequences for the patient. Even if bronchospasm occcurs, the short duration of this drug means that management of this complication is markedly facilitated. Likewise, if a patient with a failing heart needs treatment of his tachycardia, a long-acting beta blocker may result in more cardiac failure along with the bradycardic effect. If esmolol is used, then only 10 minutes of this effect will be apparent and other measurements can be taken. On the other hand, if the therapy proves to be effective, then either an infusion of esmolol or an alternative therapy with the long-acting analogue, metoprolol, can be initiated.

Perianesthetic Use

I believe that the most important perianesthetic use of beta-adrenergic blocking drugs is for treatment of tachycardia, particularly in patients with ischemic or other heart disease where increased heart rate is extremely deleterious. In patients without contraindications to beta block, either intravenous propranolol or metoprolol can be used. On the other hand, with its faster onset, it may be advantageous even in those patients without contra-indications to beta blockade to initially titrate esmolol and then switch to the longer acting drug should continued beta block be indicated. Of course, in many circumstances during anesthesia, beta block may only be desirable for short periods of time, such as tracheal intubation, sternotomy, etc. In this circumstance, esmolol is obviously the drug of choice. Although many anesthesiologists and critical care physicians choose to manage patients who have demonstrated a salutory response to esmolol with continuous infusion (100-200 g/kg/min), in fact, I believe that in terms of ease of administration and cost, it makes more sense to switch to the identical long-acting drug, metoprolol. Especially if the patient is on multiple infusions or is not to be care for in an intensive care unit, the longer acting drug is a much more satisfactory choice. Other than tachycardia, hypertension and myocardial ischemia, the most likely uses for beta blockade in the perioperative period are for treatment of atrial fibrillation and flutter where the usual responses, slowing of the ventricular rate and thyrotoxicosis, where beta blockers are uniquely effective for treating thyroid storm. I'm a strong believer in the fact that a patient who is therapeutically beta blocked should be continued on their beta blockade through surgery. As mentioned before, if a patient is on one of the long-acting drugs, then dosing in the morning of surgery may be adequate for the operative day. Most anesthesiologists will not prophylactically give beta blockers intravenously prior to the induction of anesthesia but one study suggests that even this may be advantageous (7).

There are, of course, some problems with using beta blockers. For instance, there can be little question that they decrease liver blood flow and any drug which is metabolized by the liver may have its elimination half-life lengthened when given in combination with beta blockers. The other major problem with drug interaction involves other cardioactive drugs. In particular, the combination of calcium blockers and beta blockers must be viewed with caution. This should not be surprising since the drugs have similar actions and are often prescribed for the same disease. In particular, the combination may produced unwanted prolongation in atrioventricular conduction proceeding to complete heart block. The drugs appear to be better tolerated when given orally together than intravenously. The same precautions, particularly for A-V block are true of most of the Class I antiarrhythmic drugs and digitalis. On the other hand, beta block has proved to be efficacious for treating digitalis toxicity.

TABLE 1

Beta Adrenergic Blocking Drugs

Drug	Potency	B-1 sel	PAA	MSA	Lip. Sol.	Hep. Metab.	t1/2B (hr)
Propranolol (Inderal)	1	-	-	+	High	High	2-4
Timolol (Blocadren)	6	-	-	-	Moderate	High	4-6
Nadalol (Corgard)	0.8	-	-	-	Low+	Low+	16-24+
Metoprolol (Lopressor)	1	+++	-	-	Low+	Low+	2.5-4.5
Atenolol (Tenormin)	1	+++	-	-	Low+	Low+	6-9+
Pindolol (Visken)	6	-	++++	+	Moderate	Moderate	3-5
Acebutolol (Sectral)	0.3	++	++	+	High	High	8-10*
Penbutolol (Levatol)	4-6	-	-	-	Low+	Low+	9-12+
Labetalol (Trandate, Normodyne)	0.3	-	-	-	Moderate	High	5-6
Esmolol (Brevibloc)	0.1	+++	-	-	Low	Low	0.1+

B-1 sel = beta-1 selective; PAA = partial agonist activity; MSA = membrane stabilizing activity; t1/2B = elimination half-life.

+ - significant difference from propranolol.

* - active metabolite, diacetol.

REFERENCES

1. Lands AM, Arnold A, McAuliff IJ, et al. Nature 214:597-601, 1967.
2. Bristow MR, et al. Circ Res 59:297-309, 1986.
3. Frishman WH, Teicher M. Cardiology 72:280-296, 1985.
4. Slogoff S, Keats AS. Anesthesiology 68:676-680, 1988.
5. Chung F, et al. Anesthesiology 69:343-347, 1988.
6. Merin RG. Seminars in Anesthesia 7:75-82, 1988.
7. Stone JG, Foex P, Sear J, et al. Anesthesiology 68:495-501, 1988.

AGING, AUTONOMIC FUNCTION, AND CARDIOVASCULAR HOMEOSTASIS

S. MURAVCHICK

The loss of protective laryngeal reflexes in elderly subjects was dramatically demonstrated many years ago[1]. In addition, it is now clear that virtually every measurable aspect of autonomic homeostasis is impaired progressively by advancing age. In elderly patients, even those free of cardiovascular and neurologic disease, maintenance of arterial blood pressure following assumption of the upright position (or other forms of interrupted venous return) is less precise and less predictable[2]. In fact, reduced carotid sinus baroreceptor responsiveness remains the most completely studied and well documented example of age-related autonomic dysfunction[3]. However, there are also significant reductions in autonomic responsiveness to thermal stress and to imposed hypoxemia and hypercapnia[4].

The precise mechanism by which age reduces autonomic homeostasis is not known with certainty, but several observations appear to be important. Plasma epinephrine and norepinephrine levels are consistently elevated in the elderly, even during sleep[5]. An exaggerated increase in norepinephrine release in response to orthostatic stress is particularly noteworthy, especially in individuals with systolic hypertension at rest. These high catecholamine levels should not be considered to be evidence of a "hyper-adrenergic" state because their effects are offset by reduced autonomic end-organ responsiveness. Consequently, speed, magnitude and efficacy of homeostasis fall with age because there is a corresponding decline in the affinity between catecholamines and peripheral adrenergic receptors, or

T. H. Stanley and R. J. Sperry (eds.), Anesthesiology and the Heart, 101–103.

perhaps a relative failure of adenylate cyclase activation. Although there may be a loss of beta-receptors, resistance to the effects of beta-antagonists strongly suggests that qualitative, not merely quantitative, changes in peripheral autonomic adrenoceptors are responsible for these age-related phenomena[6].

There are also significant anatomic changes in the autonomic system which appear with increasing age. Conduction velocity declines progressively in peripheral nerves. The number of sympathoadrenal fibers in the spinal cord falls, especially within the sympathetic ganglia. Cell bodies are fewer in number and tend to show accumulation of intracellular debris and reduction in dendritic elements within those areas of the hypothalmus responsible for normal autonomic function, e.g. the locus ceruleus[7].

Since anesthesia, by definition, is a state of drug-induced suspension of normal nervous system function, it also creates drug-induced denervation or "dis-integration" of the autonomic nervous system. In fact, the attenuation of cardiovascular response in sympathectomized animals is remarkably similar to that seen under moderate to deep levels of general anesthesia in clinical practice. Many anesthetics, especially potent inhalational agents, have direct depressant effects on cardiovascular function. More importantly, they suppress sympathoadrenal responses and lower the elevated plasma catecholamine levels needed to compensate for reduced end-organ responsiveness in elderly patients. Consequently, the effect of these anesthetic techniques on autonomic function is particularly impressive and elderly patients tolerate abrupt and profound reduction of autonomic tone very poorly. In a similar manner, regional anesthetic techniques which produce any degree of sympathectomy, even transiently, make cardiovascular stability in elderly patients a direct function of the degree to which external support is provided in the form of volume infusion, peripheral vasoconstriction in other areas, and myocardial stimulation.

When planning an anesthetic for an elderly patient, consider autonomic effects in terms of autonomic functional reserve.

Advancing age represents a progressive reduction in the magnitude of autonomic influences on cardiac function and an increasing dependence upon high levels of circulating catecholamines to stimulate effector organs which become increasingly refractory to beta-agonists and to vagolytic drugs. Autonomic "set-points" for homeostasis do not appear to change, but autonomic systems behave in an "underdamped" fashion in the elderly individual: they allow wider swings in blood pressure than are seen in young adults, and both hypotension and hypertension produce reflex responses in heart rate which are smaller in magnitude, less timely, and less effective in maintaining constant organ perfusion pressures than is true in young individuals. The greater the age of the patient, the greater the impact of the details of perioperative management on the outcome of geriatric surgical patients.

REFERENCES

1. Pontoppidan, H., Beecher H.K. J.A.M.A. 174:2209-2213, 1960.
2. Collins, K.J., Exton-Smith, A.N., James, M.H., et. al. Age and Ageing 9:17-24, 1980.
3. Duke, P.C., Wade, J.G., Hickey, R.F., Larson, C.P., et. al. Canad. Anaesth. Soc. J. 23:111-124, 1976.
4. Kronenberg, R.S., Drage, C.W. J. Clin. Invest. 52:1812-1819, 1973.
5. Katzman, R., Terry, R. The Neurology of Aging. Philadelphia: F.A.Davis, 1983, pp. 15-50.
6. Vestal, R.E., Wood, A.J.J., Shand, D.G. Clin. Pharmacol. Ther. 26:181-186, 1979.
7. Dorfman, L.J., Bosley, T.M. Neurology 29:38-44, 1979.

THE CARDIAC PATIENT AND ATRIAL NATRIURETIC HORMONE

EDWARD D. MILLER, JR., M.D.

We commonly think of the heart as a pump, a muscular pump that propels blood throughout the body. Recent work has now established that the heart is also an endocrine gland. It secretes a powerful peptide hormone called atrial natriuretic peptide (ANP). This hormone has an important role in the regulation of blood pressure and blood volume and in the excretion of water, sodium and potassium. The effects of this hormone on various organs are diverse and have significant implications in the care of our patients undergoing cardiac surgery.

The search for ANP has been long-standing. Research workers in the 1950's and 1960's sought a substance that would explain the natriuresis and subsequent diuresis that occurred with atrial distention. This putative hormone was also referred to as the "third factor" since it would complement the activity of two known regulators of blood pressure and blood volume: aldosterone and glomerular filtration.

Morphologic examination of atrial tissue demonstrated that the presence of a high proportion of rough endoplasmic reticulum and membrane-bound storage granules. (1,2) Subsequently, de Bold and coworkers performed the classic experiment demonstrating the importance of these granules. (3) They demonstrated that when extracts of atrial tissue were given intravenously to rats, a very

T. H. Stanley and R. J. Sperry (eds.), Anesthesiology and the Heart, 105–110.

large sodium diuresis occurred promptly. Similar extracts of ventricular tissue had no effect. These workers also showed that the atrial extracts lowered arterial blood pressure.

Since 1981 great efforts have been made to elucidate the nature of atrial natriuretic and vasoactive peptides and their precursors. Molecular biology has resulted in the cloning and elucidation of cDNA sequences and structural genes encoding for the ANP precursor. (4) It is now known that there are a variety of atrial peptides but they all contain the same core sequence of 17 amino acids in a ring formed by a cystine disulfide bridge, but differ in the lengths of their amino and carboxy termini. (5) It would appear that the various forms of the peptide may exert varying biological activity. For example the vasorelaxant properties of some forms of the peptide are not as active while the natriuretic properties are similar.

The physiological effects of the atrial peptides can be divided into four major categories. First, the atrial peptides affect renal hemodynamics and electrolyte excretion. Atrial peptides have direct effects on vascular smooth muscle, effects on blood pressure and the systemic circulation and the renin-angiotensin system. It is not surprising then that initial studies will examine blood levels of these peptides during cardiac surgery.

Atrial natriuretic peptides cause a prompt and sustained increase in glomerular filtration rate without increasing renal blood flow. This is the most striking renal effect of this peptide. The cause of this increase is not precisely known but efferent arteriolar constriction would result in such an increase in glomerular filtration. Distribution of renal blood within the kidney is altered by atrial natriuretic peptides. An increase in flow to the medullary region of the kidney causes a washout in the papillary interstitium and can contribute to the natriuresis seen. (6) The effects of ANP on transport mechanisms in the renal tubules remains to be determined.

ANP is a powerful vascular smooth muscle relaxant in isolated tissue. ANP appears to be selective in its relaxant properties. For example, ANP is more effective at antagonizing contractions induced by angiotensin than those induced by norepinephrine. (7) There is an increase in cyclic guanosine monophosphate (GMP) in vascular smooth muscle when ANP is applied. This is consistent with the notion the GMP is the second messenger for ANP, a situation not dissimilar to other vasodilators.

The decrease in blood pressure seen with the injection of ANP is not solely due to the vascular relaxing properties of the peptide however. In normotensive experimental animals, the decrease in blood pressure is due to a decrease in cardiac output since peripheral resistance does not change. Bradycardia is a consistent finding. Some experimental data suggests that the atrial natriuretic peptides may undergo conversion to or cause the release of an unidentified negative inotropic substance.

ANF has effects on other hormone systems. ANF markedly inhibits renin secretion in intact animals. Renin is an proteolytic enzyme that is released from the kidney under a variety of influences. The delivery of sodium to the distal tubule is sensed by the macula densa. With an increase in sodium delivery, as would be seen when ANP is given, renin release is inhibited. But ANP affects other portions of the renin-angiotensin system. ANP directly and selectively reduces basal secretion of aldosterone and blocks the aldosterone stimulation induced by angiotensin in the adrenal cortex. Secretion of cortisol is unaffected.

From this brief review of some of the effects of ANF, it is not surprising then that studies examining the role of ANF during cardiac surgery will now appear in the literature. Hynynen and coworkers examined plasma levels of ANP during induction of anesthesia and volume loading in patients undergoing cardiac surgery. (8)

In this study, twelve males scheduled for coronary artery surgery were studied. These patients were not in congestive failure and all received a standard fentanyl, oxygen and air anesthetic. Hemodynamic and hormonal measurements were made and then saline 10 ml/kg and leg raising was done in six patients. The other six patients served as a control.

Blood was sampled from the pulmonary artery for measurement of ANP. Radioimmunoassay for ANP was used. These authors used rabbit anti alpha ANP serum from Peninsula Laboratories. Cross-reactivity, intra and inter assay variability are reported and show that the sensitivity of the assay is such that meaningful interpretation of the data is possible. Since so much of the initial studies rely on plasma measurements, precision of the assay is critical.

These authors clearly show that volume loading results in an increase in ANP in patients anesthetized with fentanyl. There is a direct correlation between an increase in ANP and central venous pressure. However since atrial diameter was not measured, whether atrial pressure or atrial volume is the prime determinant is not known. The authors also show that there is a decrease in ANP from the awake to the anesthetized state. CVP decreased at this time and plasma renin activity also increased. Unfortunately no renal studies were done in these patients.

A variety of other studies would suggest that ANP has an important role in patients in congestive heart failure. (9, 10) There is a definite correlation between atrial pressures and the release of ANP. Why the diuretic properties of ANP do not offset the increased fluid retention in a patient with congestive failure is not clearly understood. It is known though that if the atria cannot be stretched (such as occurs in constrictive pericarditis) then ANP does not rise despite increased atrial pressure. (11)

Another area of intense study is that of the role of ANP in acute respiratory distress syndrome. Etson and coworkers examined 12 patients with ARDS and found that there was poor correlation between right atrial pressure and ANP. However, left atrial pressure, pulmonary artery systolic pressure and pulmonary artery mean pressure did correlate well. They speculated that the elevation in ANP was partially responsible for the increased capillary permeability resulting in a wet lung. (12)

Whenever a new family of hormones is discovered initial studies are done to see what influences plasma levels of the substance. Later, manipulations are done to exaggerate the response. Eventually, agonists and antagonists are produced which are able to clearly define the precise role of the hormone.

The analogy of ANP to the renin-angiotensin system is readily apparent. ANP is comprised of a series of peptides, so is the renin-angiotensin system. A variety of stimuli cause the release of both hormones. High and low molecular weight substances have been identified for both families of hormones. Both hormones are intimately involved in the regulation of volume and pressure. What is lacking for ANP are specific inhibitors. Once we had saralasin and captopril, the importance of the renin-angiotensin system could be fully appreciated. (13)

References

1. Kisch, B. Exp. Med. Surg. 14:99-122, 1956.
2. Jamieson, J.D., Polade, G.E. J. Cell Biol 23:151-172, 1964.
3. de Bold, A.J., Borenstein, H.B., Veress, A.T., Sonnenberg, H. Life Sci. 28:89-94, 1981.
4. Lewicki, J.A., Greenberg, B., Yamanaka, M., Vlasuk, G., Brewer, M., Gardner, D., Baxter, J., Johnson, L.K., Fiddes, J.C. Fed Proc 45:2086-2090, 1986.
5. Needleman, P., Fed Proc 45:2096-2100, 1986.
6. Maach, T., Camargo, M.J.F., Kleinert, H.D., Laragh, J.H., Atlas, S.A. Kidney Int. 27:607-615, 1985.
7. Burnett, J.C., Granger, J.P., Opgenorth, T.S. Am. J. Physiol. 247:F863-6, 1984.
8. Hynynen, M., Tikkanen, I., Salmenpera, M., Heinonen, J., Fyhrquist, F. J. Cardiov.Anesth. 1:401-407, 1987.
9. Raine, A.C., Erne, P., Burgissir, E., Mullen, F., et al. NEJM 315:533-37, 1986.
10. Rodeheffer, R.J., Tanaha, I., Imuda, T., Hollister, A.S., et al. J. Am. Coll. Cardiol. 8:18-26, 1986.
11. Spodich, D.H. Am. J. Cardiol. 63:1271-73, 1989.
12. Etson, H.B., Rosen, M.J., Phillips, R.A., Krahoff, L. Chest 94:1040-45, 1988.
13. Samuels, A., Miller, E., Fray, J., Haber, E., Barger, A.C. Fed. Proc. 35:2512-20, 1976.

PREOPERATIVE HYPOKALEMIA AND THE CARDIAC PATIENT

K.C. WONG, M.D., PH.D. and JOHN R. SHULTZ, JR., M.D.

Anesthetic management of the hypokalemic patient continues to be an enigma and concern for the surgical team. The primary concern is the potential risk of cardiac arrhythmias associated with hypokalemia and anesthesia. This concern has been fostered by the well known effect of cations on the electrophysiology of excitable cells[1] and of hypokalemia on the pacemakers of the heart[2] and by clinical reports which suggest that cardiac arrhythmias are made worse by respiratory alkalosis,[3,4] digitalis therapy[5] and myocardial ischemia[6] or infarction[7] in the presence of hypokalemia. Therefore, it has been traditionally taught that a surgical patient should have a serum potassium of 3.0 mEq/L (undigitalized) and 3.5 mEq/L (digitalized) before being subjected to anesthesia. In spite of this time-honored recommendation, there are no hard data to substantiate that the incidence of intraoperative arrhythmias is increased in the hypokalemic patient. In fact, two recent prospective studies in 597 surgical patients did not demonstrate a correlation between intraoperative ventricular arrhythmias and preoperative hypokalemia,[8,9] even among the high risk cardiac surgical patients.[9]

Clinical experience of anesthesiologists the world over has shown that hypokalemic patients have undergone a variety of anesthetic regimens without serious cardiac arrhythmias or instability, unfortunately such experience has not been collated and published. On the other hand, there are also circulating horror stories of malignant intraoperative arrhythmias or inability to resuscitate patients who, retrospective, were noted to be hypokalemic. Why does such a dicotomy of clinical impressions exist?

T. H. Stanley and R. J. Sperry (eds.), Anesthesiology and the Heart, 111–118.

The answer is unclear but hypokalemia is a far more complex problem both physiologically and clinically than most people appreciate. Some of these factors which confound the interpretation of clinical and/or experimental data are summarized below:

1. Clinically, hypokalemia is only a measure of intravascular potassium concentration per unit volume. Thus, hemodilution or hemoconcentration can decrease or increase serum $[K^+]$, respectively, and serum $[K^+]$ per se may not reflect the total body potassium concentration. Intracellular $[K^+]$ is around 40 times greater than extracellular $[K^+]$ (i.e. 155 to 4 mEq/L). The transmembrane $[K^+]$ gradient is responsible for the maintenance of resting membrane potential and repolarization of cardiac excitable cells. These electrophysiologic characteristics are important for the maintenance of cardiac rhythm.[1,2]
2. However, the electrophysiology of excitable cells is not solely dependent upon transmembrane $[K^+]$ gradient but is also dependent upon a complex relationship among the cations potassium, sodium, calcium and magnesium.[1,2] It is highly improbable that chronic changes in any one cation occur independent of the other cation because of their electrophysiologic inter-relationship. Thus, digitalis toxicity is potentiated by hypokalemia, hypomagnesemia and hypercalcium, a well known phenomenon which illustrates the multiple cationic involvement in cardiac function.[5,10,11]
3. Potassium hemeostasis is regulated by a multitude of factors.[12] The generalization that alkalosis induces transmembrane shift of potassium ions into the cell and acidosis induces the opposite is only valid during acute hypocapnia and hypercapnia, respectively.[13] Chronic respiratory acid-base disturbance is accompanied by renal compensatory mechanisms resulting in minimal disturbance of potassium in balance between the intracellular and extracellular compartments. The effects of metabolic acid-base disturbance on serum $[K^+]$ are more variable. Lactic acidosis produces minimal change in serum $[K^+]$ while hydrochloric acid infusion into dogs produces large increases in serum $[K^+]$. Metabolic alkalosis is associated with a marked kaliuresis without apparent effect on cellular $[K^+]$. Potassium hemeostasis is also influenced by hormones such as

insulin, mineralocorticords, catecholamines and by changes in plasma osmolality.[12]

4. The most common cause of hypokalemia in the surgical patient is diuretic therapy for the treatment of systemic hypertension. The asymptomatic hypokalemic patient may be relatively free of other concurrent diseases in addition to their systemic hypertension or may be physiologically compensated by other cationic changes, in contrast to the symptomatic hypokalemic patients.[14,15] Obviously it is inappropriate to compare these two groups of patients based upon hypokalemia alone. Preoperative assessment of the hypokalemic patient should be based upon all the factors considered for the ASA physical status classification as well as the contemplated surgery.
5. Published reports would suggest that chronic hypokalemia up to a point is reasonably well tolerated,[8,9,16,17] probably because of physiologic compensatory mechanisms and re-establishment of appropriate transmembrane electrochemical gradients of excitable cells. A chronic hypokalemic level of just below 3.0 mEq/L may be tolerated but below 2.5 mEq/L is associated with cardiovascular dysfunction.[17-20] Acute loss of potassium from the body presumably has not had sufficient time for physiologic compensatory mechanisms to take place, may produce significant cardiovascular problems. Unfortunately, the latter speculation has not been well documented in controlled studies.

In summary, serum potassium level alone is not a reliable reflection of the hypokalemic problem in a patient. Inability to control the factors that can influence hypokalemia or other concurrent cardiovascular problems that can coexist in hypokalemic patients makes comparison of results among studies difficult and increases the possibility of arriving at conflicting conclusions.

Preoperative Evaluation

From the above discussion it can be seen that hypokalemia is an enormously complex problem that can contribute to cardiovascular instability. However, experience and published data have shown that hypokalemia alone should not be the cause of alarm in the anesthetized patient. In the patient with coronary ischemic disease and unstable angina, hypokalemia may indeed be an important contributing factor to cardiac arrhythmias. Assuming all of the usual preoperative evaluations such as cardiac catheterization, chest x-ray films, blood chemistry analysis, stress tolerance tests, ECG, echocardiogram, etc. are done before surgery, hypokalemia will add to the anesthetic problems of managing the patient with low ejection fraction, ventricular arrhythmias with multifocal ectopic pacemakers, ventricular akinesis, and cardiac failure.

Anesthetic management of the cardiac patient should be aimed at cardiac ischemic and hemodynamic problems, which are discussed by other speakers in this symposium. The remarks here then will be aimed at the contribution of hypokalemia to the patient's cardiac problems. Majority of hypokalemic patients is a result of chronic potassium loss from furosemide-induced kaliuresis. Therefore, the clinician would expect there is a proportional loss of potassium from the intracellular as well as the extracellular site. The generally accepted serum potassium value of 3.0 mEq/L required for a nondigitalized patient is reasonable because assuming a total body potassium content of around 4,000 mEq/L for a 70-kg patient, a 25% loss of potassium represents about 1,000 mEq/L. In general, such a chronic loss of potassium does not produce overt cardiac arrhythmias on the ECG except for a reduction in the amplitude of the T wave and sometimes the appearance of a U wave. Without the appearance of cardiac arrhythmias on the ECG, it would not be advisable to administer intravenous potassium as a means of normalizing the serum potassium level. Acute intravenous administration of potassium is not an effective means of replenishing potassium loss from the body because of rapid elimination by the kidneys.[21] Cellular uptake of potassium can be promoted by the administration of glucose and insulin; however, I feel the latter treatment should be reserved only for more profound levels of hypokalemia or for patients who are showing cardiovascular instability and arrhythmias as symptoms of hypokalemia. The usual acceptable method of promoting potassium uptake by cells is to use up to 40 mEq/L of potassium in 10% dextrose with 25 units of regular insulin (0.5 units regular insulin per 2 gm dextrose).

Intravenous potassium administration is not innocuous. As many as 1 in 200 patients receiving potassium may suffer a morbid or fatal episode of hyperkalemia.[22] Therefore, the administration of intravenous potassium should always be accompanied by careful monitoring of the patient, by frequent checking of serum potassium level, and continuous monitoring of the ECG in the operating room. When insulin is used to facilitate cellular uptake of potassium, blood glucose values should also be monitored. Intravenous administration of potassium in other settings in the hospital must have adequate surveillance by the nursing staff.

Intraoperative Management

There are no absolute rules as to the type of general anesthetic that must be administered for the cardiac patient. Both inhalational anesthetics and a primary narcotic anesthetic have been used with equal effectiveness. More importantly, the amount of anesthetic and other intraoperative drugs administered are based upon principles of good management related to hemodynamic stability in the operating room.

Special comments are appropriate for anesthetic management of cardiac surgery. The major difference of a patient receiving coronary artery bypass grafting is that the principal problem of myocardial ischemia will be approved following the surgery. Under most circumstances hypertension rather than hypotension is the rule following cardiopulmonary bypass or during the immediate postoperative phase. Hypothermia can induce a mild degree of hypokalemia. The mechanism of this reduction in level of serum potassium is not entirely clear but may be related to cold-induced renal excretion of potassium and cellular uptake of potassium from acute respiratory alkalosis.[23] In any event, it is not unusual to observe hypokalemia as the patient is removed from cardiopulmonary bypass and is gradually rewarmed. It is conceivable that this transient hypokalemia can add to a preexisting hypokalemia, thus producing cardiac instability. Many cardiac anesthesiologists routinely will add potassium chloride in the intravenous fluid during the postbypass period. However, we do not routinely administer potassium at this time unless the serum potassium level is less than 2.9 mEq/L and there is evidence of cardiovascular instability. The clinician should be reminded that a cardioplegic agent containing high concentrations of potassium is commonly used during cardiopulmonary bypass. The routine administration of potassium following cardiopulmonary bypass without actual measurement of the serum potassium level can lead to potassium overdose or cardiovascular collapse.

In summary, hypokalemia will contribute to preexisting cardiovascular problems with regard to cardiac arrhythmias and poor contractility. A slow infusion of potassium may exert an antiarrhythmic effect in a patient who is exhibiting cardiac arrhythmias associated with hypokalemia, but it is not expected to be an effective method of replenishing cellular loss of potassium. Repletion of cellular loss of potassium should be aided by the concurrent intravenous administration of glucose and insulin. The most safe and effective way to replenish potassium loss from the body is by oral administration for at least seven days in the elective surgical patient. Intravenous administration of potassium is not innocuous. An overdose can lead to conduction block, bradycardia, and even cardiovascular collapse.

Postoperative Management

Changes in serum potassium level during the postoperative phase in the intensive care unit are common. Metabolic alkalosis is not uncommon during the immediate postoperative period from the intraoperative administration of large volumes of Ringer's lactate solution, which undergoes metabolic biotransformation to bicarbonate. Since fluid overload is fairly common, furosemide is generally administered to promote diuresis and this could also bring about the loss of potassium from renal kaliuresis. Respiratory alkalosis from continued mechanical ventilatory support is also another source of reducing serum potassium. Nasogastric suction not only enhances metabolic alkalosis from the loss of hydrochloric acid but also from the loss of potassium. For the above reasons, it is important to check the concentration of serum electrolytes frequently and to administer potassium chloride in the intravenous fluid when there is a reduction in serum potassium level.

Summary

There are a large number of factors that can produce a reduction in level of serum potassium. Acute respiratory or metabolic alkalosis can cause a shift of potassium from the serum into the cell, thus producing hypokalemia without the loss of body potassium. A chronic loss of body potassium, most commonly from the use of diuretics, would generally produce a proportional loss of potassium from the intracellular and extracellular compartments. This chronic loss of potassium may allow time for a compensatory mechanisms of the body and, therefore, does not produce overt cardiac arrhythmias or cardiovascular problems. Nevertheless, laboratory evidence suggests that the chronic hypokalemic animal is less able to tolerate severe physiologic trespass.[16,24] Present data would suggest that the acute loss of body potassium may be more harmful than the transmembrane shift of potassium or the chronic loss of potassium from the body. Hypokalemia is thus a complex problem that cannot be assessed by simply measuring the serum potassium value. The magnitude and the rate of potassium loss are important considerations. The usual limits of acceptable potassium levels for elective surgery (3.0 mEq/L for chronic hypokalemia and 3.5 mEq/L for hypokalemia with digitalis therapy) are useful but arbitrary generalizations. Other information must be utilized to modify theses guidelines. Cardiac arrhythmias are common in patients with ischemic heart disease, especially with myocardial infarction associated with hypokalemia. Therefore, special attention must be paid to the serum potassium concentration, but the clinician should not lose sight of concurrent abnormalities in changes of other cation concentrations such as sodium and magnesium. The intravenous administration of potassium should always be monitored carefully to avoid an acute overdose. Finally, the recent prospective studies in hypokalemic surgical patients,[8,9] suggest that hypokalemia per se is not reasonable to cancel an elective case; but, as can be seen from this brief review of this complex problem, these patients should not be treated the same as a normokalemic patient.

References

1. Woodbury J.W. In: Neurophysiology (Eds. Ruch T.C., Patton H.D. and Woodbury J.W., et al), W.B. Saunders, Philadelphia, 1962, pp. 2-30.
2. Surawicz B. and Gettes L.S. In: Cardiac and Vascular Disease (Eds. Conn H.L. Jr. and Horwitz O.), Lea and Febiger, Philadelphia, 1972, pp. 539-576.
3. Lawson N.W., Butler G.H. and Rat C.T. Anesth. Analg. 52:951-962, 1973.
4. Wright B.D. and DiGiovanni A.J. Anesth. Analg. 48:467-473, 1969.
5. Lown B., Black H. and Moore F.D. Am. J. Cardiol. 6:309-337, 1960.
6. Stewart D.E., Ikram H. and Espiner E.A., et al. Br. Heart J. 54:290-297, 1985.
7. Solomon R.J. and Cole A.G. Acta Med. Scand. 647(suppl):87-93, 1981.
8. Vitez T.S., Soper L.E. and Wong K.C., et al. Anesth. 63:130-133, 1985.
9. Hirsch I.A., Tomlinson D.L. and Slogoff S., et al. Anesth. Analg. 67:131-136, 1988.
10. Seller R.H., Cangiano J. and Kim D.E., et al. Am. Heart J. 79:57-68, 1970.
11. Dyckner T. and Wester P.O. Am. Heart J. 97:12-18, 1979.
12. Cox M. Med. Clin. North Am. 65:363-384, 1981.
13. Adrogue H.J. and Madias N.E. Am. J. Med. 71:456-466, 1981.
14. Holland O.B., Nixon J.V. and Kuhnert L. Am. J. Med. 70:762-768, 1981.
15. Kaplan N.M. Am. J. Med. 77:1-4, 1984.
16. Wong K.C., Tseng C.K. and Puerto B.A., et al. Anaesth. Sinica 21:139-146, 1982.
17. Albrecht , ' Am. J. Physiol. 222:555-560, 1972.
18. Simodynes E. Anesth. Analg. 60:762-763, 1981.
19. Nardone D., McDonald and Cirard D. Medicine 57:435-446, 1978.
20. Gunning J.F., Harrison C.E. and Coleman H.N. I.I.I. J. Mole. Cell. Cardiol. 4:139-153, 1972.
21. Kawamura R., Wong K.C. and Hodges M.R. Anesth. Analg. 57:108-113, 1978.
22. Kassirer J.P. and Harrington J.T. Kidney Int. 11:505-515, 1977.
23. Wong K.C. West J. Med. 138:227-232, 1983.
24. Wong K.C., Port J.D. and Steffins J. Anesth. Analg. 62:991-994, 1983.

CALCIUM CHANNEL BLOCKING DRUGS: NEW DEVELOPMENTS

R. MERIN

INTRODUCTION

Whereas the beta blocking drugs were the "drugs of the 70's", it may be fairly said that the calcium blocking drugs are the "drugs of the 80's" (1). In view of the ubiquitous nature of the calcium ion as a second or third messenger in mediating cell activity, it is not surprising that drugs which interfere in calcium homeostasis may be useful in a variety of disease states, particularly those involving excess cardiovascular activity.

Pharmacology

Although these drugs have been referred to as "calcium antagonists", in fact, they really are not pharmacologic antagonists of the calcium ion. Rather, they interfere with the passage of calcium ions through the cell membrane as the primary mode of action (there may also be some effect on calcium channels on interior cellular membranes as well, but this is still controversial). Since the influx of calcium ion from the high concentration in the extracellular fluid through the cell membrane to raise the normally low concentration intracellularly (less than 10^{-6} M) is the major event initiating contraction of all muscle, it is logical that the major use of calcium channel blocking (CCB) drugs involves interference with the contraction of various types of muscle. It is also in keeping with the physiology that effects of channel blockers on skeletal muscle are minimal since skeletal muscle does not depend to nearly as great an extent on calcium ion influx through the cell membrane for initiation of its effect.

T. H. Stanley and R. J. Sperry (eds.), Anesthesiology and the Heart, 119–123.

Consequently, CCB's primarily affect cardiac and smooth muscle contraction as the mechanism of their pharmacologic action. In addition, the calcium ion provides the major current for the automatic and conducting tissues of the heart (S-A and A-V nodes) so that these drugs also have an effective antiarrhythmic action. Inasmuch as the primary effect is not on the electrical activity of actual heart muscle, or the Purkinje fibers, the major antiarrhythmic efficacy of these drugs is in supraventricular arrhythmias, particularly paroxysmal supraventricular arrhythmias.

Unlike the beta adrenergic blocking drugs where there is practically a rigid structure activity relationship, several different chemical formations have potent calcium channel blocking activities. The original papaverine derivatives, verapamil and D-600, were the prototype CBB drugs. However, most of the recent newer drugs are dihydroperidines of the nifedipine type. The diphenyl alkylamines such as diltiazem also belong to this class of drugs. Verapamil and nifedipine are the opposite ends of the spectrum (Table 1). Nifedipine is primarily a vasodilator drug with minimal effects in intact animals and humans on cardiac muscle and electrophysiology. Verapamil, on the other hand, although possessing vasodilator properties, also is a potent antiarrhythmic and depresses cardiac muscle directly as well. Diltiazem appears to be intermediate between the two, possessing all the CCB properties but producing more prominent vasodilation than nifedipine.

Uses

The clinical uses for these drugs are remarkably similar to those of the beta blockers. As with the beta blockers, the first FDA approved indication was for the treatment of arrhythmias, in this case supraventricular arrhythmias. In particular, verapamil, and to a lesser extent diltiazem, is currently the drug of choice for conversion of paroxysmal supraventricular arrhythmias. As with the beta blockers, the second approved indication was for the treatment of ischemic heart disease. The major advantage of these drugs over the beta blockers for the treatment of IHD is that they are coronary vasodilators and hence, in addition to decreasing myocardial oxygen demand by decreasing blood pressure, heart rate and force of myocardial contraction, they may also improve supply through coronary vasodilation if coronary vasospasm is a part of the disease. The third approved use, again as with the beta blockers, is for the treatment of hypertension. Like most anti-hypertensive drugs, the calcium blockers are not a miracle drug. By trial and error, patients who appear to be particularly responsive to CCB's rather than other antihypertensive drugs can be identified. Again, like the beta blockers, if patients with hypertension also have ischemic heart disease, then the CCB's may be particularly valuable in therapy. Although not approved by the FDA, the drugs are also being used often in concert with the beta blockers to treat hypertrophic cardiomyopathies. Inasmuch as the drugs are smooth muscle relaxants, they are also under investigation for treatment of various smooth muscle spasm conditions such as bronchospasm, vasospasm and premature labor. However, their efficacy in these diseases has not been well established. However, it is important to point out that even if the drugs are not therapeutic for these smooth muscle spastic diseases, unlike the beta blockers which are relatively contraindicated in these diseases, these drugs can be used safely for other indications in patients with both bronchospasm and vasospasm.

The Drugs

As indicated above, there are basically three types of CCB's. Verapamil and diltiazem are currently the only approved drugs in their chemical category and, as indicated, are similar in their capacity with diltiazem being a somewhat better vasodilator. The dihydroperidine drugs with nifedipine as the parent now have produced two new FDA approved compounds. Both nicardipine (Cardene) and nimodipine have been released for use by the FDA. Nicardipine is a very similar drug to nifedipine. For the anesthesiologist, it was hoped that because nicardipine is not light sensitive as is nifedipine it would be released for intravenous use. However, the initial release was only for oral use. Some of the experimental investigations suggested that perhaps nicardipine was a better coronary vasodilator with less cardiac depressant properties than nifedipine, but nifedipine has minimal cardiac depressant properties anyway. The drug has been released for the treatment of both hypertension and ischemic heart disease. Nimodipine, on the other hand, appears to be a rather more specific cerebral vasodilator than some of the other dihydroperidines and it has been released specifically for cerebral protection in patients with cerebral vascular disease (2).

Preoperative Considerations

As with any drug which produces cardiovascular depression, there has been some controversy about the advisability of continuing calcium channel blocking drugs through the perioperative periods (3). Although rebound effects from withdrawal of the CCB's have not been as prominent as those seen with the beta blockers, nevertheless, the experimental evidence on the interaction between the calcium channel blocking drugs and surgery and anesthesia suggests that if the drugs are having a favorable effect in the patient, they should be continued through the perioperative period. In highly instrumented open chest animals, verapamil in particular and also diltiazem can produce major cardiovascular depression in concert with potent inhalation anesthetics. However, in less invasive closed chest preparations, clinical doses of both CCB's and anesthetics have produced minimal cardiovascular depression (3). Only with high doses of both classes of drugs have major cardiovascular effects been seen. In particular, the combination of verapamil and enflurane seems to produce a higher incidence of A-V conduction disturbances than in the other drug combinations. Chronic administration of these drugs appears to produce even less cardiovascular depression even with relatively high plasma levels of verapamil in one experimental preparation (4).

Considering the increased importance of preventing and treating perioperative myocardial ischemia and the demonstration that much of this ischemia is not related to altered hemodynamics, it would seem that the calcium blocking drugs with their prominent coronary vasodilating activity might be desirable for myocardial protection during surgery and anesthesia in patients with ischemia heart disease. Two studies, however, have suggested that in patients with ischemic heart disease treated only with calcium channel blockers that there is a higher incidence of perioperative ischemia than in comparable patients treated with beta blockers or the combination of beta blockers and calcium blockers (5,6). However, actual degree of calcium block and compliance were not assessed in these studies. Whether or not intravenous administration of calcium blockers in the perioperative period or specific immediate preop oral administration might be protective has not determined this point.

TABLE 1

Calcium Channel Blocking Drugs

Clinical Effects

	Anti-arrhythmic	Cardiac Depression	Tachy-cardia	Vasodilation		
				Syst.	Coronary	Cerebral
Verapamil (Isoptin, Calan)	+++	++	-	+	+	+
Diltiazem (Cardizem)	++	+	-	++	++	++
Nifedipine (Procardia)		+	++	+++	+++	+++
Nicardipine (Cardene)	-	-	++	+++	+++	+++
Nimodipine	-	-	++	++	++	+++

REFERENCES

1. Kapur PA. In: Advances in Anesthesia (Ed. R.K. Stoelting), Yearbook Medical Publishers, Chicago, 1985, pp 167-205.
2. Gelmers HJ, Gorter K, DeWeedt CJ, Weizer HJA. N Engl J Med 318:203-208 1988.
3. Merin RG. Anesthesiology 66:111-113, 1987.
4. Merin RG, Chelly JE, Hysing ES, et al. Anesthesiology 66:140-146, 1987.
5. Slogoff S, Keats AS. Anesthesiology 68:676-680, 1988.
6. Chung F, Huston PL, Cheng DCH, et al. Anesthesiology 69:343-349, 1988.

CARDIOVASCULAR PHARMACOLOGY: WHAT'S NEW (AND USEFUL)!

P. BARASH

Traditionally, introduction of new and potent cardiovascular drugs are accompanied by literature which focuses either on animal data or human data obtained under relatively ideal conditions. However, we as clinicians, use these drugs in an environment where many pathophysiologic, as well as pharmacologic interactions occur. We usually do not think of administering these drugs under ideal circumstances, but in relatively complex clinical situations. This lecture will present clinical scenarios under relatively typical circumstances in which anesthesiologists must make decisions regarding various therapeutic options to manage a given patient.

CASE I

A 65 year old male is scheduled for a repair of ventral hernia under general anesthesia. He has exertional angina (3/week). Medications: Nitroderm; Propranolol 40 mg q.i.d.; Nifedipine 20 mg q.i.d. Admission vital signs: BP 150/90, P 80 (NSR) R 12.

Prior to laryngoscopy and intubation:

1. Thoracic peridural
2. IV lidocaine
3. High dose narcotic
4. Esmolol

T. H. Stanley and R. J. Sperry (eds.), Anesthesiology and the Heart, 125–132.

In managing the patient with coronary artery disease, the anesthesiologist must maintain an adequate balance between myocardial oxygen supply and myocardial oxygen demand. Usually in the operating room, a greater number of therapeutic maneuvers can be directed towards reducing myocardial oxygen demand. Factors that effect myocardial oxygen consumption (demand) include wall tension (systolic pressure x radius/wall thickness), heart rate and contractility. Certain parts of anesthetic and surgical procedures are associated with increased levels of myocardial oxygen consumption. Classically, the period of laryngoscopy and intubation has been identified as such a critical period. For this patient, all four choices have been advocated as appropriate management options. Most anesthesiologists in the U.S. would not use a thoracic peridural to prevent hypertension and tachycardia in the setting of endotracheal intubation. Clinicians use IV lidocaine to blunt the sympathetic response to intubation. Although a number of reports have documented a salutary effect, there are also studies that have shown this therapy to be ineffective. Previously, high dose narcotic techniques have not been employed in high risk patients scheduled for surgical procedures of short duration, since the patient would require prolonged respiratory support postoperatively. However, with the introduction of the short acting narcotic, alfentanil, this is less of a problem and clinicians are using alfentanil in a manner similar to that in which fentanyl or sufentanil are employed in cardiac surgery. The introduction of the new cardioselective short acting beta blocker, esmolol, has now been widely used in the setting of laryngoscopy and endotracheal intubation. Investigators have documented significant reductions in the heart rate response to intubation. Further, a number of recent reports have shown the importance of maintaining an adequate level of beta blockade so that high risk patients are not at risk for developing hypertension and tachycardia during parts of surgical procedures associated with sympatho-adrenal stimulation.

<u>References:</u>

1. Chung FS, Cheng DCH, Lavelle P, et al: Calcium channel blockade does not offer adequate protection from perioperative ischemia. Anesthesiology 69:343, 1988.
2. Crawford DC, Fell D, Achola KJ, et al: Effects of alfentanil on the pressor and catecholamine responses to tracheal intubation. Br J Anaesth 59:707-12, 1987.
3. Giles RW, Berger HJ, Barash PG, et al: Continuous monitoring of left ventricular performance with the computerized nuclear probe during laryngoscopy and intubation before coronary artery bypass surgery. Am J Cardiol 50:735, 1982.
4. Gray RJ: Managing critically ill patients with esmolol an ultra short-acting beta-adrenergic blocker. Chest 93:398, 1988.
5. Laurito CE, Baughman VL, Becker GL, et al: Effects of aerosolized and/or intravenous lidocaine on hemodynamic responses to laryngoscopy and intubation in outpatients. Anesthesia and Analgesia 67:389, 1988.
6. Sill JC, Nugent M, Moyer TP, et al: Plasma levels of beta-blocking drugs prior to coronary artery bypass surgery. Anesthesiology 62:67, 1985.
7. Slogoff S, Keats, AS: Does chronic treatment with calcium entry blocking drugs reduce perioperative myocardial ischemia? Anesthesiology 68: 676, 1988.
8. Stone JG, Foex P, Sear JW, et al: Myocardial ischemia in untreated hypertensive patients: effect of a single small oral dose of a beta-adrenergic blocking agent. Anesthesiology 68:495, 1988.
9. Wattwil M, Sundberg A, Olsson J, et al: Thoracolumbar epidural anaesthesia blocks the circulatory response to laryngoscopy and intubation. Acta Anaesthesiol Scand 31:529, 1987.

CASE II

A 75 year old female with COPD undergoing permanent implantation of transvenous pacemaker. During skin closure, vital signs: BP 60/40, P 110, patient complains of chest pain.

Your plan:

1. Midazolam (1 mg)
2. Metoprolol (1 mg)
3. Esmolol infusion (300 mcg/kg/min)
4. Surgical exploration

This case is presented to demonstrate that not all patients with tachycardia intraoperatively should be treated with a beta blocker. The triad of hypotension, tachycardia and chest pain following implantation of a pacemaker mandates surgical re-exploration. The most likely etiology of the tachycardia is ventricular perforation with cardiac tamponade.

CASE III

A 48 year old male, 2 hours post CABG (fentanyl/panc). Vital signs: BP 170/100, P 100, PCWP 10, CI 3 $L/min/m^2$. You order one of the following:

1. MS (4 mg)
2. Esmolol
3. Sodium nitroprusside
4. Labetalol

A common postoperative problem is management of hypertension following coronary artery bypass surgery. The clinician has a number of options to treat the patient in this setting. Obviously, pain control should be optimized before any additional therapy is used. Once that is achieved, vasodilators, beta blockers or alpha/beta blockers can be used. Although blood pressure control can be obtained with any of these agents, each is associated with unique "side effects" that may influence the appropriate choice of therapy. For example, sodium nitroprusside, in comparison to esmolol may alter hypoxic vasoconstriction. Therefore, a patient who has borderline oxygenation may sustain significant hypoxia during administration of sodium nitroprusside. The clinician may wish to use a longer acting drug and be able to transfer the patient to oral therapy following the ICU stay. In this case, labetalol may be an appropriate alternative. Finally, in a context of poor coagulation postoperatively, a recent study has shown that sodium nitroprusside in clinically used doses adversely effects platelet aggregation. This may mandate the use of an alternative vasodilator, nitroglycerin or use of the beta blocker, esmolol.

References

1. Gray RJ, Bateman TM, Dzer LSC: Comparison of esmolol and nitroprusside for acute post-cardiac surgical hypertension. Am J Cardiol 59:887, 1987
2. Prough DS, Mills SA, Kiger J: Intravenous labetalol for blood pressure reduction following myocardial revascularization. Anesthesiology 67:A136, 1987.
3. Hines RL, Barash PG: Does clinical significant platelet dysfunction occur with sodium nitroprusside administration? Anesthesiology 70:611-615, 1989.

CASE IV

A 60 year old male for elective CABG. Stable angina and LVEF 45%. Medications include metoprolol 100 mg bid, TNG prn. During PAC insertion, BP 170/100, P 100, ST segment depression 2 mm (acute).

Your plan:

1. Immediate induction
2. TNG
3. Labetalol
4. Esmolol

Anesthesiologists have documented that arterial and pulmonary artery catheters can be placed safely, prior to induction of anesthesia in patients with coronary artery disease. A small percentage of patients may manifest ischemia during vascular catheterization. Further, recent studies have shown that patients who have not received beta blockade and/or adequate premedication may arrive in the operating holding area with myocardial ischemia. Although it may be tempting to induce anesthesia in the anxious patient and therefore, remove this as a source of sympathetic adrenal stimulation, the first priority is to diagnose the etiology of the ischemia. In this instance, the most likely cause is anxiety. Nitroglycerin forms an excellent foundation on which to base subsequent therapy. Although tempting, immediate induction may be associated with clinically significant hemodynamic instability. Therefore, if the nitroglycerin does not resolve the ischemic episode, use of a beta blocker is indicated prior to anesthetic induction.

References:

1. Chung KS, Sinatra RS, Harrison DM, et al: Does intermediate dose labetolol block the heart rate and blood pressure responses to laryngoscopy and intubation? A placebo controlled study. Anesthesiology 69:A43, 1988.
2. Harrison L, Ralley FE, Wynands JE, et al: The role of an ultra short-acting adrenergic blocker (Esmolol) in patients undergoing coronary artery bypass surgery. Anesthesiology 66:413, 1987.
3. Newsome LR, Roth JV, Hug CC, et al: Esmolol attenuates hemodynamic responses during fentanyl-pancuronium anesthesia for aortocoronary bypass surgery. Anesth Analg 65:451, 1986.

CASE V

A 49 year old female, 20 minutes post sternotomy (CABG) has following ECG trace.

<u>You administer:</u>

1. More fentanyl
2. Esmolol
3. Labetalol
4. Verapamil

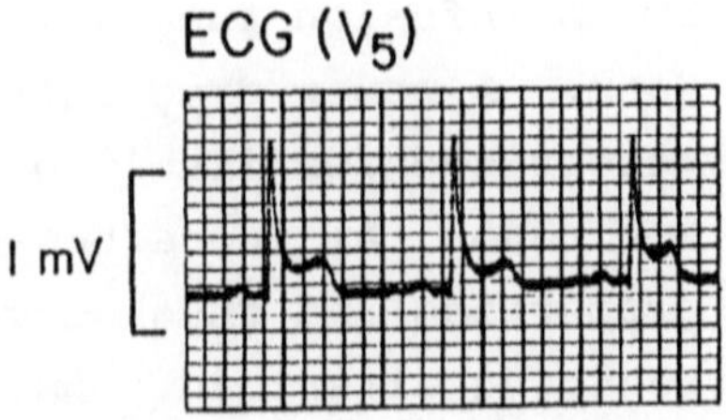

This tracing showing ST segment elevation is classic for coronary vasospasm. The calcium channel blockers are the primary therapeutic modality in managing this disorder. Of the calcium channel blockers available, only verapamil is currently recommended for parenteral use. A number of anesthesiologists prefer using sublingual nifedipine. However, this route of administration is associated with a lack of knowledge of the dose administered, as well as variability in absorption.

<u>References</u>:

1. Reves JG, Kissin I, Lell WA, et al: Calcium entry blockers: Uses and implications for anesthesiologists. Anesthesiology 57:504, 1982.

<u>CASE VI</u>

A 65 year old male undergoing CABG unable to wean from CPB. BP 60/40, P 80, PCWP 24, CI 2 $L/m^2/min$.

<u>Your management</u>:

1. Dopamine
2. Epinephrine
3. Amrinone

Various treatment strategies have been proposed in management of the patient who has cardiac failure following cardiopulmonary bypass. Unfortunately, there is a paucity of well controlled studies to document the therapeutic benefit of various treatment modalities. Epinephrine is a potent alpha-beta agonist that is an excellent primary choice for this clinical scenario. To be used effectively, epinephrine should be administered by an infusion pump which allows careful titration of the dose. A newer drug that is becoming more widely recognized for its important therapeutic advantages is amrinone. Amrinone has both inotropic and vasodilating properties and thus serves to improve contractility while reducing afterload. Amrinone works through a mechanism of phosphodiesterase inhibition. If these drugs are ineffective, thought should be given to use of mechanical devices, for example, the intra-aortic balloon pump or LV assist device.

<u>References</u>:

1. Barash P, Kopriva CJK: Cardiac pump function and how to monitor it. In: Manual of Cardiac Anesthesia, S. Thomas (ed), 1984, New York: Churchill Livingstone, pp 1-34.
2. Colucci WS, Wright RF, Braunwald E: New positive inotropic agents in the treatment of congestive heart failure. Mechanisms of action and recent clinical developments. N Engl J Med 314:290-358, 1986 Parts I and II.
3. Cohn JN, Franciosa JA: Vasodilator therapy of cardiac failure (Part I and II). N Engl J Med 297:27, 254, 1977.
4. Evans DB, Weishaar RE, Kaplan HR: Strategy for discovery and development of a positive inotropic agent. Pharmacol Ther 16:303, 1982.
5. Kemmotsu O, Hashimoto Y, Shimosato S: Inotropic effects of isoflurane on mechanisms of contraction in isolated cat papillary muscles from normal and failing hearts. Anesthesiology 39:470, 1973.
6. Durrett LR, Lawson NN: Autonomic pharmacology. In: Clinical Anesthesia. PG Barash, BF Cullen, R Stoelting, eds., 1989, Philadelphia: J.B. Lippincott Co., pp 165-226.

ANESTHETIC MANAGEMENT OF THE CHILD WITH CONGENITAL HEART DISEASE FOR NONCARDIAC SURGERY

Alan Jay Schwartz, M.D., M.S.Ed.

Introduction

Anesthesia for the child with congenital heart disease (CHD) is fundamentally the same whether for cardiac or noncardiac surgery. The anesthetic plan is predicated upon an understanding of the cardiovascular (CV) pathophysiology and its clinical presentation (see Chapter: CARDIOVASCULAR PHYSIOLOGY OF CONGENITAL HEART DISEASE). The anesthetic implications follow logically from the knowledge of the alterations of physiology.

Perioperative Management of the Child with CHD for Noncardiac Surgery

A noncardiac operation for a child with CHD may be scheduled as an inpatient or outpatient procedure. A routine preoperative evaluation is supplemented by several specific considerations of the child with CHD. The child will often have undergone one or more cardiac surgical procedures in the past. It will be important to know the types of repairs performed (palliative or totally corrective) and how these impact the CV dynamics. The palliative creation of a Blalock-Taussig (BT) shunt, for example, increases blood flow to the lungs of a child with ↓ pulmonary blood flow (PBF) in pulmonary atresia. The total correction of tetralogy of Fallot (TOF) is associated with heart block and sudden death in a small but definite group of patients.

Associated noncardiac congenital anomalies are frequently present. Approximately 25% of all children with CHD additionally

T. H. Stanley and R. J. Sperry (eds.), Anesthesiology and the Heart, 133–140.

have a noncardiac congenital anomaly which often requires surgical repair. These are looked for and the presence of clinical syndrome complexes defined. The anesthetic plan may be further restricted by the presence of additional congenital malformations.

The parents of cyanotic children may report intermittent episodes when the child has $\uparrow$ cyanosis. This indicates that a reactive pulmonary vasoconstriction is superimposed upon an anatomically $\downarrow$ PBF intensifying the hypoxia. They may report that the child squats to alleviate this. Squatting $\uparrow$ systemic vascular resistance (SVR) and counterbalances shunting away from the lungs. Episodic reactive pulmonary vasoconstriction ("Tet spell") may occur in the perioperative period and is minimized by adequate sedation and minimal stimulation. β-adrenergic blocking agents employed to reduce right ventricular outflow tract (RVOT) obstruction and its associated cyanosis, will be continued up to the time of anesthetic induction.

When cyanosis is present there is an associated polycythemia to $\uparrow$ O_2 carrying capacity. The $\uparrow$ hematocrit may predispose the child to thrombotic complications. Perioperative fluid management will be designed to prevent further hemoconcentration. In addition, there is a thrombocytosis. Platelet function, however, is abnormal and clotting factors are often reduced resulting in coagulopathies.

Congestive heart failure (CHF) is quite common in CHD. CHF is a result of the increased cardiac work load associated with shunts or obstructive lesions. Maximal medical management of CHF is recommended prior to anesthesia.

The child found to have an undiagnosed heart murmur during preanesthetic evaluation deserves consultation by a cardiologist or experienced pediatrician in order to determine whether the murmur is suggestive of organic CHD or is functional. While systolic murmurs may be innocent or pathologic, diastolic murmurs always indicate pathology. The risks of bacterial endocarditis (BE) and systemic air embolization in the presence of unrecognized cardiac defects mandate that even the asymptomatic child with a new murmur be evaluated prior to surgery.

Antibiotic prophylaxis against BE is indicated for children with CHD undergoing many noncardiac operations. Transient bactermia is common during "dirty" operations wherein the integrity of a mucosal surface is compromised. All patients who have undergone palliative or corrective cardiac surgery in the past require BE prophylaxis. The only exceptions are patent ductus arteriosus ligations, and primary closure (without a patch) of a secundum atrial septal defect (ASD). In these two instances BE prophylaxis need only be provided for the first six months postoperatively.

The selection of preanesthetic medication is based on the child's age, psychological development, and CV function and is intended to alleviate psychological and CV stress prior to and during anesthetic induction. This will reduce the likelihood of excitement and sympathetic stimulation which may predispose to ↑ pulmonary vascular resistance (PVR), ↑ SVR, or ↑ RVOT, or ↑ left ventricular outflow tract (LVOT) obstruction manifested as cyanosis or CHF. Children with compensated CHD may receive the routine institutional premedication by oral or parenteral route. Cyanotic children may be more heavily premedicated to reduce the risk of occurrence of a hypercyanotic episode. An anticholinergic alone, or combined with a reduced dose of sedative is appropriate for children with poorly compensated CV function.

The fundamental physiological deficits resulting from circulatory instability in CHD are reductions in systemic oxygenation and cardiac output (CO). Arterial O_2 saturation, heart rate (HR), and BP are parameters which reflect these hemodynamic events and each can be noninvasively quantitated. A basic monitoring setup, essential for children with CHD during noncardiac surgery, includes a stethoscope, ECG, noninvasive BP monitor, temperature probe, inspired O_2 concentration monitor, and continuous pulse oximeter for measurement of arterial O_2 saturation. End-tidal expired CO_2 measurement is increasingly used as a routine monitor. The site of BP measurement may be limited by previous cardiac surgery. A previous BT shunt, for example, prohibits use of the affected arm for accurate BP determination. More invasive monitoring is utilized when the type of surgery requires it or for children with an uncompensated CV status.

Establishment of intravenous access (IV) is a wise precaution for children with CHD no matter how minor the surgical procedure. This does introduce the problem of air bubbles. The introduction of air bubbles into the vasculature of a child with CHD who has shunting of blood may be disastrous. Bubbles in the venous blood may be shunted to the arterial circulation and result in an air embolus. Air embolus is possible even when the shunting is reported to be unfavorable to systemic embolization, i.e., ↑ PBF lesions.

The best safeguard against venous to arterial air or particulate embolus is meticulous prophylaxis. IV tubing, connection sites, stopcocks and injection ports must be free of air prior to connection to the child. Injection into an IV line is performed with care not to introduce air or particulate matter.

Fully resuscitative capabilities must be available in the perioperative locations for care of children with CHD. Resuscitation drugs may be available or mixed up in appropriate concentrations ready for use. A defibrillator must be in close proximity.

Induction of Anesthesia - Uptake and Distribution of Anesthetic Agents in the Patient with CHD

There are no specifically indicated anesthetic techniques for specific CHD lesions. Whatever anesthetic technique and agents selected, the goal remains control of hemodynamic variables within the limits imposed by the CHD lesion and state of compensation of the child at the time of anesthesia and surgery.

The choice of anesthetic induction technique depends on the child's age and psychological preparedness, whether an IV line is present, the child's CV status, and the anticipated CV effects of the anesthetic agents. Anesthetic induction may be influenced by factors which alter the uptake and distribution of inhalation or IV agents in patients with CHD.

Alveolar concentration of anesthetic ultimately determines depth of anesthesia. Increasing inspired concentration and alveolar ventilation ↑ alveolar anesthetic. Decreasing CO, blood solubility and the alveolar to mixed venous anesthetic partial pressure difference ↑ alveolar anesthetic. The uptake and distribution of anesthetic in the child with CHD and shunting of blood is the result of the interplay of all of the factors which alter alveolar anesthetic level. The following exemplifies the interdependence of all of these factors on anesthetic induction.

<u>Induction of inhalation anesthesia in a child with CHD and ↑ PBF</u>:

<u>Assumptions</u>:

1. Constant inspired anesthetic partial pressure.
2. Rapid initial rise in alveolar partial pressure approximately inspired anesthetic partial pressure.
3. Tissue groups receive normal CO.
4. Shunt results in augmentation of PBF.
5. Full anesthetic equilibration between alveoli and pulmonary blood during first circulation through lungs.

<u>Occurrences</u>:

1. Shunt blood acquires no additional anesthetic during recirculation through the pulmonary circuit.
2. Systemic arterial blood delivers anesthetic to tissues depending upon regional CO, and blood and tissue solubilities.
3. Initially, the systemic venous blood is fully desaturated upon its return to the lungs where it fully equilibrates with the alveolar partial pressure of anesthetic.

Consequence:

1. A shunt which ↑ PBF does not affect uptake and distribution of inhalation anesthetics as long as alveolar partial pressure and systemic CO do not rise.

Under different conditions of inspired anesthetic concentration, alveolar ventilation, pulmonary and systemic COs, and tissue delivery and solubility, the effect of the shunt on uptake and distribution may be quite different from the above example. With ↓ PBF lesions, there is less blood contact with alveoli reducing blood anesthetic levels. In children with ↓ PBF of an amount sufficient to result in cyanosis, the limitation of blood-alveolar contact delays uptake and distribution.

Uptake and distribution of IV agents may also be affected by shunting of blood. This is recognized by examining CO curves from children with shunt blood flow.

In clinical practice, the effect of a shunt alteration in PBF can often be offset by the appropriate dose adjustment of administered inhalation or IV agents.

Choice of Anesthetic

Volatile anesthetic agents are widely used in the management of children with CHD. Halothane and enflurane, coupled with nitrous oxide, provide a smooth mask induction. Halothane, enflurane and isoflurane, permit the delivery of 100% O_2. The CV effects of the volatile agents are dose-related and titratable, and are well tolerated by most children with CHD. The hemodynamic actions of the drugs may be used to advantage in some children. The negative chronotropic and inotropic actions of halothane may reduce the degree of ventricular outflow obstruction and promote forward ventricular output. The potential hazards of volatile anesthetics are generally related to relative anesthetic overdose. Myocardial depression resulting from excessive dose may compromise CO and produce ↓ BP or diminish PBF and systemic oxygenation.

Nitrous Oxide (N_2O) is widely used to supplement volatile anesthetics. The use of N_2O following induction in cyanotic children with ↓ PBF lesions or mixing lesions is debated. In addition to the potential hazard of air bubble enlargement, the use of N_2O precludes the administration of high concentrations of O_2. In addition, N_2O has been shown to result in ↑ PVR in children with acyanotic CHD. The ↓ PBF and ↑ R→L shunting resulting from an elevated PVR/SVR ratio suggest that this agent be used cautiously, if at all, following induction in cyanotic children and those with pulmonary vascular disease.

High dose narcotic techniques are often used during surgical repair of CHD. Fentanyl (50-75 μg/kg) and O_2 administered with pancuronium to infants with an array of CHD produces only mild reductions in BP and HR. Prolonged postoperative ventilatory depression, however, makes high dose narcotic techniques impractical for most children undergoing noncardiac operations. The effects of smaller narcotic doses during surgical stimulation are not known. Low doses of narcotics may supplement a reduced volatile anesthetic dose or can be used in conjunction with relaxants and N_2O in a balanced IV technique. Light anesthetic techniques support cardiac contractility and maintain SVR. Balanced anesthetic techniques are well tolerated by most children with ↓ PBF lesions provided excessive sympathetic tone does not result in an ↑ PVR.

Ketamine is popular among many who care for children with CHD because of its hemodynamic actions and ease of administration. Intramuscular ketamine (4-8 mg/kg) may be used to induce anesthesia in an uncooperative child. Ketamine's sympathomimetic effect maintains contractility and SVR. IV doses of 2 mg/kg have not been associated with an ↑ PVR when studied in patients with CHD, including those with pulmonary vascular disease.

Thiopental (4-6 mg/kg IV) is a well tolerated induction agent in normovolemic children with compensated CHD. Reduced doses are indicated for those patients with compromised CV function.

Postoperative recovery of the child with CHD after a noncardiac operation is routine for the anesthesia administered and surgery performed. The intraoperative monitoring, venous access, and resuscitative capabilities are continued in the recovery area until discharge. Supplemental O_2 may be administered to the child with CHD during the recovery period. Ventilation is closely monitored to recognize and avoid hypoventilation and its detrimental CV consequences.

Summary

The child with CHD for noncardiac surgery does not present a major problem to the anesthesiologist. Anesthesia is planned around the anticipated surgical procedure. Understanding the pathophysiology of the cardiac lesion will indicate which anesthetic manipulations may alter CV dynamics. The pathophysiology will also clarify potential alterations in anesthetic uptake and distribution. There are specific perianesthetic protocols which are important when caring for the child with CHD for noncardiac surgery.

Suggested Reading

1. Campbell FW, Schwartz AJ: ASA Refresher Courses in Anesthesiology, Philadelphia, JB Lippincott, 14:75-98, 1986
2. Campbell FW, Schwartz AJ: In Problems in Anesthesia, Edited by SJ Thomas, Philadelphia, JB Lippincott, 1987, pp 411-433
3. Committee on Rheumatic Fever and Bacterial Endocarditis: Pediatrics 75:603-607, 1985
4. Moore RA: Anesthesiol Rev 8(No. 12):23-29, 1981
5. Morgan BC, ed: Pediatr Clin North Am 25:721-795, 1978
6. Rosenthal A: Pediatr Clin North Am 31:1229-1240, 1984
7. Warner JC, Fripp RR, Whiteman V: Surg Clin North Am 63:1003-1015, 1983

ANESTHESIA AND THE RENIN-ANGIOTENSIN SYSTEM

EDWARD D. MILLER, JR., M.D.

It has been known since the middle of the 1800's that the kidney was an important determinant of blood pressure. Bright was the first to show that kidney disease could result in the elevation of blood pressure. It wasn't until the classic work of Goldblatt in the 1930's that a true relationship between constriction of the renal artery and elevation in blood pressure was made. Once that discovery had been made, though, many investigators thought that the renin-angiotensin system might be extremely important in control of blood pressure for a variety of circumstances. Unfortunately, once the ability to measure plasma renin activity became available in 1967,(1) the correlation between blood pressure and plasma renin activity was not as clear-cut as individuals had originally thought.(2) Some hypertensive patients, and in some other disease states, plasma renin levels were actually lower than had been anticipated, and therefore some believed that the renin-angiotensin system was not important in blood pressure control at all. However, in the early 1970's inhibitors of the renin-angiotensin system became available which specifically inhibited angiotensin II so that investigators could decide what the real role of this peptide was in blood pressure control.(3,4) The following discussion will look at some of those aspects and see how they are related to our management of patients in the operating room and in the intensive care units.

T. H. Stanley and R. J. Sperry (eds.), Anesthesiology and the Heart, 141–146.

First, let us examine the renin-angiotensin system. Renin is an enzyme that is released from the kidney under a variety of stimuli. Once released into the circulation renin acts on a substrate, angiotensinogen, formed in the liver and cleaves off ten amino acids which form the peptide angiotensin I. Angiotensin I has no known physiologic properties and is converted to angiotensin II in a single pass through the lung. The conversion of the ten amino acids, angiotensin I, to eight amino acids, angiotensin II, occurs by cleavage of two amino acids from the angiotensin I by an enzyme called converting enzyme that is located in the endothelium of the pulmonary vasculature. Angiotensin II has a variety of properties that make it important in blood pressure control. These include constriction of arterioles, stimulation of aldosterone secretion, potentiation of thirst, potentiation of catecholamine release, and a variety of other stimulatory properties. The interaction of the renin-angiotensin system with atrial natriuretic peptide is complex at best, and since there are no specific inhibitors of atrial natriuretic peptide at this time, the relative role of each of these series of peptides remains to be investigated.

The mechanisms that are known to release renin from the afferent arteriole of the kidney include: a decrease in efferent arteriolar pressure (called the baroreceptor theory), changes in sodium which is delivered to the distal nephron, (called the macula densa theory) and neurogenic control, that is stimulation of the nerves that cause the kidney to release renin. As can be seen, these mechanisms all are involved in the regulation of volume and pressure status of the animal or the human.

Over the past twenty years, a variety of inhibitors of the renin-angiotensin system have now been produced. Saralasin, a competitive inhibitor of angiotensin II was the first of such peptides, but had to be used intravenously. It also had the property of causing agonist properties before its antagonist properties became apparent. In some patients this resulted in significant increases in blood pressure to extremely dangerous levels. Subsequently, captopril a substance that is known to inhibit the conversion of angiotensin I to angiotensin II was produced and is one of the most widely used inhibitors of the renin-angiotensin system. Enelapril and other inhibitors of converting enzyme have recently been introduced onto the market and have the advantage that these agents have an intravenous form. It should be remembered that these agents are effective because they block the formation of angiotensin II and since angiotensin I has no pressor properties, the blockade of the system can be appreciated.

But what are those clinical areas where the renin-angiotensin system may have significant control of blood pressure? First, it is known that in patients who are either hypovolemic or in hemorrrhagic shock there are significant elevations of plasma renin activity in an effort to restore circulation. Patients who have been salt restricted, or patients who have been subjected to dehydration prior to coming to the operating room, can also be expected to have high levels of plasma renin activity. The intense vasoconstriction that goes on in such states causes a maldistribution of blood flow to vital organs in an effort to preserve flow to the heart and brain. One can imagine that by restoration of either blood or volume, plasma renin activity will decrease. Inhibition of the renin-angiotensin system in hemorrhage or dehydration is not suggested since this is a compensatory mechanism attempting to maintain blood pressure. Restoration of volume is of prime importance.

Deliberate hypotension is known to stimulate the renin-angiotensin system significantly.(5,6,7) Early studies showed that not only was there an increase in plasma renin activity when sodium nitroprusside was used to induce hypotension, but there was also rebound hypertension that occurred with the discontinuation of sodium nitroprusside. This rebound hypertension was due to circulating levels of angiotensin II. Subsequent studies have shown that with blockade of the renin-angiotensin system there is no significant rebound hypertension.(8) It has also been demonstrated that propranolol can significantly decrease renin release from the kidney. Both by pretreatment and by intravenous treatment, during controlled hypotension, plasma renin activity is markedly lowered and there is a tendency for less sodium nitroprusside to be used to provide the same degree of hypotension. More recent studies have shown that with the pretreatment of patients with 3 mg/kg of captopril, the dose of sodium nitroprusside can be markedly decreased and the same degree of hypotension achieved with ease.(9)

Another area in which converting enzyme inhibition has proven effective is in the cross-clamping of the thoracic aorta. With surgical operations on the thoracic aorta, blood supplied to the various organs may be markedly diminished during the time of cross-clamp. One of the major concerns is blood flow to the kidneys, the liver, and the spinal cord. Initial studies suggest that blood flow can be markedly improved to these regions after the cross-clamp on the thoracic aorta is removed. This would suggest that locally active angiotensin II produces an intense vasoconstriction that persists after the release of the cross-clamp. Pretreatment with converting enzyme inhibitors seems to improve blood flow to these organs. Whether this improved flow will result in improved function, has not been determined.(10,11)

The period of the 1970's was marked by an explosion of information concerning the family of peptides called the angiotensins. Not only could we measure these peptides in tissue and blood, but the important specific inhibitors were synthesized. As can be seen from this discussion, these inhibitors allowed us to better understand the role of the renin-angiotensin system in a host of disorders. It was also seen from these studies that the measurement of plasma renin activity alone was not a reliable index of the role of the renin-angiotensin system. For example, most patients with essential hypertension have either low or normal plasma renin activity. However, most hypertensive patients treated with captopril have a marked decrease in their blood pressure which is sustained for long periods of time. Such a response suggests that inhibition of the renin-angiotensin system does play an important role in blood pressure control despite normal plasma renin activity. It was also not surprising that with studies such as the ones with captopril, that new information was gleaned which suggested other peptides or other substances might be important in blood pressure control. Certainly the interaction with the sympathetic nervous system, the parasympathetic nervous system, antidiuretic hormone, the prostaglandins, and endothelial derived relaxing factor and atrial natriuretic peptide all suggested that these substances worked in concert to control blood pressure. It would be foolhardy to believe that the renin-angiotensin system alone is responsible for blood pressure control. However, it does play an important role in certain situations, while in others, it acts as a back-up for the normal moment-to-moment regulation of blood pressure. With the introduction of more inhibitors of these peptides we will have a better appreciation of how these substances interact to control blood pressure.

REFERENCES

1. Haber, E., Sancho, J., Re, R., and Barger, A.C. Clin. Sci. Mol. Med. 48:495-502, 1975.
2. Bumpus, F.M., Sen, S., Smeby, R., Sweet, C.S., Ferrario, C.M., and Khosla, M.C. Circ. Res. 32 (Suppl. 1):150-160, 1973.
3. Miller, E.D., Samuels, A., Haber, E., and Barger, A.C. Science 117:1108-1109, 1972.
4. Samuels, A. Miller, E.D., Fray, J., Haber, E., and Barger, A.C. Fed. Proc. 35:2512-2520, 1976.
5. Miller, E.D., Longnecker, D.E., and Peach, M.J. Anesthesiology 48:399-403, 1978.
6. Miller, E.D., Gianfagna, W., Ackerly, J.A., and Peach, M.J. Anesthesiology 50:88-92, 1979.
7. Miller, E.D. Ackerly, J.A., Vaughan, E.D., Peach, M.J., and Epstein, R.M. Anesthesiology 47:257-263, 1977.
8. Miller, E.D., Delaney, T.J., and Beckman, J.J. Anesthesiology 54:199-203, 1981.
9. Woodside, J.R., Garner, L., Bedford, R.F., Sussman, M.D., Miller, E.D., Longnecker, D.E., and Epstein, R.M. Anesthesiology 60:413-417, 1984.
10. Joob, A.W., Harmen, P.K., Miller, E.D., Ayers, C.R., and Mentzer, R.M. Society of Cardiovascular Anesthesiologists, May, 1986, Montreal, Canada.
11. Joob, A.W., Harmen, P.K., Freelander, A.E., Miller, E.D., and Kron, I.L. Surg. Forum 35:318-319, 1984.

CONTROVERSIES IN CARDIAC MONITORING

P. BARASH

Nearly 90 years since Cushing and Codman advocated the use of heart rate and blood pressure to monitor the anesthetized patient, controversy still surrounds the appropriate selection of cardiovascular monitoring. Currently, standards are being promulgated for the minimal level of monitoring required for all patients (1). However, the authors concede that the standards are not comprehensive, but serve to reduce the risk of untoward events for which the cardiovascular and neurologic systems are the final common pathway.

Cardiovascular monitoring facilitates the diagnosis and treatment of complex hemodynamic derangements. These can be categorized in terms of pump function, intravascular volume, and vascular resistance. Monitoring is an extension of the physical examination. Conservative clinicians may argue that clinical experience and physical examination are adequate to diagnose and treat hemodynamic abberations. However, "routine" clinical assessment has proven to be a poor predictor of the patients' hemodynamic status (2-4). Accurate diagnosis for the anesthetized patient may be impaired by the patients' disease process, pharmacologic interventions, sedation, muscle relaxation, etc. Thus, the current debate surrounds the issue of the precise indications for more extensive evaluation.

T. H. Stanley and R. J. Sperry (eds.), Anesthesiology and the Heart, 147–161.

Although the benefit of these monitoring techniques is important for patient care, their limitations are now becoming obvious. Perhaps the easiest way to highlight the current controversy in cardiovascular monitoring is to select a patient with a clinically significant cardiac history and expose him to two different surgical procedures: (1) TURP, and (2) repair of an abdominal aortic aneurysm.

> A 65 year old (70 kg) male is admitted for elective TURP. He had a myocardial infarction four months prior to admission which was complicated by congestive heart failure. At present, he has two to three anginal attacks per week precipitated by exercise, e.g. walking more than 10 blocks. The anginal attacks are relieved by sublingual nitroglycerin. He has no signs or symptoms of congestive heart failure. Current medications include: nifedipine (10 mg q.i.d.), isosorbide (20 mg q.i.d.) and TNG sublingual prn. Physical examination is within normal limits. Laboratory data is within normal limits except for the electrocardiogram which shows an old, inferior wall myocardial infarction.

1. Is the patient the "best" monitor of myocardial ischemia?

A notion exists that an "awake" patient, who has a TURP under regional anesthesia (spinal or peridural), is a sensitive indicator of myocardial ischemia. Recent evidence suggests that this concept is incorrect and may lead to significant morbidity. A number of studies have documented the incidence of "silent ischemia" or asymptomatic coronary artery disease (5-7). This entity can be defined as: the absence of angina (or its equivalents) in the presence of objective evidence of transient myocardial ischemia (EKG, radionuclear or echocardiographic studies, etc.). Three groups of patients may present with this disease process:

(a) Totally asymptomatic patients

(b) Asymptomatic patients post-myocardial infarction (MI) who have active ischemia

(c) Patients with angina who are asymptomatic with some ischemic episodes, but not with others.

At present, approximately two to four percent of asymptomatic males (greater than 45 years of age) and 20-30% of asymptomatic post MI patients have episodes of silent ischemia (5). The incidence of "silent" S-T segment depression (EKG) is quite high. More than 2/3 of ischemic events are undetected by "awake" patients (6-7). To further complicate matters, many of these events are not accompanied by significant alterations in heart rate or blood pressure. Slogoff and Keats have reported similar findings in a group of anesthetized patients undergoing coronary artery bypass surgery (8-9). Only one third of these ischemic events were associated with hemodynamic abnormalities. A number of awake patients with silent ischemia have a "defective anginal warning system" (10). It appears they have an altered perception of pain. On a theoretical basis, treatment with sedative or analgesic medications may further decrease their ability to perceive angina.

Similar to studies in the cardiology literature, recent anesthesiology investigations have documented the high incidence of silent ischemia in the perioperative period. Wilton et al, reported that 6/18 patients scheduled for elective CABG had significant periods of ischemia unaccompanied by angina. These six patients had 37 episodes with a mean duration 40 min (range 15-561 min)(11). More recently Knight et al, reported that 87% (108/124 episodes) of preoperative myocardial ischemia was silent (12). However, a note of caution was sounded by Epstein et al who advised against early enthusiastic acceptable of ambulatory ECG monitoring (AECG) for diagnosis and management of myocardial ischemia. They stated the diagnosis of coronary vasospasm was the only area in which AECG was a superior diagnostic tool than stress testing (13). More recently, the American Heart

Association has published extensive guidelines for use of AECG (14). These criteria classify currently acceptable and non-acceptable use of AECG in management of patients with coronary artery disease.

In my opinion, although the patient undergoing a regional anesthetic may help to contribute to the diagnosis of acute myocardial ischemia, other monitoring modalities that are more objective and detect ischemia earlier are required.

2. How is the diagnosis of myocardial ischemia enhanced by the use of the electrocardiogram?

The EKG supplies an enormous amount of information regarding the status of the coronary circulation (15). By use of the calibrated electrocardiogram in the diagnostic mode (10 mm = 1 mv) employing leads V_5/II 96% of EKG ischemic events can be detected. However, a recent study evaluating electrocardiography (during angioplasty procedures) reported that, significantly more patients with ischemia were detected by a 12 lead than with a 3 lead system (86% vs. 57%) (16). The importance of detecting myocardial ischemia has been highlighted by the studies of Slogoff and Keats, in which the amount of S-T segment depression was directly related to the incidence of postoperative MI (8-9). Interestingly enough there are no accepted standards for the electrocardiographic diagnosis of ischemia. However, most investigators use one or a combination of the following (17):

(1) greater than 1 mm ST segment depression
(2) greater than 1 mm "J" point depression
(3) greater than 1 mm ST segment elevation (coronary artery spasm)
(4) inverted T waves
(5) pseudonormalization of T waves
(6) the onset of new dysrhythmias, especially bundle branch block or ventricular ectopy.

Digitalis effect, left ventricular hypertrophy and electrolyte abnormalities must be considered in the differential diagnosis. If these factors are not present, then ST segment changes seen on the electrocardiogram should be considered acute ischemia and appropriate therapy started immediately. New technology will improve detection of intraoperative ST segment changes. Biagini and colleagues have discussed the difficulty in diagnosing myocardial ischemia by oscilloscopic presentation (18). CCU nurses identified only 31/213 ischemic episodes. A cardiologist analyzing the same oscilloscopic traces, diagnosed less than half the events correctly (102/213)! Thus, computer assisted analysis of ST segments, as well as arrhythmia detection may be an important contribution to patient care. Kotrly, et al. have demonstrated the utility of computerized ST segment analysis (19).

3. <u>Is an arterial catheter required?</u>

Placement of an arterial catheter facilitates measurement of:

(1) blood pressure

(2) chemistries of pH, pCO_2 and pO_2

(3) indirect indices of cardiac "pump" function.

For this patient who does not have a history of labile blood pressure, the use of a non-invasive monitor will probably be sufficient. Although beat-to-beat blood pressure obtained from an intra-arterial catheter would be "nice to have", it probably will not add more to clinical care than an automated blood pressure monitor obtaining measurements every 30-60 seconds (if required) (20-21). Alternatively, a new non-invasive blood pressure monitor using the Penaz method allows inscription of the arterial wave on a beat-to-beat basis (22). Information regarding oxygenation and ventilation may be obtained with a pulse oximeter and capnograph (or mass spectrometer) respectively.

Finally, although the arterial waveform may supply data relative to the cardiac pump function, a recent study suggests that this may be of limited value. Gerber, et al. evaluated the relationship of the dicrotic notch (radial artery) to systemic vascular resistance and cardiac output (23). They were unable to find any correlation.

4. Is insertion of a PA catheter warranted?

This issue is probably the most controversial for the patient undergoing a TURP. Changes in LV compliance (PCWP/cardiac output) and the presence of an AC wave (PCWP trace) are much earlier indicators of myocardial ischemia than the presence of angina or EKG changes (see below) (15,24). The presence of new "v" waves on the PA trace are indicative of papillary muscle dysfunction, most likely secondary to ischemia or acute LV dilatation.

In summary for this patient undergoing TURP, early recognition of ischemia is a high management priority. Monitoring strategies must meet this requirement. At a minimum a calibrated EKG with leads II/V_5 displayed should be available. Diagnosis may further be enhanced by use of the awake (sedated) patient. The PA catheter may also make important contributions to earlier recognition of ischemia. Obviously, measurements made with the use of this catheter will also guide fluid therapy. The patient may not be able to withstand the normal absorption of irrigating fluid. Here again, monitoring may enhance the anesthesiologist's physical examination aimed at evaluating the appropriateness of intravascular volume expansion (color, presence of rales, S_3 gallop, etc). Recently, Rosenbaum et al conducted a study to determine the incidence of silent ischemia and complications of TURP (25). They did not find any intraoperative episodes of ischemia. Further, ventricular ectopy was related to age only. In a comparison of open prostatectomy vs TURP, Roos et al reported a higher long term mortality rate with TURP. The etiology of this difference is unknown (26).

Let us now consider the same patient for resection of an abdominal aneurysm under general anesthesia.

> A 65 year old (70 kg) male is admitted for resection of abdominal aortic aneurysm. He had a myocardial infarction four months prior to admission which was complicated by congestive heart failure. At present, he has two to three anginal attacks per week precipitated by exercise, e.g. walking more than 10 blocks. The anginal attacks are relieved by sublingual nitroglycerin. He has no signs or symptoms of congestive heart failure. Current medications include: nifedipine (10 mg q.i.d.), isosorbide (20 mg q.i.d.) and TNG sublingual prn. Physical examination is within normal limits. Laboratory data is within normal limits except for the electrocardiogram which shows an old, inferior wall myocardial infarction.

1. <u>What are the best clinically available indicators of myocardial ischemia? Is echocardiography useful?</u>

Much of the foregoing discussion is also applicable for this surgical procedure. Since the patient will have a general anesthetic and endotracheal intubation for this procedure, a transesophageal echosocope could be inserted. The strength of echocardiography lies in the ability to make combined anatomic and physiologic diagnosis (27). Echocardiography requires a transducer which is an emitter and receiver of ultrasound (greater than one million Hz). Since the speed of sound (1,540 m/sec) is constant for the heart and surrounding tissues, the distance between the reflecting surface and the transducer can be derived from the elapsed time between propragation and reception of the signal by the transducer (similar to sonar). Two dimensional echocardiography overcomes inherent problems associated with M mode (motion mode) echo which usually uses an "ice pick view" of the heart. The most commonly used intraoperative approach is 2D transesophageal echocardiography (TEE) in which the transducer is mounted on a gastroscope. Detection of ischemia is facilitated by the analysis of abnormal regional wall motion and decreased systolic wall thickening. Roizen, et al. studied 12 patients undergoing supra-celiac cross clamping (28). Ninety-two percent (92%) of the patients developed regional wall motion abnormalities detected by TEE which were consistent with ischemia. These early changes were not detected by EKG. Similarly, Smith, et al. compared TEE and EKG in patients undergoing vascular or coronary artery surgery (29). Regional wall motion abnormalities (ischemia) were seen in 24/50 patients; only 6/24 had EKG changes. Myocardial infarction occurred in 4/24 of the patients; 3 patients had no EKG signs of ischemia. Parenthetically, a recent investigation by Haggmark et al compared hemodynamic, ECG, mechanical (PAC and cardiokymogram) and metabolic indications of myocardial ischemia in a high risk population (30). The concluded that ventricular wall motion abnormalities were not most common and earliest indicator of ischemia. Intraoperative echocardiography, another imaging modality, is being clinically used in a number of hospitals. In comparison to the Wells and Kaplan report, these investigators were unable to find any utility of the PAC to aid in diagnois of ischemia (24,30). However, at present, its high cost has limited its widespread spread application as a monitor.

2. Is a pulmonary artery catheter required?

Although the preceding case emphasized the use of the PA catheter (PAC) for ischemia detection, the major application of this device in the present case is evaluation of hemodynamic responses to guide pharmacologic and fluid therapy. One can argue on the basis of Del Guercio and Cohen's work that the patient should have extensive preoperative hemodynamic evaluation (2). In their study all patients (N=148) had been "cleared" by their internist. However, pre-operative physiologic assessment (arterial and pulmonary artery catheterization) uncovered physiologic aberrations indicative of a higher risk in 64% of the patients. Studies also suggest that it is difficult to accurately predict hemodynamic abnormalities in critically ill from physical examination alone. In ICU patients, for example, Iberti, et al. reported that in one third of patients a diagnosis was changed and that 60% of the physicians made at least one therapeutic change based on PAC derived data (3). In another report, using data obtained from ICU patients, a predictive accuracy of only 44% was achieved for cardiac index and pulmonary capillary wedge pressure when physical examination (and lab data) were the foundation of the data base (4). In an OR study, physicians "blinded" to PAC data were unaware of 65% of severe hemodynamic abnormalities in a group of patients undergoing coronary artery bypass surgery (31). The use of continuous mixed venous oximetry ($Sv0_2$) may further enhance care (32-33). Abrupt and serious decreases in $Sv0_2$ may occur initially without corresponding decreases in other hemodynamic parameters. Shoemaker, et al. have shown in a randomized ICU study, that PA monitoring combined with pharmacologic therapy to a given hemodynamic endpoint results in a significant cost benefit ratio (34).

Apropos to the patient under discussion, Rao, et al. also reported that the use of PA monitoring, in conjunction with appropriate pharmacologic therapy, and ICU stay results in a significant reduction in postoperative myocardial infarction (35).

Although PCWP and cardiac output serve as an important hemodynamic "landmarks" for guiding diagnosis and therapy (e.g. ventricular function curves) a number of limitations to the use of this catheter are present. These may have an important impact for patient care. First and foremost, according to the Starling hypothesis, muscle stretch (LV end diastolic volume) <u>not</u> LV end diastolic pressure (LVEDP) determines cardiac output. A number of studies have shown a poor correlation between LVEDV and LVEDP or PCWP (36-39). On the basis of a reduced LV compliance (seen with ischemia), PCWP may be a poor predictor of LVEDV.

LVEDV $\propto$ LVEDP $\propto$ LAP $\propto$ PCWP $\propto$ PAEDP $\propto$ RAP

↑	↑	↑	↖	↖
ventricular compliance	mitral valve	airway pressure	pulmonary vascular resistance	right ventricular compliance
				tricuspid valve

Further PCWP may not correlate with LVEDP (or LAP) under the following circumstances:

1. <u>PCWP greater than LVEDP</u>
   a. mitral stenosis
   b. elevated airway pressure (e.g. PEEP)
   c. left atrial myxomia
2. <u>PCWP less than LVEDP</u>
   a. stiff left ventricle
   b. LVEDP greater than 25 mmHg
   c. premature mitral valve closure (e.g. aortic insufficiency)

Finally, at present cardiac output can be obtained on intermittent basis by thermodilution techniques. New technology including venous oximetry (SvO_2) and doppler may provide cardiac output data on a continuous basis (40-41).

I have not discussed complications which are an important part of the "monitoring equation" (42). Both invasive <u>and</u> noninvasive monitors pose hazards to the patient. Selection of appropriate monitors must weigh benefit to risk for the individual patient. The indications for monitoring, perhaps, should be stated as follows. The use of these devices should complement the etiologic and functional diagnosis; define temporal progression of the disease process (and response to therapy) and modify therapy on the basis of this data. Unfortunately, there is a dearth of randomized prospective controlled studies to support the use of sophisticated monitors for the anesthetized patient (43-45).

In conclusion, common sense prevails in certain decisions, while controversy surrounds others.

REFERENCES

1. Eichhorn JH, Cooper JB, Cullen DJ, Maier WR, Philip JH, Seeman RG. Standards for patient monitoring during anesthesia at Harvard Medical School. JAMA 1986;256:1017-1020.
2. Del Guercio LRM, Cohn JD. Monitoring operative risk in the elderly. JAMA 1980;243:1350-1355.
3. Iberti TJ, Fisher CJ. A prospective study on the use of the pulmonary artery catheter in a medical intensive care unit - its effect on diagnosis and therapy. Crit Care Med 1983;10:238.
4. Connors Jr AF, McCaffree DR, Gray BA. Evaluation of right heart catheterization in the critically ill patient without acute myocardial infarction. N Engl J Med 1983;308:263-267.
5. Cohn PE. Silent myocardial ischemia: Clinical significance and relation to sudden cardiac death. Chest 1986;90:597-600.
6. Pepine CJ. Silent myocardial ischemia: Definition, magnitude, and scope of the problem. Cardiol Clin 1986;4:577-581.
7. Cohn PF: Silent ischemia and myocardial infarction. New York: Marcel Dekker, 1986.
8. Slogoff S, Keats AS. Further observations on perioperative myocardial ischemia. Anesthesiology 1986;65:539-542.

9. Slogoff S, Keats AS. Does perioperative myocardial ischemia lead to postoperative myocardial infarction? Anesthesiology 1985;62:107-114.

10. Glazier JJ, Chierchia S, Brown M, Maseri A. Importance of generalized defective perception of painful stimuli as a cause of silent myocardial ischemia in chronic stable angina pectoris. Am J Cardiol 1986;58:667-672.

11. Wilton NCT, Luckoff C, Sachdev M, et al: Silent pre-operative myocardial ischemia in surgical patients with ischemic heart disease. Anesthesiology 1987;67:A591.

12. Knight AA, Hollenberg M, London MJ, et al: Perioperative myocardial ischemia: Importance of preoperative pain pattern. Anesthesiology 1988;68:681-688.

13. Epstein SE, Quyyumi AA, Bonow RO: Current concepts: Myocardial ischemia - silent or symptomatic. N Engl J Med 1988;318:1038-1043.

14. Knoebel SB, Crawford MH, Dunn MI, et al: Guidelines for Ambulatory Electrocardiography. Circulation 1989;79:206-215.

15. Barash PG. Monitoring myocardial oxygen balance: Physiologic basis and clinical application. Refresher Courses in Anesthesiology 1985;13:21-32.

16. Wohlgelernter D, Clemans M, Highman HA, et al. Regional myocardial dysfunction during coronary angioplasty; evaluation by two-dimensional echocardiography and 12 lead electrocardiography. JAAC 1986;7:1245-1254.

17. LaMantia K, Barash PG. Monitoring myocardial ischemia. In: Estafanous FG, ed. Anesthesia and the Heart, 1989. Massachusetts, Butterworth Publishers, pp 257-268.

18. Biagini A, L'Abbate AL, Testa R, et al. Unreliability of conventional visual electrocardiographic monitoring for detection of transient ST segment changes in coronary care unit. Europ Heart J 1984;5:784-791.

19. Kotrly K, Kotter GS, Mortara D, Kampine JP. Intraoperative detection of myocardial ischemia with ST segment trend monitoring system. Anesth Analg 1984;63:343-345.

20. Bruner JM, Krenis LJ, Kunsman JM, Sherman AP. Comparison of direct and indirect methods of measuring arterial blood pressure. Med Instr 1981;15:11-21, 97-101, 182-188.

21. Loubser PG. Comparison of intra-arterial and automated oscillometric blood pressure measurement methods in postoperative hypertensive patients. Medical Instr 1986;20:255-259.

22. Smith NT, Wesseling KH, de Wit B. Evaluation of two prototype devices producing noninvasive, pulsatile, calibrated blood pressure measurement from a finger. J Clin Monit 1985;1:17-29.

23. Gerber MJ, Carp D, Hines R, Barash PG: Arterial waveforms and systemic vascular resistance: Is there a correlation? Anesthesiology 1987; 66:823-825.

24. Kaplan JA, Wells PH. Early diagnosis of myocardial ischemia using the pulmonary artery catheter. Anesth Analg 1981;60:789-793.

25. Mathew J, Rosenbaum S, Barash P: Incidence of etiology and reintubation in the postanesthesia care unit: Physician error or patient disease? Anesth Analg 1989; 68:S186.

26. Roos NP, Wennberg JE, Malenka DJ, et al: Mortality and reoperation after open and transurethral resection of the prostate for benign prostatic hyperplasia. N Engl J Md 1989; 320:1120.

27. LaMantia KR, Lehmann KG, Barash PG. Echocardiography in the Perioperative period. Acute Care 1985;11:106-116.
28. Roizen MF, Beaupre PN, Alpert RA, et al. Monitoring with two-dimensional transesophageal echocardiography. Comparison of myocardial function in patients undergoing supra-celiac, suprarenal infraceliac or infrarenal aortic occlusion. J Vasc Surg 1984;1:300-305.
29. Smith JS, Cahalan MK, Benefiel DJ, et al. Intraoperative detection of myocardial ischemia in high-risk patients: Electrocardiography versus two-dimensional transesophageal echocardiography. Circulation 1985;72:1015-1021.
30. Haggmark S, Hohner P, Ostman M, et al: Comparison of hemodynamic, electrtocardiographic, mechanical and metabolic indicators of intraoperative myocardial ischemia in vascular patients with coronary artery disease. Anesthesiology 1989;70:19-25.
31. Waller JL, Johnson SP, Kaplan JA. Usefulness of pulmonary artery catheters during aortocoronary bypass surgery. Anesth Analg 1982;61:221-222.
32. Baele PL, McMichan JC, Marsh HM, Sill JC, Southorn PA. Continuous monitoring of mixed venous oxygen saturation in critically ill patients. Anesth Analg 1982;61:513-517.
33. Waller JL, Kaplan JA, Bauman DI, Craver JM. Clinical evaluation of a new fiberoptic catheter oximeter during cardiac surgery. Anesth Analg 1982;61:676-679.
34. Shoemaker WC, Appel PL, Kram HB, Lee TS: Prospective trial of supranormal as therapeutic goals in high risk surgical patients. Chest 94:1176-111186, 1988.

35. Rao TLK, Jacobs KH, El-Etr AA. Reinfarction following anesthesia in patients with myocardial infarction. Anesthesiology 1983;59:499-505.

36. Calvin JE, Driedger AA, Sibbald WJ. Does the pulmonary capillary wedge pressure predict left ventricular preload in critically ill patients. Crit Care Med 1981;9:437-443?

37. Mammana RB, Hiro S, Levitsky S, et al. Inaccuracy of pulmonary capillary wedge pressure when compared to left atrial pressure in the early post surgical period. J Thorac Cardiovasc Surg 1982;84:420.

38. Ellis R, Mangano DT, VanDyke DC. Relationship of wedge pressure to end-diastolic volume in patients undergoing myocardial revascularization. J. Thorac Cardiovasc Surg 1979;78:605

39. Hansen RM, Viquerat CE, Matthay MA, et al. Poor correlation between pulmonary arterial wedge pressure and left ventricular end diastolic volume after coronary artery bypass graft surgery. Anesthesiology 1986;64:764-770.

40. Mark JB, Steinbrook RA, Gugino LD, et al. Continuous noninvasive monitoring of cardiac output with esophageal doppler ultrasound during cardiac surgery. Anesth Analg 1986;65:1013-1020.

41. Nishimura RA, Miller FA, Callahan MJ, Benassi RC, Seward JB, Tajik AJ. Doppler echocardiography: Theory, instrumentation, technique, and application. Mayo Clin Proc 1985;60:321-343.

42. Keefer JR, Barash PG. Pulmonary artery catheterization: A decade of clinical progress? 1983;84:241-242.

43. Cohen MM, Duncan PG, Pope WDB: A survey of 112,000 anaesthetics at one teaching hospital (1975-83). Can Anaesth Soc J 1986;33:22-31.

NITROUS OXIDE AND THE COMPROMISED HEART

P.Foëx

Since its introduction in the midle of the last century, nitrous oxide has been used almost universally in anaesthesia and for analgesia and its effects on the circulation have often been considered negligible. However, because of the increase in the number of anaesthetics given to patients with a severely compromised cardiovascular system, the effects of nitrous oxide on the heart and the circulation, deserve re-examination.

Nitrous oxide and the normal heart.

As late as 1955, Fieldman and his colleagues (1) explained the decreases in cardiac output, blood pressure and stroke volume observed under thiopental sodium and nitrous oxide anaesthesia entirely in terms of the effects of thiopental sodium, tacitly assuming that nitrous oxide had no effect on the circulation. Similarly, Heller and co-workers, (2) on the basis of their observations of "excellent cardiovascular homeostasis" under anaesthesia with nitrous oxide, oxygen and curare, concluded that "nitrous oxide does not produce myocardial depression ... and interferes minimally with the integrity of the peripheral vascular bed". A number of recent reports, however, have demonstrated that nitrous oxide has significant cardiovascular effects particularly in patients suffering from coronary artery disease.

Information concerning the effect of nitrous oxide on the normal heart has been gained from studies of isolated heart muscle preparations, heart-lung preparations, intact animals, and man.

T. H. Stanley and R. J. Sperry (eds.), Anesthesiology and the Heart, 163–176.

Studies of isolated heart muscle preparations have the advantage that the effect of drugs, including anaesthetic agents, can be observed without interference from neurogenic or hormonal responses. However, in the case of nitrous oxide, such experiments have their limitations. As the concentration of nitrous oxide increases, the effects of hypoxia may be superimposed to those of nitrous oxide because oxygenation of the preparation is solely by diffusion. This problem is particularly important when preparations are tested at 37°C, as opposed to room temperature, because of the higher oxygen consumption. Using papillary heart muscle preparations tested at 37°C, Goldberg and his colleagues (3) found that cardiac performance was reduced to almost the same extent by the addition of nitrous oxide and that of nitrogen; these authors concluded that nitrous oxide did not by itself depress myocardial contractility. In more controlled studies, carried out at room temperature and after eliminating heart muscle preparations that could not contract normally in a mixture of 50% nitrogen in oxygen, Price (4) demonstrated that the replacement of nitrogen by nitrous oxide caused a significant reduction in contractile performance. The severity of myocardial depression was greatest when the ionised calcium concentration was lowest, (Fig.1).

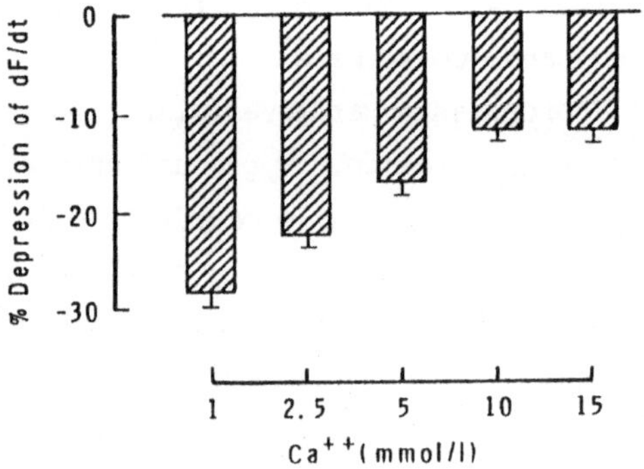

Figure 1. Depression of cardiac performance induced by nitrous oxide is a function of calcium ion concentration (after Price, 1976).

Because the nitrous oxide depression was a function of the ionised calcium concentration, Price concluded that nitrous oxide interfered with calcium fluxes in the heart muscle.

Using heart-lung preparations Fisher and his colleagues (5) found that nitrous oxide caused slight cardiac dilatation without changing pulmonary or right atrial pressures in the dog. The cardiac dilatation may have reflected negative inotropy or a change in myocardial compliance. Price and Helrich (6) constructed right ventricular function curves for the dog's heart and found nitrous oxide to depress myocardial contractility.

In intact animals, the addition of nitrous oxide to halothane anaesthesia causes an immediate reduction of myocardial contractility (7) accompanied within a few seconds by an increase in peripheral vascular resistance. The latter may reflect a direct effect of nitrous oxide on the vascular smooth muscle or an increase in sympathetic activity at the alpha-adrenergic receptors. The association of reductions of stroke volume, stroke work and left ventricular dP/dt_{max} with increases in left ventricular end-diastolic pressure caused by the substitution of nitrogen by nitrous oxide confirms the negative inotropy of nitrous oxide (8). The addition of nitrous oxide under pentobarbitone anaesthesia has also been shown to cause increases in systemic vascular resistance and in left ventricular end-diastolic pressure, and to reduce cardiac output. The cardiac depression, however, was not accompanied by a reduction in coronary blood flow (9), probably because heart rate and arterial pressure remained unchanged. Indirect evidence for the role of the sympathetic nervous system in the haemodynamic response to nitrous oxide can be obtained by comparing the haemodynamic values under nitrous oxide anaesthesia, supplementing pentobarbitone, with or without beta-adrenergic blockade. Cardiac output, aortic blood acceleration, and heart rate were substantially higher before beta-adrenoceptor blockade than after administration of propranolol (10). More direct evidence of sympathetic stimulation has been obtained in animals by studying the preganglionic sympathetic discharge (11) and the splanchnic nerve discharge (12), both of which are increased by nitrous oxide.

Depression of the normal heart has also been observed in volunteers. In a study of the effect of 40% nitrous oxide in oxygen, Eisele and Smith (13) observed gradual reductions in heart rate and cardiac output accompanied by substantial increases in systemic vascular resistance. Contractile performance, estimated by ballistocardiography, was significantly reduced. In three of five subjects plasma adrenaline levels rose, while in all five plasma noradrenaline levels increased. This is corroborative evidence, in man, that nitroous oxide increases sympathetic activity.

In healthy subjects, the addition of nitrous oxide to halothane anaesthesia with spontaneous ventilation has been extensively examined by Hornbein and his colleagues (14). At approximately equi-anaesthetic potencies, halothane-nitrous oxide anaesthesia caused less cardio-respiratory depression than halothane-oxygen anaesthesia. When nitrous oxide was added to 0.8% halothane, cardiac output, arterial pressure and heart rate increased, suggesting that nitrous oxide caused sympathetic overactivity. However, when nitrous oxide was added to 1.5% halothane, cardiac output, arterial pressure and heart rate decreased. In these studies, the responsiveness of the circulation to carbon dioxide was examined and nitrous oxide was found to decrease or even suppress the hyperdynamic response of the circulation to hypercarbia.

When artificial ventilation is used, the addition of nitrous oxide to halothane anaesthesia causes some peripheral vasoconstriction (15), which does not occur with the addition of nitrous oxide under enflurane anaesthesia. At equipotent anaesthetic concentrations (1.5 MAC) nitrous oxide-enflurane may cause less depression than enflurane alone (16). However, in another study involving enflurane anaesthesia, Bennett and his colleagues (17) observed that nitrous oxide caused dose-dependent reductions in cardiac output (Fig.2) and arterial pressure associated with an increase in systemic vascular resistance.

When the heart and the circulation are normal, nitrous oxide appears to cause direct myocardial depression which is compensated by sympathetic activation. Depending upon the depth of anaesthesia and upon the level of arterial PCO_2, the sympathetic response may mask the direct depression of the myocardium, and nitrous oxide may appear to have little effect on the circulation. Because of the peripheral vasoconstriction, the haemodynamic variable most commonly measured, arterial pressure, may remain unchanged, even though cardiac output is reduced.

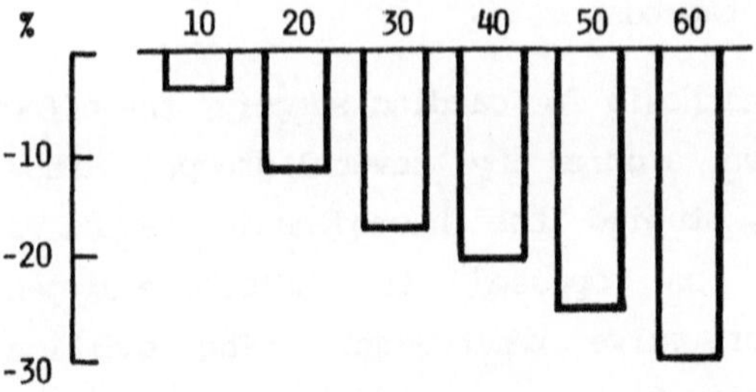

Figure 2. Over the range of 10 to 60 % inspired nitrous oxide, cardiac output is reduced up to 30% during enflurane anaesthesia (after Bennett et al, 1977).

Nitrous oxide and the compromised myocardium.

The administration of nitrous oxide for sedation and analgesia in the postoperative period is relatively common practice. One of the first studies of the effects of nitrous oxide analgesia in patients after myocardial infarction demonstrated that effective analgesia could be obtained without circulatory depression (18). However, in a study of the effect of nitrous oxide during cardiac catheterization, Eisele and his colleagues (19) found that nitrous oxide decreased left ventricular contractility, increased left ventricular end-diastolic pressure and decreased cardiac output in patients with coronary artery lesions. The depressant effect of nitrous oxide appeared to be more marked in the presence of severe coronary artery disease than in its absence since in patients with angina but free of coronary artery lesions, cardiac performance was maintained. Similarly, Wynne and his colleagues (20) examined the effects of nitrous oxide in thirty patients undergoing cardiac catheterization. Small but significant reductions in cardiac index, LV dP/dt_{max} and stroke work index were observed, together with an increase in end-systolic volume index. However, associated with this mild cardiac depression there was a significant reduction of the rate-pressure product which may be considered advantageous.

During anaesthesia for cardiac surgery, the effects of nitrous oxide have been studied by several groups. Stoelting and his colleagues (21), studied the haemodynamic responses to nitrous oxide-halothane as opposed to halothane-oxygen anaesthesia immediately before valve replacement. The addition of nitrous oxide caused significant increases in right and left ventricular filling pressures, while other haemodynamic variables remained unaltered. This observation is at variance with those made in patients with coronary artery disease, in whom, under morphine anaesthesia, nitrous oxide caused dose-dependent reductions in cardiac output accompanied by dose-dependent increases in systemic vascular resistance while heart rate remained essentially unchanged and systolic arterial pressure was reduced, (22). In another study, during which left ventricular pressure was measured, Lappas and his colleagues (23) observed a significant reduction in cardiac output and LV dP/dt_{max} when nitrous oxide was added to morphine anaesthesia. In the absence of changes in systemic vascular resistance, the major effect of nitrous oxide in these patients was myocardial depression.

In patients studied under fentanyl anaesthesia, nitrous oxide also caused substantial reductions in cardiac output accompanied by fairly large increases in systemic vascular resistance (24). While most studies have examined the effects of nitrous oxide on the systemic circulation, the studies by Lappas and his colleagues (23) and those of Lunn and his co-workers (24), have demonstrated that nitrous oxide causes substantial increases in pulmonary vascular resistance, the mechanism of which has yet to be elucidated.

In an attempt to rationalise the use of nitrous oxide in patients with coronary artery disease, Balasaraswathi and his colleagues (25), have examined the influence of the level of left ventricular end-diastolic pressure on the response to 50% nitrous oxide in patients anaesthetised with fentanyl. They found that nitrous oxide exerted no significant effect in those with left ventricular end-diastolic pressure less than 15 mm Hg, whereas it significantly decreased cardiac output in those with left ventricular end-diastolic pressure greater than 15 mmHg. In the latter group systemic vascular resistance rose significantly.

Nitrous oxide, regional wall function and myocardial metabolism.

Most of the studies reviewed so far have examined global cardiac performance and paid little or no attention to regional cardiac function and to myocardial metabolism, although these aspects of heart function are of considerable importance in patients with coronary artery disease. Some recent studies, including our own, have addressed these questions either in experimental models or in patients with coronary artery disease.

The majority of experimental studies of the effects of nitrous oxide have been carried out on normal hearts. However, studies of the effect of anaesthesia on myocardium supplied by a narrowed coronary artery may be more relevant to the problem of anaesthesia for patients with coronary artery disease than studies carried out in normal hearts.

In a series of studies based on an experimental model of critical coronary constriction (26,27,28), we have examined the effects of nitrous oxide on global and regional left ventricular function. In the first group of studies, (Fig.3,4) the addition of nitrous oxide to fentanyl or sufentanil anaesthesia was shown to cause significant reductions in systolic shortening, associated with early diastolic dysfunction (post-systolic shortening) in the compromised territory (26) in contrast nitrous oxide did not modify global and regional function in the normal myocardium.

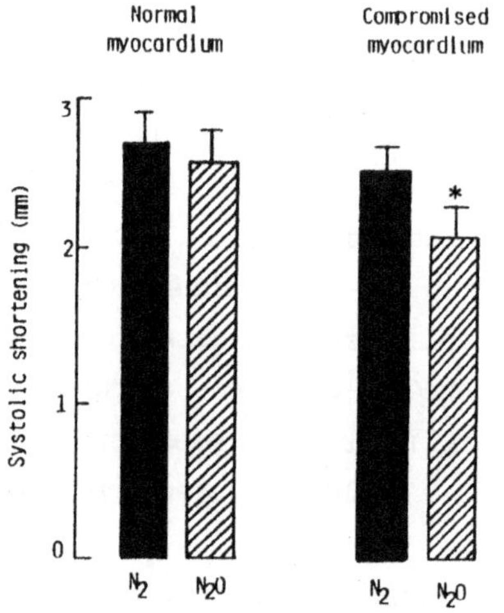

Figure 3. The replacement of nitrogen-oxygen (N_2) by nitrous oxide-oxygen (N_2O) decreases systolis shortening significantly only in compromised myocardium (after Philbin et al, 1985).

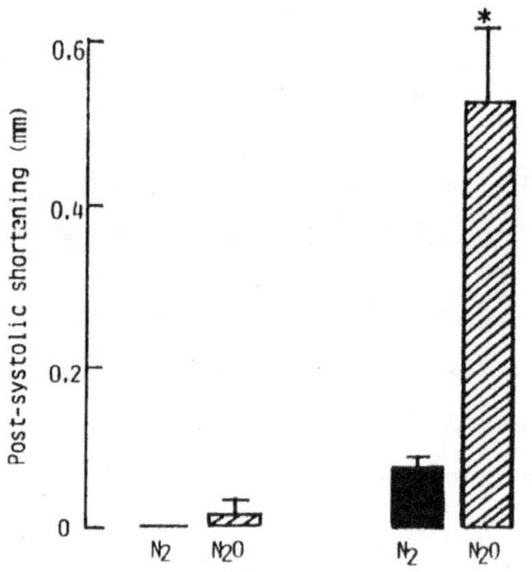

Figure 4. Post-systolic shortening, an indicator of wall dysfunction occurs only in the compromised myocardium when nitrous oxide-oxygen (N_2O) replaces nitrogen-oxygen (N_2). After Philbin et al, 1985.

A subsequent study showed that dysfunction may already develop when 40% nitrous oxide was added to fentanyl anaesthesia (27). Somewhat greater degrees of selective depression of compromised myocardium have been reported during halothane anaesthesia (28) and more recently, during propofol anaesthesia (29). Such selective changes in function are suggestive of myocardial ischaemia. However, they occurred in the absence of significant reductions in coronary perfusion pressure and coronary blood flow, in coronary blood flow over and above that due to critical coronary constriction. Thus, the cause of the ischaemic dysfunction remains uncertain. Close examination of arterial blood gases has made it possible to rule out hypoxia due to second gas effect (27). This aspect of the study is particularly important as nitrous oxide has been shwon to inhibit the hypoxic pulmonary vasoconstriction in a number of animal models. However, recent studies of the pulmonary pressure/flow relationships suggest that pulmonary vascular effects of nitrous oxide are too small to be clinically relevant and are unlikely to be responsible for hypoxaemia during anaesthesia (30). Several other hypotheses can be put forward. Firstly, a modification in the distribution of coronary blood flow away from the subendocardium. This would remain undetected in our model because only total flow, not its distribution across the myocardium, was measured. Secondly, nitrous oxide may have modified the oxyhaemoglobin dissociation curve and oxygen availability. While a leftward shift of the oxyhaemoglobin dissociation curve had been previously reported in man (31), recent studies have shown that nitrous oxide does not alter the affinity of haemoglobin for oxygen (32), Moreover, dissociation curves obtained in our laboratory have failed to reveal a leftward shift in the dog. Thirdly, nitrous oxide could modify oxygen usage at cellular level in the absence of impairment of oxygen supply. However, recent studies using nuclear magnetic resonance spectroscopy have failed to show any effect of nitrous oxide on high energy phosphates in normal myocardium (33).

A drawback of our own studies is that the depth of anaesthesia was not kept constant when nitrous oxide was added. However, in the face of compromised coronary blood flow, the replacement of 1.8% isoflurane in 50% O_2 (balance nitrogen) by 1.4% isoflurane in 50% O_2 (balance nitrous oxide), has been shown to reduce systolic function and cause maldistribution of myocardial blood flow at a constant anaesthetic depth (34). Thus the adverse effect of nitrous oxide cannot be ascribed purely to changes in depth of anaesthesia.

The interest of these experimental observations would be limited in the absence of evidence that nitrous oxide can have deleterious effects in patients with coronary artery disease. Such adverse effects have been reported by two groups. Reiz and colleagues have reported decreases in heart rate, systemic arterial pressure, myocardial oxygen consumption and myocardial oxygen extraction when nitrous oxide was added to isoflurane, (35,36). This was associated with depressed myocardial lactate extraction and worsening of electrocardiographic signs of ischaemia. Similarly, Moffitt and his colleagues (37) have observed adverse effects when nitrous oxide was added to halothane. In their patients, the reductions of heart rate, arterial pressure and rate pressure product may have benefited the ischaemic myocardium by reducing myocardial oxygen consumption; however, the substantial reduction of myocardial lactate extraction and the reduction of coronary sinus oxygen content indicates that myocardial oxgenation was compromised. It is likely that the significant depression of the myocardium caused by nitrous oxide reduced the coronary perfusion pressure to such an extent that coronary blood flow decreased more than oxygen demand. In another study, Moffitt and his colleagues (38) reported adverse responses when nitrous oxide was added to 0.5% enflurane: coronary sinus oxygen content and lactate extraction decreased. In contrast, the addition of nitrous oxide to fentanyl anaesthesia caused reductions in heart rate, arterial pressure cardiac output and coronary sinus blood flow without reductions of coronary sinus oxygen content and lactate extraction.

The significance of alterations of the oxygen balance of the myocardium brought about by nitrous oxide should not be underestimated. There is not only experimental evidence but also clinical data to support the view that nitrous oxide may have deleterious effects on the ischaemic myocardium. Even brief periods of ischaemia can cause prolonged alterations in high energy phosphates, myocardial ultrastructure and function. Not only can the myocardium be "stunned" as described by Braunwald and Kloner (39) but infarction may occur (40). In this respect it is interesting to note that Rao and his colleagues (41) found a significantly higher incidence of myocardial reinfarction in patients anaesthetised with oxygen, nitrous oxide, relaxants and narcotics than in patients anaesthetized with oxgyen relaxants and narcotics.

Conclusion

Nitrous oxide exerts relatively moderate effects on the heart and the circulation in normal subjects. However, in the compromised heart the effects are more pronounced and alterations in regional cardiac function and in the electrocardiogramme suggest that ischaemia may be induced. Maybe we should reconsider the place of nitrous oxide in the anaesthetic management of patients with severe coronary artery disease.

References:

1 Fieldman EJ, Ridley RW, Wood EH. Anesthesiology, 1955; **16**: 473-489.

2 Heller ML, Watson TR jr, Storrs RC, Hanover NM. J Am Med Assoc, 1956; **161**: 1543-1542.

3 Goldberg AH, Sohn YZ, Phear WPB. Anesthesiology, 1972; **37**: 373-380.

4 Price HL. Anesthesiology, 1976; **44**: 211-215.

5 Fischer CW, Bennett LL, Allahwala A. Anesthesiology, 1951; **12**: 19-26.

6 Price HL, Helrich M. J Pharmacol Exper Ther, 1955; **115**: 206-216.

7 Eisele JH, Trenchard D, Stubbs J, Guz A. Br J Anaesth, 1969; **41**: 86-93.

8 Lundborg RO, Mile JM, Theye RA. Can Anaesth Soc J, 1966; **13**: 361-367.

9 Thorburn J, Smith G, Vance JP, Brown DM. Br J Anaesth, 1979; **51**: 937-942.

10 Foëx P, Prys-Roberts C. Br J Anaesth, 1974; **46**: 397-404.

11 Millar RA, Warden JC, Cooperman LH, Price HL. Br J Anaesth, 1970; **42**: 366-378.

12 Fukunaga AF, Epstein RM. Anesthesiology, 1973; **39**: 23-36.

13 Eisele JH, Smith TN. Anesth Analg, 1972; **51**: 956-962.

14 Hornbein TF, Martin WE, Bonica JJ, Freund FG, Parmentier P. Anesthesiology, 1969; **31**: 250-260.

15 Smith NT, Eger EI II, Stoelting RK, Whayne TF, Cullen DJ.(1970) Anesthesiology, 1970; **32**: 410-421.

16 Smith NT, Calverley RK, Prys-Roberts C, Eger EI II, Jones CV. Anesthesiology, 1978; **48**: 345-349.

17 Bennett GM, Loeser EA, Kamamura R, Stanlet TM. Anesthesiology, 1977; **46**: 227-229.

18 Kerr F, Ewing DJ, Irving JB, Kirby BJ. Lancet, 1972; **i**: 63-66.

19 Eisele JH, Reitan JA, Massumi RA, Zelis RF, Miller RR. Anesthesiology, 1976; **44**: 16-20.

20 Wynne J, Mann T, Alpert JS, Green LH, Grossman W. J Am Med Assoc, 1980; **243**: 1440-1443

21 Stoelting RK, Reis RR, Longnecker DE. Anesthesiology, 1973; **37**: 430-435.

22 McDermott RW, Stanley TH. Anesthesiology, 1974; [41]: 89-91.

23 Lappas DG, Buckley MJ, Laver MB,et al.(1975) Anesthesiology, 1975; **43**: 61-69.

24 Lunn JK, Stanley TH, Eisele J, Webster L, Woodward A. Anesth Analg, 1979; **58**: 390-395.

25 Balasaraswathi K, Kumar P, Rao TLK, El-Etr AA. Anesthesiology, 1981; **55**: 708-709.

26 Philbin DM, Foëx P, Drummond G, Lowenstein E, Ryder WA, Jones LA. Anesthesiology, 1985; **62**: 166-174.

27 Leone BJ, Philbin DM, Lehot J-J, Foëx P, Ryder WA. Anesth Analg, 1988; **67**: 814-822.

28 Ramsay JG, Arvieux CC, Foëx P, Philbin DM, Jeavons P, Ryder WA, Jones LA. Anesth Analg, 1986; **65**: 431-436.

29 Diedericks J, Leone BJ, Sear JW, Foëx P, Ryder WA. Br J Anaesth, 1989; **62**: 224P.

30 Lejeune P, Deloof T, Leeman M, Melot C, Naeije R. Anesthesiology, 1988; **68**, 92-99.

31 Fournier L, Major D. Can Anaesth Soc J, 1982; **29**: 498.

32 Lanza V, Mercadante S, Pignatoro A. Anesthesiology, 1988; **68**: 591-594.

33 Ramsay JG, Rajagopalan B, Harmsen E, Bore P, Foëx P, Radda G. Can Anaesth Soc J, 1987; **34**: S59.

34 Nathan HJ. Anesthesiology, 1988; **68**: 407-415.

35 Reiz S. Acta Anaesth Scand, 1983; **27**: 464-469.

36 Reiz S, Ostman M. Anesth Analg, 1985; **64**: 570-576.

37 Moffit EA, Sethna DH, Gary RJ, Raymond MJ, Matloff JM, Bussels JA. Can Anaesth Soc J, 1983; **50**: 5-9.

38 Moffit EA, Scovil JE, Barker RA, Imrie DD, Glen JJ, Cousins CL, Sullivan JA, Kinley CE. Anesth Analg, 1984; **63**: 1071-1075.

39 Braunwald E, Kloner RA. Circulation, 1982; **66**: 1146-1149.

40 Geft IL, Fisbein MC, Ninomyia K, Hasida J, Chaux E, Yano J, Y-Rit J, Genov T, Shell W, Ganz W. Ciculation, 1982; **66**: 1159-1153.

41 Rao TLK, Jacobs KH, El-Etr AA. Anesthesiology, 1983, **59**: 499-505.

Inhalation Anesthetics in Patients With Cardiac Disease

John H. Tinker, M.D.

Basic Coronary Physiology

Before we can discuss the effects of anesthetics on the coronary circulation, it seems pertinent to discuss the basic control mechanisms involved in the coronary circulation. It is fair to say that the coronary circulation is one of if not the most "responsive" circulations in the body. Obviously, the final determinant of flow to any given region of myocardium is the metabolic demand of that region. Unfortunately, although the metabolic demand of a given region might be posing a certain requirement, at any given time, numerous factors may stand in the way of that metabolic demand being totally satisfied. These factors include coronary artery disease, excessive heart rate, rapidly changing afterload, dysrhythmias, as well as various external "tonal" influences such as from sympathetic nerve endings "playing upon" various regions of the heart, plus hormonal influences from the adrenal glands and elsewhere.

It was commonly taught in the past that coronary oxygen extraction was nearly complete i.e. the maximal amount of oxygen that could be extracted, on a given passage through the myocardium, would be extracted on that pass. In other words, coronary mixed venous oxygen saturation was considered to usually if not always be as low as it was practically possible to go in the body namely below 50% i.e. with a PO_2 in the low 20's. It turns out that resting coronary venous oxygen saturation is not usually that low and therefore it is fair to say that the "first line of defense" against a sudden increase in oxygen demand of the myocardium is simply for the

T. H. Stanley and R. J. Sperry (eds.), Anesthesiology and the Heart, 177–190.

myocardium to increase extraction of oxygen from the blood already passing through it at that moment. Obviously, this first line of defense only goes so far.

Next, coronary vasodilation occurs. The final common determinant of coronary vasodilation in a particular cardiac region is local demand. The local demand produces adenosine, and this is certainly one of the agents important in this regional dilatation. There are also other factors such as "endothelial relaxant factor" etc. Anyway, local demand determines the state of vasodilation in a given region. On the other hand, external influences play an extremely important part. Most anesthesiologists know that the carotid sinus reflex is a tachycardic stimulus in response to a lowered carotid arterial pressure. It is also true that this same reflex produces a large decrease in coronary vascular resistance when arterial pressure decreases. This is important in interpretation of the studies we mention below, because it is difficult clinically to hold arterial pressure constant. The question always arises as to whether peripheral vascular effects, namely lowered arterial pressure, or intrinsic pharmacologic properties of the anesthetic itself, contribute to the coronary vasodilation observed. Suffice it to say here that these reflexes which play upon the heart are the most important external determinants of overall coronary blood flow and exert second by second control over coronary vascular resistance to a large degree at least in a global fashion.

Local factors, reflexes, and neuro influences as well as endocrine influences all play roles in the regulation of the coronary circulation.

Coronary Steal

Coronary steal is a term which is a catchy one and has unfortunately several shades of meaning. If there is a collateral dependent zone of myocardium, in other words blood must flow to that collateral dependent zone through another zone which is more directly connected to a coronary artery, then it is conceivable that a direct pharmacologic vasodilator might decrease the normal tone of the "primary" area of myocardium thus "stealing" blood away from the collateral dependent zone.

Another "model" of coronary steal is slightly different. In this conceptual model, one myocardial zone is supplied by an artery which has multiple stenoses, such that the vascular tone in that zone is minimal, but no ischemia is present. The other zone is supplied by an artery which has considerably fewer stenoses and so there is vascular tone in that zone. Both of these small arteries are branches of the same larger vessel and therefore, after a pharmacologic direct vasodilating stimulus, the zone which can dilate, theoretically might dilate, in turn again stealing blood away from the other zone despite the absence of much in the way of functioning collaterals. Coronary stealing has been demonstrated with nitroprusside and with adenosine. Regional blood flows are usually measured, in these models, with radioactive microspheres. It is probably impossible to definitively demonstrate actual coronary steal in vivo in man, because of the invasive nature of the methods that need to be used to determine regional coronary blood flow. In the absence of actual determinations of coronary blood flow, it is not possible to be certain that a given occurrence of myocardial ischemia was necessarily due to the prior development of coronary steal. After all, hypotension combined with tachycardia, reflex or otherwise, can reduce myocardial blood supply in a particular critical region to the level of the production of myocardial ischemia, without invoking any such exotic mechanism as coronary steal. Also, it is becoming increasingly obvious that some if not much of the development of ischemia in the presence of critical coronary stenoses is probably due to the formation of small thrombi. In future years, we may look back on our frantic attempts to control "demand" with somewhat of a jaundiced eye. It is possible that our future therapeutic and preventive efforts will be focused on the problem of microvascular thrombi.

Anesthesia and Coronary Steal

In 1983, Reiz et al,[1] in a study involving 21 unpremedicated patients scheduled for coronary bypass surgery who had severe coronary artery disease of varying types, speculated that isoflurane anesthesia might have been associated with the production of signs of ischemia in 10 of these 21 patients, by a mechanism involving pharmacologic indiscriminate coronary vasodilation i.e. steal. In this study, unpremedicated patients, with a group average mean arterial pressure on arrival in the operating room of 110 mmhg, were then given a protocol anesthetic which reduced the group average mean arterial pressure to 68 mmhg, over a relatively short period of time. The authors contended that this led to ischemia because of a mechanism involving coronary steal. The drop in mean arterial pressure, and the reflex tachycardia induced thereby, not to mention the fact that such a rapid drop in arterial pressure, via the reflex mechanisms mentioned above, is exactly a massive stimulus for coronary vasodilation. Despite all these other possibilities, the authors contended that the mechanism of the resultant ischemia was indeed coronary steal. They based this contention on the fact that coronary sinus flow was better maintained during this relatively hypotensive anesthetic than they would have expected based on indices of oxygen demand. This led to their conclusion that isoflurane was a direct coronary vasodilator. Other explanations include the possibility that such a precipitous drop in perfusion pressure, even if it would normally elicit a massive reflex coronary vasodilation, might be inhibited from so doing by the other kinds of anesthetics. Indeed there is evidence that halothane and enflurane are considerably more effective in blocking carotid sinus baroreflexes than is isoflurane. In summary of this study, the problem is as stated above, namely that we need to figure out a way to separate direct pharmacologic actions of an anesthetic from its peripheral and/or reflex effects.

At first glance, the above contention might not seem too important, because if the anesthetic is going to have these peripheral and reflex effects, then wouldn't it be deleterious whether the coronary vasodilation was due to these reflex effects or to the anesthetic itself? The answer to that is no. If the coronary vasodilation is due to the anesthetic itself, then one would indeed expect coronary steal. If the coronary vasodilation is due to peripheral dilation-induced hypotension, and/or baroreflex induced coronary vasodilation, then one would not expect such indiscriminate vasodilation as to cause clinically relevant steal.

Four "Models" for the Study of Coronary Steal vs. Anesthetics

A. The Human Model

The Reiz et al[1] paper, described above, did indeed stimulate other human studies, including most importantly, those of Moffitt et al[2] and Tarnow et al[3]. In the Moffit et al studies, again coronary sinus flow and oxygen contents were measured. Again it was observed that isoflurane anesthesia appeared to produce coronary dilation in excess of that produced by relatively equivalent concentrations of halothane and enflurane. To put it another way, with halothane and enflurane, the studies of both Reiz et al[1] and Moffitt et al[2] tend to show that as these two agents reduce oxygen demand, both of the whole body and the myocardium, coronary blood flow decreases approximately appropriately. In contrast, this does not seem to be the case with isoflurane. Although most of these studies have not found increased coronary blood flow during situations of less oxygen demand created by anesthesia with isoflurane, they have found greater preservation of control coronary blood flows seen during the awake state, indicating that isoflurane is somewhat of a direct coronary vasodilator. There is little dispute about this. The dispute lies in the area of whether or not such apparent preservation of coronary blood flow i.e. a greater decrease in coronary vascular resistance with isoflurane for a given set of oxygen demand conditions compared to halothane or enflurane, constitutes a direct coronary vasodilatory stimulus sufficient to produce clinically relevant coronary steal.

A study by Tarnow et al[3], also in humans, illustrates the difficulty of this dilemma. In that study, patients with coronary artery disease who had angina pectoris were electrically paced to tachycardia induced angina while awake. The heart rate level at which each patient developed clinical angina was recorded, as was the electrocardiogram at that point. Next, the patients were anesthetized with isoflurane to a clinically relevant level, and then paced to tachycardia again. During pacing induced tachycardia under isoflurane anesthesia, ECG changes similar to those which occurred during awake angina did not appear until significantly higher levels of tachycardia were induced. Obviously, the patients couldn't complain of angina but the patients during isoflurane anesthesia did indeed seem to tolerate considerably greater levels of tachycardia. Tarnow et al[3] concluded, in sharp contrast to the studies of Reiz et al[1] and Moffitt et al[2], that isoflurane protected patients with coronary artery disease against the development of ischemia.

There are numerous difficulties with human studies. First, coronary blood flow must be measured with a reverse thermodilution coronary sinus catheter. This catheter has some potential problems. First it is pushed into the coronary sinus an arbitrary distance by the operator. The further one pushes it into the coronary sinus, the more it occludes the flow in that vessel. There are no valves in the coronary venous system, so that if you impede flow in the coronary sinus, said flow will be diverted elsewhere, usually to the right ventricular thebesian venous channels. This means that you will not measure that diverted flow with the coronary sinus catheter. Another problem with this catheter is that, in some patients, the great coronary vein does not empty into the coronary sinus but rather empties directly separately in the right atrium and thus its flow would not be measured. Under the best of circumstances, the coronary sinus only contains about 70-75% of the total coronary blood flow. Another problem with this method of measuring is that the atrium gets in the way. When the atrium beats, it not only pushes blood down into the right ventricle, but also backward into the coronary sinus. This means that the reverse thermodilution mechanism of the coronary sinus catheter will have atrial blood washed over it at intervals corresponding to heart rate. If heart rate at the beginning of the study period is not the same as it is during the experimental part i.e. the anesthetic, then the accuracy of the coronary sinus blood flow measurements will be in question. This is important because it is based on these apparently better preserved coronary blood flows that Reiz et al[1] and Moffitt et al[2] contend that isoflurane is a direct coronary vasodilator. These patients did have some degree or other, with great variability, of reflex tachycardia.

Please do not get the idea that I am unappreciative of the massive efforts involved in these human studies. They are fascinating, they have raised questions which now probably need to be addressed in the laboratory. I do not, believe that the weight of evidence from the human studies has thus far been convincing that isoflurane, in clinical concentrations, with the usual clinical efforts to prevent hypotension and tachycardia, can lead to myocardial ischemia via a mechanism of coronary steal. There is no doubt in my mind that the old internists' adage "keep the blood pressure up, don't let the heart rate go up, keep the oxygen levels up", is true and I am certain that we all try to do this. I think it is well understood by anesthetists that if you fail in the above objective, in a patient with reduced coronary vascular reserve, you do run the risk of induction of severe ischemia and its consequences. I don't think you necessarily must invoke a mechanism of coronary steal.

B. The Dog Model of Buffington et al[4,5]

Dogs have a naturally collateralized coronary circulation, which is different from the human condition. This fact has elicted much criticism of the use of dogs for experiments involving coronary physiology, but it does permit studies of coronary steal. In other animals which have more human-like coronary circulations, such as the pig, inducing the animal to produce disease-related coronary collaterals, is difficult and problematic, although it can be done. In any event, in the dog, Buffington's group produced a gradual (approximately 1 week) occlusion of a major coronary artery using an ameroid (a casein-like substance inside an rigid metal ring) constrictor. This gradual constriction either produces an infarct in the distal area, in which case the animal is excluded from further study, or it produces a collateral-dependent zone distal to the occlusion. This collateral dependent zone does not have perfect oxygen delivery and therefore not perfect mechanical reserve, but indeed it is alive and functioning. Flow to this collateral dependent zone is therefore originating in another major coronary artery, flowing through that artery's normal area and then, via collaterals, into the collateral-dependent zone. Buffington's experiments were conducted as follows. Using a cannula in the non- occluded coronary mentioned above, flow in that coronary was held constant at a value determined previously by pilot studies to be consonant with maintenance of normal resting function during "basal" anesthesia with chloralose. During this "basal" anesthetic, control regional blood flows were measured by injecting microspheres into the cannulated coronary artery. This allowed determination, eventually, of relative flow in the normal area and the collateral area and the determination of a collateral to normal flow ratio. Next, at this same overall flow, either halothane or isoflurane was added to the "basal" chloralose anesthetic in concentrations of 1 MAC only. When steady state 1 MAC halothane or isoflurane anesthesia was achieved, a different type of microspheres were again injected to determine the collateral to normal flow ratios again. It is important to point out that this experiment was done during constant flow, produced via an external pump. During the basal anesthesia conditions, the collateral to normal flow ratios were approximately 0.7, i.e. approximately 70% as much flow as going to the collateralized zone as was going to the normal zone. During 1 MAC halothane anesthesia, this ratio was not significantly reduced. During 1 MAC isoflurane anesthesia, the collateral to normal flow ratio dropped to about 0.4. Because overall flow was constant, this is incontrovertible evidence that steal had occurred i.e. that more of the same flow was being diverted to the normal area and less was going to the collateral dependent zone.

Unfortunately, the perfusion pressures at which these two experiments i.e. halothane vs. isoflurane, were done, were not the same at all. Control perfusion pressures were approximately 55 mmhg and were only reduced to 51 mmhg with halothane, but were reduced to 41 mmhg with isoflurane. The authors chose "equiMAC" concentrations, 1 each of halothane and isoflurane, rather than producing a "dose response" curve. Obviously, if pressures had been held constant between the two anesthetics, then flow could not have been. The fact that the authors chose to hold flow constant and let pressures vary with the anesthetics, may have influenced the relative outcome of the experiment. It is possible that at equal perfusion pressures, there would be little difference between the collateral to normal flow ratios between halothane and isoflurane, though this experiment has not yet been done (it is underway in my laboratory).

So what can we say from the Buffington experiments? It is true that these experiments represent the only actual demonstration of coronary steal with any anesthetic. Unfortunately, they show that at relatively low perfusion pressures, isoflurane is capable of inducing steal. They do not show whether halothane would or would not induce steal at these same low perfusion pressures. Obviously, I am in disagreement with the use of "equiMAC" concentrations of anesthetic when studying the coronary circulation. If equiMAC concentrations represent equal cerebral depressive doses, this is not actually the way anesthetics are clinically administered, indeed instead they are used to control hemodynamics. My thought would be to study them at equal levels of hemodynamic depression, in this case, coronary perfusion pressure. I think this is very important if we are to condemn one anesthetic relative to another.

C. The In Vitro Experiments

These are the simplest seeming experiments of all. All you need to do is take a coronary artery, cut a tiny slice of it, mount it in a bath and measure the tension on that slice after you constrict it with potassium. Next, you add your suspected coronary vasodilator and measure the effect of that drug, in clinical concentrations, on the previously constricted coronary artery ring. Actually, these experiments are anything but simple, and the work of Bollen et al[6], and Blaise et al[7], is elegant and complex. Suffice it to say here that this is a model which is widely used for testing drugs for their ability to either constrict or dilate coronary and/or other arteries. When clinically relevant concentrations, in dose response fashion, of halothane vs. isoflurane are tested in this model, using either dog coronary arteries (Blaise et al)[7] or pig coronary arteries (Bollen et al)[6], surprising results are obtained. Neither halothane or isoflurane are really vasodilators of these coronary arteries. If anything, halothane is a slightly better vasodilator (though not much of one) than is isoflurane.

Criticism of these studies comes from the fact that these are relatively large vessels. Actually, these investigators are very sophisticated and these vessels are not all that large, many of them are as small as 1 or 2 mm in diameter. Nonetheless, these are epicardial vessels and therefore the fact that halothane and isoflurane are not direct pharmacologic vasodilators of these vessels does not mean that some other vessel, probably at a much smaller level, is not being dilated by isoflurane (or halothane for that matter). These studies lead me to conclude that if direct pharmacologic vasodilation is occurring with isoflurane, it is occurring at the resistance (arteriolar) level. Nonetheless, these studies do not lend support to the idea that isoflurane might cause coronary steal via direct pharmacologic coronary dilation.

D. Studies of Reactive Hyperemia[8-10]

If you temporarily (10-15 seconds) but completely occlude a coronary artery, then release the occlusion suddenly and measure either flow or flow velocity distal to the occlusion, you will see a remarkable degree of reactive hyperemia. The coronary circulation is immensely reactive and the height of the reactive hyperemia has been contended by Marcus et al[11] and others to be indicative of the state or reserve of the coronary circulation distal to the point at which occlusion was produced. Actually, Marcus et al[11] believed that the height of the reactive hyperemic curve, divided by the depth of the so called "debt", measured by observing mean coronary flow velocity and noting its value before dropping it to zero with the temporary occlusion, this reactive hyperemic height divided by the previously noted debt is a measure of "coronary vascular reserve".

Using this concept, we (Gilbert, Roberts, and myself) conceptualized that if isoflurane (or halothane) was a direct pharmacologic vasodilator then as incrementally increased concentrations of the agent were delivered, the height of the reactive hyperemia after a 10 second coronary occlusion would be diminished because the agent would have already caused direct pharmacologic coronary vasodilation.[8-10] Our contention was, therefore, that if either of these agents was associated with relative <u>preservation</u> of the ability of the coronary circulation to dilate in response to a temporary total occlusion, <u>then that agent could not have been very much of a direct pharmacologic vasodilator</u>. It is important to note that a 10-15 second coronary occlusion does not damage the myocardium if repeatedly done in careful fashion. Also, this 10-15 second coronary occlusion is the most powerful coronary dilating stimulus known. In short, if there was "anything left to dilate" this stimulus will dilate it.

To our surprise, when we incrementally increased the steady state end tidal anesthetic concentrations, 0.5 MAC at a time, in pigs, measuring the coronary vascular reserve at each of these incremental steady state concentrations of either halothane or isoflurane, we found that <u>isoflurane preserved coronary vascular reserve at least twice as well as did halothane</u>. We do not see how isoflurane could therefore have been acting as a direct coronary vasodilator.

These studies can be criticized as follows. First, we were measuring coronary flow velocity, not coronary flow. It is conceivable that dilation could have increased coronary flow while decreasing the measured velocity. We controlled for this and this study has now passed extensive peer review so we do not believe that criticism particularly valid. Our experimental model was the previously normal pig, not with diseased coronary arteries.

Nonetheless we conclude from this study that we could find no evidence whatsoever that isoflurane was an indiscriminate coronary pharmacologic vasodilator. We also believe that the reactive hyperemic method we used is an excellent way to cancel out the peripheral and reflex effects of these anesthetics, again because a 10-15 second total coronary occlusion is the most powerful coronary dilation stimulus known.

Summary and Conclusions

I have tried to summarize above extensive and complex experimental work in humans and various animal models. This work is complex and difficult to interpret. It is possible to take this literature and selectively use it to bolster one's point of view. Clinicians should not take isolated experimental studies and jump to conclusions about clinical use of anesthetics. Experimenters should not arrive at sweeping conclusions based on a particular experimental study performed under some or other carefully or not so carefully controlled conditions. Editorialists, such as Becker[12] in a recent issue of Anesthesiology, should not conclude that an anesthetic is "dangerous", based on these kinds of studies. It is especially invalid to use the term "dangerous" unless the author is willing to present us with a viable, experimentally proven, safer alternative. To tell us that isoflurane is "dangerous" implies that we should switch to some unspecified other agent.

What conclusions can we arrive at based on these studies? #1. It is possible to produce coronary steal, in dogs, at constant coronary flow, with isoflurane at 41 mmhg perfusion pressure. The comparison between halothane and isoflurane is suspect because it was performed at two markedly different coronary perfusion pressures. #2. Myocardial ischemia can be induced in humans with coronary artery disease when hypotension and tachycardia is permitted during isoflurane anesthesia. During these conditions, relative preservation of coronary blood flow greater than that which would be expected because of measured or calculated demand, has been interpreted as meaning that mechanism was that of coronary steal. I am not convinced that this mechanism needs to be invoked here, but we can conclude from these studies that if you allow hypotension and tachycardia to occur in patients with coronary artery disease, ischemia is possible. #3. In isolated in vitro studies, direct pharmacologic vasodilation of the coronary vessels cannot be demonstrated in either dogs or pigs with either isoflurane or halothane. #4. Studies of coronary reactive hyperemia i.e. "coronary reserve" show considerably better preservation of said reserve with isoflurane compared to halothane. These studies were done in previously normal pigs.

Summarizing, it seems to me that it is still valid to do what we have always tried to do in the operating room in patients with coronary artery disease, namely preserve myocardial oxygen supply and not let demand get too far out of hand. It is increasingly clear to me that supply is more important than demand in these patients. This is why I work hard to keep subendocardial perfusion pressure as normal as possible by preventing or treating acute increases in pulmonary capillary wedge pressure. I do this while trying to preserve reasonable levels of mean arterial pressure. It is also important to keep hemoglobin content in mind.

Finally, let me speculate a bit about the future. A well known study by Slogoff and Keats[13] contended that occurrence of myocardial ischemia in the operating room, in patients with coronary artery disease, was associated with an increased incidence of perioperative myocardial infarction. Indeed their data can be interpreted this way. As Dr. Jerry Reves has pointed out, their data can be interpreted almost exactly oppositely, namely that a perioperative myocardial infarction will result only about 6% of the time, despite the fact that ischemia occurred in the operating room. This is fascinating to me because one must ask why did the infarct occur in those 6% and not in the other 94% of patients? Increasingly, based on a large weight of evidence from numerous directions, I think the answer is thrombosis. I think we must become much more sophisticated about understanding, measuring and treating the coagulation states of our patients perioperatively. I think we must understand what it is that the stress response actually does to the blood's coagulability in each patient and develop methods of treating it. We went through a whole decade of intense worries about myocardial oxygen demand. Countless lectures were given showing the famous scale between myocardial oxygen supply demand balance. Since the bottom line is really not ischemia but infarction, I think our focus must now turn toward what it is that produces the actual infarction. By this I do not mean that we should ignore ischemia, obviously it must be treated, and I think we know how to treat it now very well. I think we also are getting better and better at preventing it from occurring in the operating room, but I am less sure that we are getting any better at preventing perioperative myocardial infarction. Therefore, I will close with a (always dangerous) prediction for the future, namely watch for new developments in the area of studies of the coagulation state of patients in the postoperative period. In the meantime, I remain unconvinced that "coronary steal" induced by any anesthetic, isoflurane or otherwise, will be an important part of our future clinical considerations.

References

1. Reiz S, Balfors E, Sorsensen M, et al. Anesthesiology 59:91-97, 1983.
2. Moffitt E, Barker RA, Glenn JJ et al. Anesth Analg 65:53-61, 1986.
3. Tarnow J, Markschies-Hornung A, Schulte-Sasse U. Anesthesiology 64:147-156, 1986.
4. Buffington C, Levine A. Anesthesiology 65:A6, 1986.
5. Buffington C, Romson JL, Levine A, et al. Anesthesiology 66:280-292, 1987.
6. Bollen B, Tinker JH, Hermsmeyer K. Anesthesiology 66:748-752, 1987.
7. Blaise G., Sill J, Nugent M et al. Anesth Anal 65:S20, 1986.
8. Gilbert M, Roberts S, Blomberg R, Tinker J. Anesthesiology 63:A15, 1985.
9. Roberts SL, Gilbert M, Tinker JH. Anesth Analg 66:485-491, 1987.
10. Gilbert M. Anesthesiology (in press).
11. Marcus M, Wright C, Doty D et al. Circ Res 49:877-891, 1981.
12. Becker L. Anesthesiology 66:259-261, 1987.
13. Slogoff S, Keats A. Anesthesiology 62:107, 1985.

OPIOIDS IN PATIENTS WITH CARDIAC DISEASE

THEODORE H. STANLEY, M.D., and PETER L. BAILEY, M.D.

INTRODUCTION

Opioids have been administered for hundreds of years to allay anxiety and reduce the pain associated with surgery (1). Many of these compounds are not only used as premedicants and analgesics during and after anesthesia and surgery, but also as primary or sole intravenous anesthetics. Some investigators suggest that, with minor modifications, a number of new synthetic opioids may qualify as the "ideal intravenous anesthetic" (2). Others state that it is unrealistic to expect newer opioids to be markedly different or more efficacious than older compounds (3). In this chapter, we discuss the pharmacology and use of naturally occurring and synthetic intravenous opioids in contemporary anesthetic practice. The terms "opioid," "opiate," "narcotic," "narcotic analgesic," and "narcotic anesthetic" are used to describe drugs that specifically bind to any of several subspecies of opioid receptors, and share some of the properties of one or more of the naturally occurring endogenous opioids.

Are Opioids Anesthetics?

Although opiate narcotics have achieved prominence as principal or sole anesthetics in cardiac and other selected surgeries, whether or not opioids alone are capable of producing anesthesia is a question that continues to be vigorously debated (3,4,5). To date there is no study demonstrating that an opioid alone can reliably produce anesthesia in man in the absence of all other supplements, including muscle relaxants and premedicants.

The most popular model used to examine whether or not opiate narcotics can serve as anesthetics has been to assess their ability to substitute for a potent inhalation agent in dogs (6,7,8,9,10,11) and rats (12,13) subjected to tail-clamp MAC evaluations. A consistent 60 to 70 percent re-

T. H. Stanley and R. J. Sperry (eds.), Anesthesiology and the Heart, 191–229.

duction in the MAC of enflurane or isoflurane has been shown in dogs with morphine, (9) fentanyl (10), alfentanil (6,8), and sufentanil (7). The fact that further increases in narcotic doses and plasma levels often resulted in no additional MAC reductions after a certain MAC reduction was achieved has led to the conclusion that maximum opioid narcotic effects reach a ceiling which is subanesthetic (9,10).

Studies in rats have shown a greater ability of opioid narcotics to reduce the MAC of inhalation agents: 84 percent for morphine (13) and 90 percent for sufentanil without a plateau or ceiling effect noted (12) (Fig. 1). In contrast to investigators using the dog model, these authors concluded that "sufentanil is essentially a complete anesthetic" (12). Other reports demonstrating lower thiopental requirements for loss of consciousness after sufentanil than fentanyl support the greater anesthetic capabilities of sufentanil over fentanyl (14) (see Fig. 2).

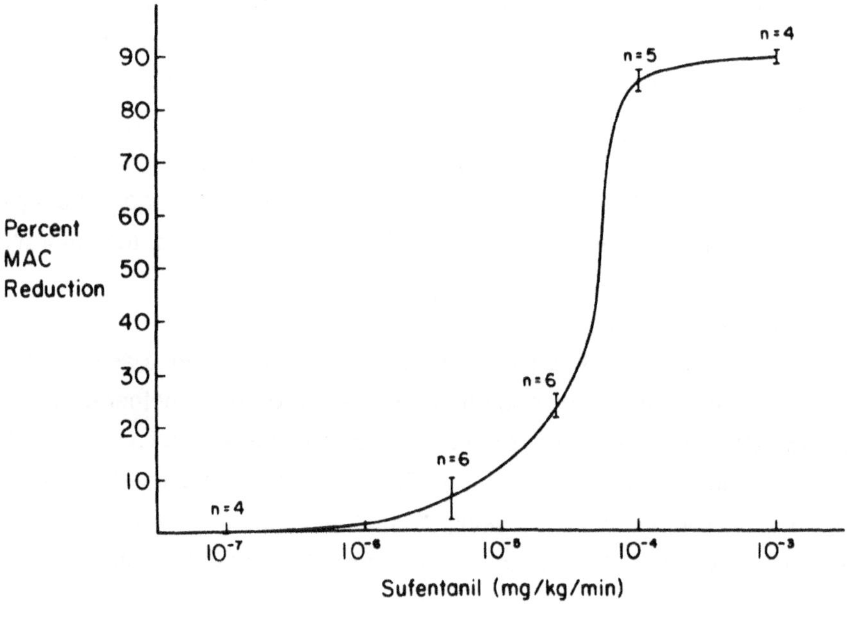

Fig. 1. Reduction of halothane minimum alveolar concentration in the rat observed with progressively increased sufentanil dosage. (Hecker B.R., Lake, C.L., DiFazio, C.A., Moscicki, J.C. and Engle, J.S.: Anesth Analg 62:987, 1983.)

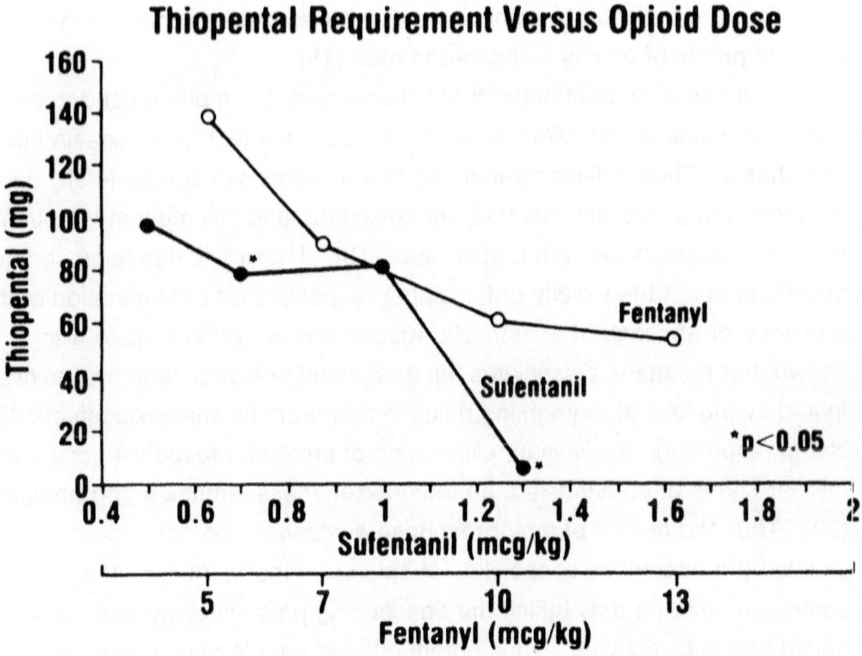

Fig. 2. Thiopental was administered IV in 25 mg increments every 30 sec until the patient was unconscious. The thiopental requirement was plotted against the opioid dose. Sufentanil and fentanyl doses were plotted on the same scale, using a potency ratio of 1:8. The thiopental requirement was significantly smaller ($P < 0.0001$) for sufentanil, 0.7 and 1.3 $\mu g \cdot kg^{-1}$, compared to equipotent doses of fentanyl (5 and 10 $ug \cdot kg^{-1}$, respectively). Only one of the ten patients receiving sufentanil, 1.3 $ug \cdot kg^{-1}$ required any thiopental, compared to 10 of 10 in the fentanyl, 10 $ug \cdot kg^{-1}$ group, and 8 of ten in the fentanyl, 13 $ug \cdot kg^{-1}$ group ($P < 0.0001$). (Bowdle T. and Ward R. Anesthesiology. 70:26, 1989.)

For numerous reasons, MAC reduction studies have significant limitations. Species differences, although minimal in terms of MAC determinations with inhalation agents, are significant with opioids (9,13,15,16) and render extrapolation of results to man questionable. Some authors argue that a similarity between opioids and associated cardiovascular effects in man and the dog supports the conclusion that responses of the two species to narcotic analgesics are similar (6,17). Others have found that dogs are not only more resistant to opioid narcotics but also demonstrate a markedly different profile of effects compared to man (15).

It has also been noted that tail clamping, the method used to elicit a motor response during MAC reduction studies may test for analgesia but not anesthesia. Thus, tail-clamp-induced motor responses can be totally absent in opioid narcotized animals that are conscious and still present in animals rendered unconscious with barbiturates (18). These findings raise serious questions about the validity of tail-clamp responses for determination of the presence or absence of anesthesia. Kissen and Brown (19) have also shown that reserpine dissociates the anesthetic effects of fentanyl (as manifested by the loss of the righting reflex in rats) from its analgesic effects (tail-clamp response). In addition, elimination of the motor response occurs at deeper levels of anesthesia than unconsciousness, amnesia and analgesia (20). Thus the results of motor response evaluations do not necessarily indicate the anesthetic capabilities of opioids. Finally, inhalation agents, such as halothane may inhibit the descending pain inhibitory pathways that opioid narcotics activate. Thus potent inhaled agents may antagonize opioid effects (21).

Nevertheless, the presumed specific mechanism by which opioid narcotics act has led to the opinion that they should not be expected to produce anesthesia (5). In addition, receptor occupation theory and the demonstration of a ceiling to opioid effects in MAC reduction studies in dogs has led some investigators to question whether titrating additional narcotic after an apparent ceiling is reached can produce additional CNS depression (anesthesia) (22). However, the ability of a drug to produce analgesia in subanesthetic concentrations and loss of consciousness in higher concentrations may be mediated, at least in part, by different processes (see above) (23). A dual mechanism in the anesthetic action of opioids has been proposed and requires that in addition to receptor mediated effects, an opioid must be lipid soluble enough to function as a general anesthetic (24). Interestingly, a biphasic response has been noted with sufentanil (12)(Fig. 1) and fentanyl (15).

Awareness Under General Anesthesia

The problem of patient awareness under general anesthesia is as old as the specialty itself. However, it was with the introduction of muscle relaxants that the importance of the problem became fully recognized.

Muscle relaxants permitted greater flexibility for the anesthesiologist and surgeon. Different techniques, e.g., "balanced anesthesia," could be tailored to permit more patients to undergo a variety of procedures. Prior to the advent of muscle relaxants the constraints of using a potent inhalation agent such as ether as the sole anesthetic often precluded the undertaking of "high risk" operations in some patients. Thus, the development and clinical application of muscle relaxants permitted "lighter levels" of general anesthesia and simultaneously encouraged the search for and use of many other drugs as anesthetics or anesthetic adjuvants.

Opiate narcotics have played an increasingly important role as anesthetics. While in the clinical realm the use of an opiate narcotic as a primary or sole anesthetic has received wide acceptance, it is still argued by some that opioids should not be expected to produce unconsciousness (5) and, therefore, they are not complete anesthetics. The question of whether or not opiate narcotics produce unconsciousness is most important to the practicing anesthesiologist who, among many things, needs to provide amnesia and a lack of awareness for his or her patients.

While various definitions of consciousness and awareness have been proposed, the simplest and most practical definition of awareness is "the spontaneous recall of events occurring during general anesthesia." A key word in this definition is spontaneous for there are numerous studies documenting that the registration or retention of mental images or information under general anesthesia commonly occurs and can be demonstrated or elicited postoperatively by hypnosis (25) and word or picture recognition tests (26). In addition, it has been well documented by EEG and auditory evoked responses that auditory functioning is left largely intact even under inhalational anesthesia (27). Intraoperative suggestions made to fully anesthetized patients can also impact their postoperative course in such ways as decreasing the need for urinary bladder catheterization (28). It is, therefore, not necessary or perhaps even possible to block the registration or retention of all information in patients who undergo general anesthesia irrespective of the anesthetic used. It is rather the consolidation of such material and the recollection or recall of intraoperative events that should concern the anesthesiologist most.

Whether or not the use of opiate narcotics in anesthesia is associated with an increased incidence of awareness is debatable. Awareness has been reported with many anesthetic techniques (29,30,31,32,33,34). While some feel the reported frequency of awareness with high dose fentanyl and other opioids compares favorably with inhalation techniques (29) others feel there has been an ascending trend in the occurrence of awareness over the past decades. There is little confirmative data for either position.

While the reported incidence of awareness during anesthesia varies greatly (1-25 percent) (35) a 1 to 2 percent incidence is generally accepted as accurate. Utting (36) published data comparing nitrous oxide alone or with halothane. Patients were premedicated with promethazine (25 to 50 mg), induced with thiopental (100 to 350 mg) and tubocurarine (30 to 45 mg). Anesthesia was maintained with either nitrous oxide (70 percent) in oxygen (30 percent) alone (500 patients) or with 0.5 percent halothane added. No patient receiving halothane experienced awareness while 0.4 percent of patients receiving nitrous oxide alone experienced definite awareness. An additional 1.8 percent may have experienced some awareness. While it is not clear that adding opiate narcotics to nitrous oxide reduces awareness, opiates do reduce the MAC requirements of inhalation agents (6,7,8,9,10,11,12,13). Opiate narcotics differ in their effects as supplements to nitrous oxide/oxygen anesthesia. Fentanyl, and in particular sufentanil, may be superior to less potent narcotics (morphine and meperidine) (37).

Regardless of the anesthetic technique, several measures can be taken to minimize the occurrence of awareness under general anesthesia, or the problems which can arise when a patient has such an experience. Preoperative evaluation of the patient allows decisions as to the role an opiate narcotic should play in intraoperative management. Nonetheless, predicting the appropriate drug and dose remains difficult. Generally, healthier patients with normal or high cardiac outputs prior to anesthesia require larger doses of narcotics for anesthesia than do patients who have serious metabolic disease, or cardiovascular limitations, especially reduced cardiac output (2,38,39). Older patients experience higher blood and presumably brain concentrations of opioids than do younger patients after a similar dose. This probably explains the ease with which older patients are rendered anesthetic with opioids (40) (Table 1). Patients' habits (e.g.,

Table 1. Unconsciousness As a Function of Age in 72 Patients Given Fentanyl (30 mg•kg-1) for Induction of Anesthesia

Age (years)	Rendered Unconscious (%)
18-39	57
31-45	77
46-60	53
>60	100

$c^2 = 4.787$; $p = 0.0287$

(Bailey P.L., Wilbrink J., Zwanikken P., et al. Anesth. Analg. 64:48, 1985)

smoking, alcohol consumption) may also influence anesthetic requirements (41). Undoubtedly, differences in plasma protein binding, fat solubility, hepatic metabolism, renal excretion, and regional perfusion influence requirements for opioids as well. How and why all these factors influence opioid and analgesic and anesthetic requirements in humans is complex. However, if data obtained in rat receptor-binding studies are applicable, part of the answer may lie in determining and ensuring that the percentage of CNS opioid-receptor occupation necessary for anesthesia is achieved in every patient (42). This will undoubtedly be difficult for many reasons, not the least of which relates to variability of opioid requirements. In addition, acute tolerance, as seen with barbiturates, may occur with opioids, further complicating the issue. For example, awakening or absence of analgesia can take place at higher plasma opioid levels than are associated with initial loss of consciousness or onset of analgesia (43).

In selected cases (cardiac anesthesia, trauma) where opiate narcotics may be the sole agent, preoperative discussion of the possibility of awareness is recommended. Although pain does not often accompany awareness, the results of a national inquiry in Great Britain suggest this is not always the case (27). In that survey 41 percent of patients felt pain during their awareness episode.

The ability to monitor for intraoperative awareness remains limited. Although monitoring CNS activity (EEG, sensory evoked potentials) or esophageal contractility may be of assistance in evaluating depth of anesthesia, reliably producing a level of CNS depression consistent with lack of awareness remains a clinical art. Signs suggestive of the possibility of awareness are limited to movement and increased autonomic activity. Hypertension, tachycardia, pupil dilation, tearing, sweating or salivation may indicate too light a level of anesthesia. Eye lid motion, swallowing increased spontaneous respiratory effort and extremity or head motion are other signs often assumed to indicate inadequate amnesia. Monitoring for muscle activity as an indicator of awareness is in fact quite valuable because muscle movements usually occur before the threshold for awareness is reached. Indeed, motor signs (muscle movements) frequently occur prior to changes in hemodynamics or activation of the sympathetic nervous system (37). Unfortunately, the use of muscle relaxants during narcotic based anesthesia removes this important clinical sign. Limiting muscle relaxant use during nitrous narcotic anesthesia to appropriate indications (e.g., intraabdominal or ophthalmic surgery) improves the detection of possible awareness.

Some clinicians reduce awareness episodes by adding one or more sedative-hypnotics during premedication, induction and/or maintenance of anesthesia. While administration of supplements (nitrous oxide, diazepam, droperidol) or larger doses of narcotics will increase the likelihood of amnesia (44) they do not guarantee it (32,40). Furthermore, undesirable side effects such as prolonged postoperative respiratory depression and cardiovascular depression are frequent after administration of most supplements (45,46,47). Many clinicians use 0.3 to 0.6 MAC or "MAC awake" concentrations of potent inhalation agents in the hope of ensuring amnesia. Unfortunately, the hemodynamic stability sought with a narcotic technique may be compromised with this approach as well.

In light of current understanding of awareness and CNS function under anaesthesia, intraoperative conversation, especially that which contains material meaningful to the patient, should be curtailed during anesthesia and surgery. Although potent stimuli such as laryngoscopy, intubation, skin incision, sternotomy, and aortic root dissection are considered to be the events most frequently associated with awareness, comments about a patient's size or discussion of clinical aspects of the patient's case can also cause EEG arousal and be recalled (27). On the other hand, intraoperative therapeutic suggestion, which can be used to significantly improve patient outcome (28) remains underutilized.

Intraoperative awareness may or may not be reported by patients postoperatively. The absence of spontaneous recall, therefore, does not ensure a lack of awareness under anesthesia. Traumatic neurosis consisting of nightmares, anxiety, preoccupation with death and reluctance to discuss the incident is a symptom complex often associated with awareness during surgery (32,48). Awareness associated with anesthesia is best dealt with by informing patients of its possibility preoperatively and by frank and open discussion of such an episode after an occurrence. Direct explanation is considered to be the most helpful approach to a reluctant and fearful patient (48).

CARDIOVASCULAR ACTIONS

Although hypotension, hypertension, bradycardia, and numerous other cardiovascular problems were reported following morphine administration, these side effects seem to occur less frequently after fentanyl (2,49). The newer, more potent opioid, sufentanil, also produces minimal changes in cardiovascular dynamics (50,51). Likewise, alfentanil provides superior cardiovascular stability when compared to non-opioid induction agents (52), however, in certain patients significant hemodynamic fluctuations can occur (53).

Slow administration of morphine, 1 $mg{\cdot}kg^{-1}$ over 5 to 10 minutes IV, usually does not cause significant circulatory changes in supine patients with or without cardiac disease (49). In patients with aortic valvular disease, stroke volume and cardiac output may be increased after morphine administration, probably because the compound does not result in myocardial depression but does decrease systemic vascular resistance, at least transiently (49,54,55). Vasko and co-workers (56) found that morphine has a significant positive inotropic effect that is dependent on endogenous catecholamine release in dogs. Morphine increases blood and urine catecholamine concentrations in a dose-dependent manner in patients with cardiac disease (57,58,59). The release of catecholamines by morphine and meperidine follows and parallels histamine release (60,61).

Although large doses (0.5 to 30 $mg{\cdot}kg^{-1}$) of fentanyl produce significant increases in plasma catecholamines in dogs (62) anesthetic doses of fentanyl (24 to 75 $\mu g \cdot kg^{-1}$) decrease rather than increase plasma catecholamine and cortisol concentrations in humans (63). The effect of fentanyl on plasma catecholamines may be dose dependent. Hicks et al (64) noted elevated plasma norepinephrine levels after 15 $\mu g \cdot kg^{-1}$ of fentanyl, but normal (baseline) values after 50 $\mu g \cdot kg^{-1}$ in human subjects. Similarly, anesthetic doses of sufentanil usually do not change circulating catecholamine concentrations. Most investigators have reported that fentanyl has no effect on myocardial contractility or cardiac output (2,65,66). However, others have reported negative (64) or positive (67) inotropic effects, and still others a myocardial depression-sparing action of fentanyl during halothane and enflurane anesthesia (68,69).

Despite the minimal cardiovascular effects of opioids, significant hypotension, hypertension, and cardiac dysrhythmias have been reported after the administration of virtually all opioid compounds in some patients. Therefore, certain precautions should be observed during the induction and maintenance of anesthesia with morphine and other opioids.

<u>Hypotension</u>

<u>Common Mechanisms</u>. Most opioids reduce sympathetic and enhance vagal and parasympathetic tone, particularly when administered in a large bolus dose. If not countered by indirect effects (e.g., catecholamine release) or the co-administration of drugs with anticholinergic or sympathetic activity (e.g., atropine or pancuronium) opioids can cause hypotension. Patients depending on high sympathetic tone or exogenous catecholamines to maintain cardiovascular function are more predisposed to hypotension after opioids. These and other specific cardiovascular effects of the opioid analgesics, e.g., histamine release, venodilation, will be addressed.

<u>Morphine</u>

Hypotension can occur during and after administration of even small doses of morphine (5 to 10 mg IV) (70). With anesthetic doses (1 to 4 $mg \cdot kg^{-1}$ IV) hypotension occurs more frequently and is more profound (4,71). Indeed, Conahan et al (71) found an incidence of hypotension (systolic blood pressure <70 mm Hg) of 10 percent during anesthetic induction with morphine in patients about to undergo cardiac valvular surgery. Several mechanisms may contribute to the hypotension associated with morphine (Table 2). Rate of morphine infusion also appears to be important in producing and/or avoiding hypotension. Hypotension is not uncommon when the infusion rate is 10 mg•min^{-1} or greater but is rare when it

Table 2. Potential Mechanisms Underlying Morphine Induced Hypotension

1. Histamine release
2. Centrally mediated decrease in sympathetic tone
3. Vagal induced bradycardia
4. Direct and indirect venous and arterial vasodilation
5. Splanchnic sequestration of blood

is $\leq$ 5 mg•min^{-1} (72). Rate of infusion seems to have less of an effect on blood pressure after fentanyl and sufentanil but may still be important with alfentanil.

Morphine, 1 mg•kg^{-1}, produces marked increases in plasma histamine in some patients (Table 3). These changes usually result in an increase in cardiac index and decreases in arterial blood pressure and systemic vascular resistance (73). Similar cardiovascular changes occur when patients are pretreated with diphenhydramine (a histamine H_1-antagonist) or cimetidine (a histamine H_2-antagonist) before morphine. However, in patients pretreated with both H_1 and H_2-antagonists, the cardiovascular responses are significantly attenuated despite comparable increases in plasma histamine concentrations. These data and other reports (60,61,74) strongly suggest that many of the hemodynamic effects of morphine are caused by histamine and indicate a possible means of their prevention.

Increases in plasma histamine after morphine cause dilation of terminal arterioles. Histamine also produces direct positive cardiac chronotropic and inotropic actions that are receptor mediated. Finally, histamine also causes sympathoadrenal activation secondary to catecholamine release. Hypotension is less frequent with high-dose fentanyl anesthesia in part because, unlike morphine, fentanyl does not produce increases in plasma histamine (73). Likewise, sufentanil and alfentanil do not produce changes in plasma histamine (75).

Morphine has been shown to reduce venous and arterial tone both in experimental animals and in human subjects. These changes often result in a decrease in venous return to the heart and may contribute to hypotension (49,76,77,78,79,80,81,82). Arterial dilation occurs sooner and is of shorter duration than venodilation after morphine (80,83). Venodilation after morphine is dose related and necessitates an increase in the volume of blood and/or crystalloid fluids administered to maintain adequate ventricular filling (76,80). Patients anesthetized with morphine, as compared to halothane, have increased blood requirements during and after operation (Table 4). Venodilation and increased blood requirements apparently do not occur with lower doses of morphine (<0.5 mg•kg^{-1}) plus N_2O.

Table 4. Blood Requirements During Operation (Aortic Valve Replacement or Coronary Artery Bypass Operation) and for the First Postoperative Day in 61 Patients Anesthetized with Morphine (1.0-4.0 mg•kg-1) plus Oxygen or Halothane (0.1 - 1.5%) Plus 30% Nitrous Oxide and Oxygen

		Mean blood requirements (ml)	
Pathology	Anesthetic	Intraoperative	Postoperative
Aortic valvular disease	Morphine	2.800*	1,652*
	Halothane	1,010	757
Coronary artery disease	Morphine	2,705*	1,417*
	Halothane	1,750	722

*P 0.05. Student's paired t-test when compared to halothane values. (Modified and preprinted with permission from Stanley TH, Gray NH, Isern-Amaral JH, et al: Comparison of blood requirements during morphine and halothane anesthesia for open-heart surgery. Anesthesiology 41:34, 1974)

Although morphine reduces venous return to the heart in the dog by causing hepatic sequestration of plasma, there is no evidence that this mechanism is of any significance in humans (81,82). Others have suggested that venous vasodilation after large doses of morphine is the primary cause for decreased venous return (76,80,83). Venodilation is not caused by the preservatives present in commercial preparations of morphine (83) but may be related to a reflex mechanism(s). Zelis and co-workers (84) found that morphine selectively impairs certain sympathetic reflexes involving peripheral veins. Their data suggests that this response is due to a CNS action of the drug with secondary withdrawal of sympathetic tone. Vasodilation after morphine may also be due to a direct effect of morphine on vascular smooth muscle (73,77,83). At high doses morphine inhibits the presynaptic release of norepinephrine in saphenous vein rings resulting in a decreased contractile response to electrical stimulation (83). This effect is not reversed by naloxone nor attenuated by histamine blockers. In dogs, hypotension after large doses of morphine (1 $mg \cdot kg^{-1}$) has been attributed to changes in the distribution of blood flow (85). Although not associated with sustained decreases in cardiac output, blood pressure, or total peripheral resistance, Priano and Vatner (85) found 1 and 3 $mg \cdot kg^{-1}$ of morphine produces significant decreases in mesenteric and renal blood flow in dogs.

Hypotension after morphine is not related to myocardial depression, although in healthy volunteers morphine (2 $mg \cdot kg^{-1}$) does cause a prolongation of the preejection period, an estimate of isovolumetric cardiac contractility (86,87). High doses of morphine (3 $mg \cdot kg^{-1}$) activate the sympathoadrenal system (while producing peripheral vasodilation) (88). These changes could counteract myocardial depressant effects of the opioid. On the other hand, increases in sympathetic activity could be detrimental in some patients. Moffitt et al (55) showed that 1 $mg \cdot kg^{-1}$ of morphine does not inhibit lactate production and can produce ischemia with surgical stimulation in patients undergoing coronary artery bypass operations. In summary, hypotension from morphine can be minimized or eliminated by pretreatment with H_1- and H_2-histamine antagonists, use of a slow drug-infusion rate, volume loading, and/or placement of patients in a Trendelenburg (head-down) position.

<u>Meperidine</u>

Meperidine, in contrast to most other opioids, decreases myocardial contractility in isolated cardiac preparations and intact animals (89). Equianalgesic doses of meperidine are 20 times more depressant to the contractile element of the isolated cat papillary muscle than morphine (89). In man, meperidine-N_2O anesthesia has been found to produce greater cardiovascular depression than morphine-N_2O anesthesia (90,91). Even in relatively low doses (2 to 2.5 $mg \cdot kg^{-1}$), meperidine causes a decrease in arterial blood pressure, peripheral resistance, and cardiac output and an increase in heart rate (91,92,93,94,95,96). Anesthetic doses of meperidine

(10 mg•kg1 IV) are associated with marked decreases in cardiac output and frequently cause cardiac arrest in dogs (92) (Fig. 3).

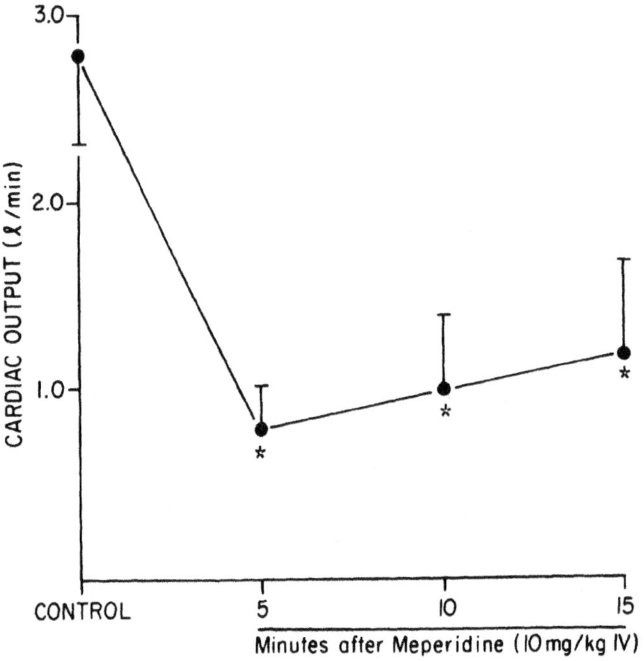

Fig. 3. Cardiac output (mean ± SD) before and after meperidine (10 mg•kg-1 IV) in nine basally anesthetized (sodium thiopental) mongrel dogs. *P <0.0.1, one-way analysis of variance. (TH Stanley, unpublished data.)

Meperidine also causes histamine release more frequently than most other opioids, including morphine, fentanyl, sufentanil, or alfentanil. Flacke et al (61) found that 5 of 16 patients experienced increased plasma histamine concentrations after meperidine whereas only 1 of 10 patients receiving morphine had similar changes. Increases in plasma histamine occur most often in females and are highly correlated to the magnitude of subsequent hypotension (61).

Meperidine, in contrast to morphine, rarely results in bradycardia but can cause tachycardia. Some have attributed tachycardia after meperidine to its structural similarity to atropine. Others (De Castro G, personal communication) believe meperidine associated increases in heart rate are related to early manifestations of its toxic CNS effects. Meperidine's ability to increase plasma histamine, depress myocardial contractility and increase heart rate has reduced its popularity as an anesthetic agent. Meperidine also has little value as a "complete anesthetic" and may be detrimental, even in small doses, in patients who have little cardiovascular reserve.

Fentanyl

Fentanyl, in analgesic (2 to 10 $\mu g \cdot kg^{-1}$) or anesthetic (30 to 100 $\mu g \cdot kg^{-1}$) doses, infrequently causes significant decreases in blood pressure when given alone, even in patients with poor left ventricular (LV) function (2,64,65,97,98,99). Some investigators believe that absence of hypotension after fentanyl is chiefly related to its lack of effect on plasma histamine concentrations (73).

Most evidence indicates that fentanyl produces little or no change in myocardial contractility (2,65,66,68,100) although a few investigators have reported a small negative inotropic effect (64,73,101). Virtually all hemodynamic variables, including heart rate, arterial blood pressure, cardiac output, systemic and pulmonary vascular resistance, and pulmonary artery occlusion or wedge pressure, remain unchanged after large (anesthetic) doses of fentanyl (2,65,73,98,99,101).

Most recently, Miller et al (102) compared anesthetic inductions (in patients premedicated with lorazepam scheduled for coronary artery surgery) with fentanyl (75 $\mu g \cdot kg^{-1}$), sufentanil (15 $\mu g \cdot kg^{-1}$) and alfentanil (125 $\mu g \cdot kg^{-1}$ followed by 5 $\mu g \cdot kg^{-1} \cdot min^{-1}$). Anesthetic induction with fentanyl was associated with the least change in mean arterial pressure and myocardial performance. While sufentanil did not produce hemodynamic instability, it did cause myocardial depression. Those authors and others have suggested that fentanyl may be preferred over sufentanil in patients with poor left ventricular function. On the other hand, other investigators have found better hemodynamic stability and less hypotension after sufentanil than fentanyl in patients undergoing valvular heart surgery (103). In contrast, most available data suggests that alfentanil is associated with more hypotension, bradycardia and surgically induced hypertension than either fentanyl or sufentanil.

Hypotension after fentanyl is probably most related to associated bradycardia and can be prevented or treated with anticholinergics, ephedrine, or even pancuronium (104,105). Patients with high sympathetic tone are more likely to experience hypotension after fentanyl. Flacke et al (106) have postulated that cardiovascular depression after fentanyl is due to inhibition of central sympathetic outflow that is apart from analgesia or other sensory depressant effects of the narcotic. They found that naloxone reversal of fentanyl-induced cardiovascular depression is blocked by clonidine, an alpha-2 agonist. Thus, some central cardiovascular regulating mechanisms, are opioid sensitive. After eliminating all autonomic tone in dogs Flacke et al (107) found minimal hemodynamic changes after fentanyl or fentanyl plus large doses of diazepam. Thus they concluded that hypotension induced by fentanyl was indirect in nature, i.e., mediated by a decrease in CNS sympathetic vasoregulatory outflow.

Sufentanil

Sufentanil, which is 7 to 10 times more potent than fentanyl, causes hypotension with equal or greater frequency than the latter. Since sufentanil is available in similar concentrations as fentanyl (50 $\mu g \cdot ml^{-1}$) a possible cause of hypotension is relative overdose. Sufentanil does not produce increases in plasma histamine but does cause vagal-induced bradycardia (75). Ablation of sympathetic tone and enhanced parasympathetic tone are the most likely mechanisms for sufentanil associated hypotension. Sufentanil induced hypotension may also be mediated by a direct depression of vascular smooth muscle (108).

Several studies suggest that sufentanil is not only more potent than fentanyl but is also closer to a "complete anesthetic." These claims are supported by greater MAC reduction during co-administration of inhalation anesthetics in laboratory animals and less hemodynamic responses to stimuli such as intubation than fentanyl (102). Sufentanil causes more hypotension than equipotent doses of fentanyl. Mathews et al (109) found sufentanil (5 $\mu g \cdot kg^{-1}$) produced lower mean arterial blood pressures than fentanyl (25 $\mu g \cdot kg^{-1}$) during induction of anesthesia in patients having coronary artery surgery. Sebel et al (51) also found that sufentanil (15 $\mu g \cdot kg^{-1}$, injected over 2 minutes) caused significantly lower blood pressures during induction of anesthesia in patients premedicated with lorazepam and scheduled for coronary artery surgery than equipotent doses of fentanyl. Two of these authors' patients had marked decreases in their systolic blood pressure (116 to 60 and 150 to 70 mm Hg). Miller et al (102) showed that although sufentanil (15 $\mu g \cdot kg^{-1}$) attenuated the hemodynamic response to intubation better than fentanyl (75 $\mu g \cdot kg^{-1}$), it impaired myocardial function and depressed systolic blood pressure more. On the other hand, Lake and DiFazio (103) found sufentanil (5 $\mu g \cdot kg^{-1}$) produced more complete, reliable anesthesia and less hypotension than fentanyl (25 $\mu g \cdot kg^{-1}$). Careful titration to effect may be even more warranted with sufentanil, in order to minimize significant hypotension, especially in patients dependent on high intrinsic sympathetic tone or with poor left ventricular functioning.

Alfentanil

Alfentanil, a rapidly and particularly short-acting agent with a high therapeutic index (1,080) in rats (110) is approximately one-fifth to one-third as potent as fentanyl. Studies in dogs have demonstrated little change in hemodynamics with moderate does (160 $\mu g \cdot kg^{-1}$) of alfentanil and transient cardiac stimulation (increases in LV contractility, aortic blood flow velocity and acceleration) with very large doses (5 $mg \cdot kg^{-1}$) (94). Heart rate, cardiac output, and pulmonary and systemic vascular resistance increased following 5 $mg \cdot kg^{-1}$ of alfentanil. Others have reported transient increases in myocardial contractility, mean aortic, pulmonary artery, left and right atrial pressures, and systemic vascular resistance with lower doses (200 $\mu g \cdot kg^{-1}$) of alfentanil in dogs (111,112).

Some authors have found that alfentanil causes similar decreases in heart rate, blood pressure and cardiac index as fentanyl (29,113,114) while others have reported that alfentanil produces the least desirable hemodynamic profile (more hypotension as well as myocardial ischemia) of fentanyl, alfentanil and sufentanil in patients undergoing coronary artery grafting (53,102,115,116,117).

Alfentanil's rather unique pharmacokinetic properties (see below) may contribute to the hemodynamic fluctuations clinicians observe with its use. On the other hand, its pharmacodynamic properties are quite similar to the other opioids and proper precautions and titration when administering the compound can make it a desirable agent, especially for short or medium length procedures. Cardiovascular stability is improved by avoiding indiscriminant use of adjuvants, e.g., benzodiazepines. Titration to specific endpoint (e.g., loss of consciousness) rather than the administration of a precalculated bolus will also provide for improved cardiovascular stability.

Hypertension

Common Mechanisms. Sudden increases in arterial blood pressure, especially during endotracheal intubation or profound surgical stimulation, has been a common problem associated with narcotic anesthesia and is most often attributed to "light anesthesia." Wynands et al (99) have also shown that patients with good left ventricular function will more frequently become hypertensive than patients with poor left ventricular function during fentanyl anesthesia for coronary artery surgery. The authors did not attribute this phenomenon to differences in depth of anesthesia but rather to the fact that patients with preserved myocardial function were more able to increase cardiac index in response to increases in systemic vascular resistance induced by surgical stimuli. Patients with limited myocardial reserve could not always maintain cardiac output in the face of an increased SVR and thus their blood pressure did not increase and might even decrease.

Two other mechanisms (sympathetic activation and cardiogenic reflexes) may underlie hypertension associated with opioid based anesthesia. Thomson et al (118) reported the occurrence of a hyperdynamic cardiovascular response to anesthetic induction with high-dose fentanyl in 10 percent of patients and attributed it to central sympathetic activation. Opioids, may increase catecholamine levels even without increases in plasma histamine. Fentanyl increases norepinephrine release from some sympathetic nerve endings and it may also inhibit its neuronal uptake in dogs. Both increases and decreases in serum catecholamines have been reported in man after fentanyl. Gaumann and Yaksh (119) have also recently reported that sufentanil produced 6- to 20-fold increases in adrenal vein concentrations of catecholamines and parallel increases in arterial blood pressures in cats. Interestingly, sufentanil and the accompanying increase in catecholamine levels prevented the hypotension that normally occurred in these animals after a 25 percent loss of blood volume.

A number of authors have suggested that aortic root dissection causes hypertension via stimulation of a specific cardiogenic reflex (120). Many authors have found that aortic root manipulation is the most provocative stimulus for intraoperative hypertension. Hypertension after aortic root dissection is not associated with increases in plasma catecholamine concentrations or light levels of anesthesia (29). Although higher doses of fentanyl or sufentanil can decrease its occurrence, no dose of any opioid has been shown to reliably prevent hypertension during surgery in man.

Morphine

Hypertension during cardiovascular surgery was also a problem in patients anesthetized with morphine (121,122). Arens et al (121) reported a 36 percent incidence of hypertension, defined as a rise in systolic blood pressure to >200 mm Hg or an increase of 60 mm Hg above preoperative pressure, in patients undergoing coronary artery surgery with 1.5 to 3.0 $mg\cdot kg^{-1}$ of morphine. Hasbrouk (122) using up to 595 mg of morphine found blood pressure to rise about 15 percent above baseline and documented simultaneous increases in plasma epinephrine and norepinephrine. Conahan (71) found more severe hypertension in cardiac valve surgery patients anesthetized with morphine compared to halothane anesthesia. These episodes were attributed to increases in systemic vascular resistance.

Hypertension during morphine anesthesia has been variously attributed to light or inadequate anesthesia (123) reflex mechanisms (4) stimulation of the renin-angiotensin mechanism (124) and sympathoadrenal activation (88).

Fentanyl

Although hypertension is rare before endotracheal intubation or surgical stimulation with high-dose fentanyl anesthesia during cardiac surgery, it is the most common cardiovascular disturbance during or after sternotomy and aortic root manipulation (98,125,126,127). The reported incidence of hypertension with fentanyl-based anesthesia varies widely. Stanley et al (2,39) reported no change in cardiovascular variables following surgical stimulation. Other investigators have reported incidences of hypertension specifically related to sternotomy from 0 to 100 percent in patients given fentanyl 50 to 100 $\mu g\cdot kg^{-1}$ (2,98,125,126,127,128,129,130). The reason for this variability between investigators is not clear. Possible explanations include the type of premedication, the rate of fentanyl administration, the induction and subsequent dose(s) of fentanyl, the timing of its administration, and the type, dose and rate of administration of various muscle relaxants used for endotracheal intubation and surgical relaxation. Other factors include the degree of β-adrenergic and/or calcium channel blockade present at the time of surgery, preoperative ventricular function, volume status, patient habits, and the presence or absence of awareness (32,41,126,127,129,130).

Although satisfactory control of hemodynamics can be achieved by increasing the dose of fentanyl (126,129) use of extremely high doses of the opioid is not always warranted considering associated side effects and the availability of alternative techniques. Doses of fentanyl of 140 $\mu g \cdot kg^{-1}$ or more are likely to result in prolonged respiratory depression during the postoperative period and an increased need for vasopressor support (129,131). Satisfactory blood pressure control can be achieved with fentanyl (50 to 120 $\mu g \cdot kg^{-1}$) plus vasodilator therapy (125,126,128,129,132). However, with lower doses of fentanyl ($\leq$50 $\mu g \cdot kg^{-1}$), and no supplements, there may be an increased risk of intraoperative awareness that is virtually eliminated with doses of > 120 $\mu g \cdot kg^{-1}$ but has occasionally been reported with lower doses (32,33,34).

The total amount of fentanyl used is often limited to 100 $\mu g \cdot kg^{-1}$. When hemodynamic control is not achieved with this dose, vasodilator therapy is begun with sodium nitroprusside or nitroglycerin. Other clinicians may supplement anesthesia with a potent inhaled anesthetic and/or an intravenous sedative-hypnotic (2,32) to control episodes of hypertension. Mixing inhaled anesthetics with high doses of fentanyl can decrease stroke volume, cardiac output, and mean arterial blood pressure and increase ventricular filling pressure (133,134). Yet fentanyl and potent inhaled anesthetics (enflurane or halothane) can be given together without decreasing myocardial contractility or blood pressure, cardiac output, and stroke volume (68,69). Furthermore, some inhaled anesthetics (halothane or isoflurane) may be protective of the myocardium during periods of ischemia (135,136). On the other hand, some clinicians avoid any use of isoflurane in patients at significant risk for myocardial ischemia because of the risk of coronary artery steal. In addition, the effects of adding inhaled anesthetics to large doses of fentanyl or other opioids on the myocardial oxygen supply-demand ratio in patients with coronary artery disease are not always predictable.

Fentanyl, like other opioids, and indeed all anesthetics, is never completely predictable in terms of its ability to eliminate hemodynamic responses to painful stimuli. Indeed, some have concluded that plasma fentanyl concentrations that reliably block hypertensive responses to noxious stimuli may not exist (Fig. 4) (131).

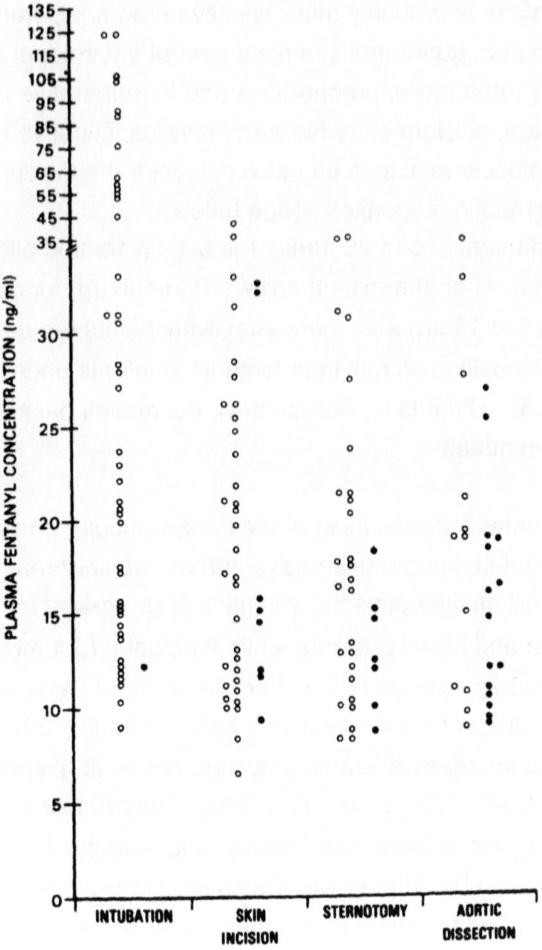

Fig.4. The plasma fentanyl concentration and number of patients with a hypertensive response at each event studied. • Hypertensive. o Normotensive. (Wynands JP, Wong G, Townsend J, et al. Anesth. Analg.. 63:101, 1983.)

Sufentanil

While some investigators find little difference between fentanyl and sufentanil when used as primary anesthetics for cardiac surgery (109,137) many feel that sufentanil provides better control of the hemodynamic responses to intubation (102) sternotomy and sternal spread (130). They also claim sufentanil decreases the need for vasodilators during cardiopulmonary bypass, the postbypass period and postoperatively (130). While sufentanil alone is probably more effective than equipotent doses of fentanyl, it does not guarantee complete control of intraoperative blood pressure (51). Furthermore, preoperative and intraoperative use of beta-adrenergic blockers, calcium entry blockers, nitrates, sedative/hypnotic premedicants and muscle relaxants can also influence the incidence of intraoperative hemodynamic responses. (See below.)

Sufentanil, 15 to 25 $\mu g \cdot kg^{-1}$ is usually titrated either by infusion (25 to 200 $\mu g \cdot min^{-1}$) or intermittent bolus (10 to 100 µg) for cardiac surgery. Sufentanil (5 to 10 µg) also more effectively blunts the hemodynamic response to noxious stimuli than fentanyl in infants undergoing cardiac surgery (138). Sufentanil, like fentanyl, decreases pulmonary vascular resistance in infants.

Alfentanil

Alfentanil shares most of the cardiovascular properties of fentanyl and sufentanil at comparable doses. When administered alone to unpremedicated healthy patients, alfentanil (175 $\mu g \cdot kg^{-1}$) eliminates increases in heart rate and blood pressure while thiopental (3-4 $mg \cdot kg^{-1}$) plus lidocaine (1.5 $mg \cdot kg^{-1}$) does not. Others have found cardiovascular stimulation during and after anesthetic induction with alfentanil (139). The ED_{50} for loss of consciousness following induction doses of alfentanil usually lies between 100 and 125 $\mu g \cdot kg^{-1}$ (139,140). Unfortunately, alfentanil has proved to be less reliable than fentanyl and sufentanil in blocking increases in heart rate and blood pressure during anesthetic induction, sternotomy, sternal spread and aortotomy in patients with ischemic heart disease having coronary artery surgery (141). A higher incidence of ischemia during alfentanil anesthesia than with comparable doses of fentanyl or sufentanil.has also been reported (102). Although some investigators believe alfentanil is a suitable anesthetic for cardiac surgery (29) alfentanil will probably not supplant fentanyl or sufentanil as a sole agent during cardiac surgery.

Heart Rate, Rhythm and Baroreceptor Function

With the exception of meperidine, all µ-receptor stimulating opioid analgesics usually produce decreases in heart rate. Fentanyl-induced bradycardia is more marked in anesthetized than conscious dogs or human subjects (142,143). When used for induction of anesthesia, there is a higher incidence of bradycardia when patients or dogs breathe pure oxygen than when nitrous oxide is used with oxygen (144,145). This may be due to the increase in sympathetic nervous system activity associated with nitrous oxide anesthesia (146,147). Second and subsequent doses of fentanyl cause less bradycardia than do initial doses (62,144). Infusions in dogs decrease heart rate after the first 50 $\mu g \cdot kg^{-1}$ of fentanyl (135). Administration of additional fentanyl (up to 2 $mg \cdot kg^{-1}$) is required to duplicate the initial percentage decrease in heart rate (62). The degree of bradycardia after infusion of opioids may be dose related (135,142,148), although opioids have not always been found to produce dose dependent effects on heart rate (139). An equally important factor may be the speed of injection. While a well-controlled experimental investigation has not been published, clinical experience in human subjects and animals studies with numerous species (144,148,149,150,151) suggest that bradycardia can be minimized by slow administration of potent opioids. Premedication with atropine or glycopyrrolate attenuates bradycardia induced by morphine, fentanyl, and other highly potent opioids but does not always eliminate it (2,39,40,62,144,149). Atropine is often effective in treating opioid-induced bradycardia, although even large doses (1 to 2 mg) are occasionally ineffective. Administration of small to moderate doses of intravenous pancuronium (0.5 to 2.0 mg) prior to induction of anesthesia with fentanyl or other potent narcotics attenuates bradycardia (149,152,153).

The mechanism of fentanyl-induced bradycardia, while not completely understood, is most likely due to stimulation of the central vagal nucleus (142). Bradycardia is almost totally prevented by bilateral vagatomy (142) or pharmacologic vagal block with atropine (144). Blockade of sympathetic chronotropic action may also play a minor role (142). Similar mechanisms have been proposed for morphine (154,155). Morphine is also thought to have a direct effect on the sinoatrial (SA) node (156,157) and to depress atrioventricular (AV) conduction (158). Morphine, through histamine release, can cause increases in heart rate. Histamine has positive chronotropic effects and can cause sympathoadrenal activation. Meperidine can cause a tachycardia which may be related to its structural similarity to atropine, the release of histamine, hypotension or normeperidine, its principal metabolite.

Asystole may follow opioid induced bradycardia and several case reports illustrate predisposing factors (Table 5) (159,160,161,162). Sufentanil and alfentanil appear to be more likely than fentanyl to result in asystole. Opioid-induced decreases in sympathetic tone coupled with vagal stimulation may predispose certain patients to this problem. Severe bradycardia and asystole often appear prior to or during laryngoscopy and intubation. Laryngoscopy can relieve or exacerbate bradyarrhythmias or asystole. Asystoles of 10 to 12 secs may resolve on their own but usually respond to atropine, 0.4 to 0.8 mg IV. On occasion much larger doses of atropine (>1.0 mg), isproterenol or a precordial thump may be required to treat severe bradycardia/asystole.

Table 5. Factors Predisposing Patients to Bradycardia and Asystole During Induction of Anesthesia With Large Doses of Narcotics

1.	Presence of beta-adrenergic and/or calcium entry blockade
2.	Premedication with or concomitant use of benzodiazepines
3.	Muscle relaxants with little or no vagolytic properties (vecuronium)
4.	Muscle relaxants with vagotonic properties (succinylcholine)
5.	Added vagal stimuli, e.g., laryngoscopy
6.	Rapid administration of the opioid

Fentanyl prolongs the R-R interval, AV node conduction and the AV node refractory period (163). Although these effects could theoretically lead to the development of reentry-type dysrhythmias, in practice this rarely occurs. The overall effect of narcotic anesthesia may be antiarrhythmic. Although doses of epinephrine sufficient to induce dysrhythmias in dogs are the same during narcotic-nitrous oxide anesthesia and halothane or enflurane plus nitrous oxide anesthesia, the incidence of malignant dysrhythmias (ventricular tachycardia and ventricular fibrillation) was less with narcotics plus nitrous oxide (164). Sufentanil prolongs action potential duration in isolated canine cardiac Purkinje fibers. This may be related to enhanced Ca^{+2} entry during the plateau phase of the action potential (164). Opioids can also prolong the OT interval. However, the risk of opioid use in patients with QT abnormalities or on medications such as quinidine is unknown (165).

Supraventricular tachycardia is the most common dysrhythmia, other than bradycardia, noted during narcotic anesthetic techniques (166). Supraventricular tachycardia usually occurs during or immediately after endotracheal intubation or surgical stimulation. This suggests that inadequate anesthesia rather than a direct effect of the narcotic is responsible for these abnormalities. Increases in heart rate often parallel increases in blood pressure when narcotic dosage or anesthesia is inadequate.

Opioids are often used to prevent increases in heart rate during anesthesia particularly during the induction-intubation sequence. The use of fentanyl (3 to 7 $\mu g \cdot kg^{-1}$), alfentanil (15 to 30 $\mu g \cdot kg^{-1}$) or sufentanil (0.2 to 0.8 $\mu g \cdot kg^{-1}$) decreases sodium thiopental, etomidate and other induction agent requirements. In addition, increases in heart rate and arterial blood pressure that occur during laryngoscopy and intubation are better controlled when agents like thiopental are used after narcotic pretreatment. Opioids also blunt or prevent increases in heart rate that accompany isoflurane(166) or other inhalation anesthetic (167).

Low pressure baroreceptors at the junction of the great vessels and atria are sensitive to decreases in filling pressure. Their stimulation causes reflex increases in systemic vascular resistance in order to maintain arterial blood pressure. Fentanyl-diazepam-N_2O anesthesia does not attenuate this reflex; whereas potent inhalation agents such as halothane do (168). Opioids may depress arterial baroreflex control of the heart rate induced by hypotension or hypertension (169,170) but other reports suggest this reflex is preserved under opioid anesthesia (169,171). Infants, after receiving 10 $\mu g \cdot kg^{-1}$ of fentanyl, demonstrate significant depression of baroreflex responses (172). The significance of this phenomenon is all the more important because cardiac output is quite dependent on heart rate in infants.

<u>Myocardial Ischemia and Coronary Blood Flow</u>

Cardiac anesthesiologists attempt to control hemodynamics in order to minimize increases in myocardial oxygen consumption, maintain oxygen supply to the heart and avoid ischemia. While opioids do not protect against ischemia in animal models (173,174) potent inhalation agents may offer some protection. In addition, some studies suggest that fentanyl and sufentanil do not provide adequate hemodynamic control in humans during coronary artery surgery (175,176) especially when compared to a potent inhalation agent (55,177,178). A major problem with many of these studies is that a fixed dose of opioid, e.g., 1 mg•kg^{-1} of morphine (55) is routinely given. Lack of flexibility of such protocols is not consistent with the clinical necessity and practice of titrating narcotics to an endpoint. Others have found that high does of opioids maintain myocardial perfusion and the oxygen supply/demand ratio as well or better than inhalation based techniques (179,180).

Alfentanil is associated with more myocardial ischemia (as indicated by reversal of myocardial lactate extraction to production and worsening ventricular diastolic compliance) than fentanyl or sufentanil in patients having coronary artery surgery (102). Sufentanil causes more depression of systolic function than fentanyl but also may offer greater hemodynamic control in patients with good left ventricular function (LVF).. On the other hand, fentanyl is probably easier and safer to use than sufentanil in patients with poor LVF. Interestingly, hemodynamics are often stable and do not reliably indicate ischemia. Kleinman et al (181). reported that hemodynamic changes were most often absent during ischemia in patients anesthetized with either fentanyl or halothane. Recent data from a prospective randomized comparison of sufentanil versus enflurane, isoflurane and halothane for coronary artery surgery revealed no difference in new intraoperative ischemia, the incidence of postoperative myocardial infarction or death (182). These results occurred in spite of a greater (two-fold) incidence of hypotension associated with the inhalation agent techniques and a greater (two-fold) incidence of hypertension associated with sufentanil. Tachycardia, the only hemodynamic parameter significantly related to ischemia, occurred with the same frequency with all agents. Slogoff et al (182) and others have suggested that other factors (e.g., recent infarction, presence or absence of beta-adrenergic or calcium entry blockade, prolonged aortic cross clamp time, serious preoperative dysrhythmias) are significantly more important than anesthetic technique as determinants of outcome after coronary artery surgery (183).

Opioids, or at least fentanyl, appear to have no significant effect on coronary vasomotion and do not diminish ability of large coronary arteries or coronary arterioles to respond to vasoactive agents (184,185). This lack of effect of fentanyl on coronary autoregulation compares distinctly with the potent inhalation agents which are coronary vasodilators.

SUPPLEMENTS

A variety of adjuvant drugs have been used as supplements in combination with opioids. Rationales for this approach include attempts to reduce awareness, control hypertension, and decrease the total dose of opioid to minimize postoperative respiratory depression. On the other hand, certain premedicants, especially the benzodiazepines, may predispose patients to hypotension when high-dose opioid anesthesia is used. In addition, although some suggest a reasonable approach to controlling hemodynamics to be a combination of opioids and inhalation agents (177). supplementation of opioid anesthesia with a variety of agents, including inhalation anesthetics, often results in a loss of cardiovascular stability.

Nitrous Oxide.

Nitrous oxide is probably the most common supplement used with narcotic based anesthesia. Nitrous oxide has minimal effects on cardiovascular dynamics when administered alone in dogs (186) but can depress myocardial contractility in humans (187). In addition, nitrous oxide in combination with opioids is associated with significant cardiovascular depression. After administration of morphine (2 mg•kg^{-1}), McDermott and Stanley (188) found that nitrous oxide produced concentration-dependent decreases in stroke volume, cardiac output, and arterial blood pressure and increases in systemic vascular resistance. (Table 6). While fentanyl alone produces no ventricular dysfunction

Table 6. Cardiovascular Effects of 0-50% Nitrous Oxide During Morphine Anesthesia

	Percent (Mean) N_2O					
Parameter	0	10	20	30	40	50
Stroke volume (ml)	57.0	51.0*	50.0*	46.0*	42.0*	36.0*
Cardiac output (L•min^{-1})	5.2	4.6*	4.3*	4.0*	3.7*	2.9*
Systolic arterial blood pressure (mm Hg)	124.0	119.0*	117.0*	109.0*	104.0*	94.0*
Peripheral resistance (PRU)	159.0	176.0*	183.0*	204.0*	259.0*	312.0*

*P < 0.05. Student's paired t-test when compared to control value.
(McDermott R. and Stanley T.H. Anesthesiology 41:89, 1974)

(even in the presence of significant coronary artery stenosis), the addition of nitrous oxide can yield significant cardiovascular depression (97). These changes occur in man and animals with all opioids in virtually all studies (93,95,97,144,188,189,190,191,192). It has also been suggested that a lower FiO_2 rather than the presence of nitrous oxide is primarily responsible for the changes in cardiovascular performance (193). Myocardial ischemia and dysfunction may occur during inhalation of N_2O as coronary blood flow decreases from hypotension and an increase in coronary vascular resistance (192). Increases in systemic vascular resistance associated with N_2O supplementation of opioids may in part cause the deterioration in cardiac output and function (65,86). Myocardial dysfunction with N_2O may not be evident with routine monitoring, i.e., blood pressure, because of the elevated systemic vascular resistance (194). In spite of these potential problems, nitrous oxide remains a popular supplement. In children undergoing repair of congenital cardiac defects, N_2O may still be valuable and safe as a supplement to opioid anesthesia (195).

Inhalation Agents. In light of the potential for adverse effects of N_2O in patients anesthetized with opioids, potent inhalation agents may be a better alternative. Their intrinsic ability to depress the myocardium in a dose-dependent fashion often allows the titration of agents such as halothane or enflurane to control hemodynamics when high dose opioids are inadequate (196,197,198). Low concentrations of isoflurane have been safely used to treat intraoperative hypertension during high dose sufentanil anesthesia for coronary artery surgery (199). However, undesirable cardiovascular depression (decreases in blood pressure and cardiac index) has been reported during halothane supplementation of high-dose fentanyl anesthesia, and may occur with other potent inhalation agents as well (200). In addition, ongoing ischemia may not necessarily be ameliorated by such approaches in spite of good hemodynamic control (200). Others have shown that adding halothane to a sufentanil (10 to 20 $\mu g \cdot kg^{-1}$) anesthetic to control increases in blood pressure may produce hemodynamic alterations (decreased blood pressure, cardiac output, PCWP and SVR) that exacerbate regional myocardial hypoperfusion and increase lactate production (201). Cautious titration of potent inhalation anesthetics to control increases in blood pressure during a high dose opioid anesthetic may be most successful when techniques to assess regional myocardial function are available (e.g., transesophageal echocardiography). The risk of inducing a maldistribution in the coronary circulation exists with isoflurane and enflurane as well (202). Nevertheless, and in spite of the potential problems, the ease of administration and titration of potent inhalation agents makes them a useful adjunct during opioid anesthesia.

Benzodiazepines

Benzodiazepines produce few significant hemodynamic alterations when administered alone. This, combined with their potent amnestic properties, make them a desirable supplement to high dose opioid anesthesia, where awareness is a potential problem. Benzodiazepines potentiate the effects of opioids and thus decrease narcotic requirements for loss of consciousness (2,40,203). However, combinations of benzodiazepines and narcotics, while occasionally preserving ventricular function (203) often cause profound decreases in blood pressure and cardiac index. Some investigators have found intravenous lorazepam and high dose fentanyl anesthesia to cause less hemodynamic changes than other benzodiazepines (204,205). These findings are encouraging but need additional clarification.

Unfortunately, most studies indicate that benzodiazepines, even administered as premedicants (2,40,47,157,206,207,208) consistently produce lower blood pressures, heart rates, cardiac outputs and systemic vascular resistances with opioid-based techniques than benzodiazepine-free premedicants (e.g., morphine-scopolamine) or no premedicant. Sudden dramatic hypotension has also been reported with some combinations (midazolam and sufentanil) (209,210). In patients with poor left ventricular function, this drug regimen may prove particularly hazardous (207).

Several mechanisms underlie the cardiovascular depression produced when benzodiazepines are added to opioids. Benzodiazepines produce a transient depression of arterial baroreflex function and a sustained decrease in sympathetic tone (211). Catecholamine levels are lower with a diazepam/morphine combination than morphine alone (88). Combinations of fentanyl and diazepam result in a negative inotropic effect (212). Decreases in systemic vascular resistance are also usually noted and are probably related to diminished sympathetic tone. Some have suggested that fluid loading may attenuate decreases in blood pressure, ventricular filling, and cardiac output when benzodiazepines are combined with opioids (213).

Other Supplements

Beta-Adrenergic Blockers Since the 1970's it has been recognized that sympathetic responses to surgery are better controlled by continuing beta-adrenergic blockade therapy through the perioperative period. During high-dose opioid anesthesia for coronary artery surgery, beta blockade reduces opioid requirements and the need for supplements, improves hemodynamic stability and decreases intraoperative and postoperative myocardial ischemia (214,215,216). A decrease in arrhythmias has also been observed (216). Esmolol, an ultra short-acting beta blocker is becoming increasingly popular for use during operation (216,217).

Alpha2 Adrenergic Agonists. The role of α_2-adrenergic blockers in anesthesia are just beginning to be explored (218). Clonidine and its congeners reduce anesthetic requirements in animal models and in man (219,220) probably by decreasing central sympathetic outflow and nociception (221). The need for other supplements is also decreased, although bradycardia requiring the administration of atropine may be an occasional problem. Postoperative benefits can include higher cardiac outputs, earlier extubation, reduced plasma catecholamines, and less shivering (220). Most studies have evaluated clonidine as a premedicant though postoperative infusion may allow continuation of its favorable effects (222). Respiratory function is preserved when clonidine (.2 to .4 mg) is combined with morphine (0.21 mg•kg^{-1}) as a premedicant (Bailey P, unpublished data).

Calcium Entry Blockers (CEB's). While CEB's can significantly depress cardiac function and cause regional wall motion abnormalities during potent inhalation anesthesia, opioid-CEB interactions appear to be mild. Fentanyl and pancuronium anesthesia does not effect verapamil pharmacokinetics. Mean arterial pressure and cardiac function and conduction also do not change appreciably in dogs when opioids and verapamil are combined (223,224). Fentanyl anesthesia causes minimal decreases in cardiac index and only modest decreases in blood pressure and SVR in patients receiving verapamil (225). On the other hand, the presence of beta-adrenergic blockade, the quality of left ventricular function, and the presence of other anesthetics will influence the response to CEB's. In addition, CEB's have different profiles of effects and can result in persistent hypotension or unpredictable responses when used as an adjunct to opioid anesthesia for controlled hypotension (226).

Nitroglycerin (NTG). Nitroglycerin is often used with high dose narcotic anesthesia to treat increases in blood pressure and ischemia. Opinions differ as to whether or not the routine use of a nitroglycerin infusion during high-dose fentanyl anesthesia for coronary artery surgery can reduce ischemia. Thomson et al (227) reported that 0.5 $\mu g \cdot kg^{-1} \cdot min^{-1}$ of NTG did not significantly alter the incidence of ischemia (50 percent) they found in patients undergoing coronary artery surgery during fentanyl-pancuronium anesthesia. Coriat et al (228) on the other hand reported that 1.0 but not 0.5 $\mu g \cdot kg^{-1} \cdot min^{-1}$ did significantly reduce intraoperative ischemia. These or larger doses of NTG may also result in hypotension, tachycardia and decreases in ventricular filling pressures. The optimal doses of NTG during narcotic anesthesia has not been determined.

REFERENCES

1. Foldes, F.F., Swerdlow, M. and Siker, E.S. Narcotics and Narcotic Antagonists. Charles C Thomas, Springfield, IL, 1964.
2. Stanley, T.H. and Webster, L.R. Anesth. Analg. 57:411, 1978.
3. Lowenstein, E. and Philbin, D. Anesthesiology. 55:195, 1981.
4. Lowenstein, E. Anesthesiology. 35:563, 1971.
5. Wong, K.C. Anesth. Analg. 62:625-626, 1983.
6. Hall, R.I., Szlam, F. and Hug C.C., Jr. Anesth. Analg. 66:1287-1291, 1987.
7. Hall, R.I., Murphy, M.R. and Hug, C.C., Jr. Anesthesiology. 67:518-525, 1987.
8. Hall, R.I., Szlam, F. and Hug, C.C. Anesth. Analg. 66:S76, 1987.
9. Murphy, M.R. and Hug, C.C. Anesthesiology. 57:489-492, 1982.
10. Murphy, M.R. and Hug, C.C. Anesthesiology. 57:485-488,, 1982.
11. Murphy, M.R. and Hug, C.C. Anesthesiology. 59:A338, 1983.
12. Hecker, B.R., Lake, C.L., DiFazio, C.A., et al. Anesth. Analg. 62:987-990, 1983.
13. Lake, C.L., DiFazio, C.A., Moscicki, J.C. and Engle, J.S. Anesth. Analg. 64:807-810, 1985.
14. Bowdle, T.A. and Ward, R.J. Anesthesiology. 70:26-30, 1989.
15. Bailey, P.L., Port, D.J., McJames, S., et al. Anesth. Analg. 66:542-548, 1987.
16. Port, J.D., Stanley, T.H., Steffey, E.P., et al. Anesthesiology. 61:A378, 1984.
17. Arndt, J.O., Mikat, M. and Parasher, C. Anesthesiology. 61:355-361, 1984.
18. Shingu, K., Eger, E.I., II., Johnson, B.H., et al. Anesth. Analg. 62:51-54, 1983.

19. Kissen, I. and Brown, P.T. Anesthesiology. 62:597-600, 1985.
20. White, D.C. In: Lunn, J.N. and Rosen, M. (eds.) : Consciousness, Awareness and Pain in General Anesthesia. Butterworth, Boston, 1987, p. 1-9.
21. Kissin, I. and Jebeles, J.A. Anesthesiology. 61:671, 1984.
22. Eisele, J.H., Jr and Steffey, E.P. Anesthesiology. 60:60:392, 1984.
23. Dundee, J.W., Nichol, R.M. and Black, G.W. Br J Anaesth. 34:158-160, 1962.
24. Dodson, B.A. and Miller, K.W. Anesthesiology. 62:615-620, 1985.
25. Levinson, B.W. Br J Anaesth. 37:544-546, 1965.
26. Bennett, H.L., Davis, H.S. and Giamnini, J.A. Br J Anaesth. 57:174-179, 1985.
27. Jones, J.G. In: Lunn, J.N. and Rosen, M. (eds.) : Consciousness, awareness and pain in general. Butterworth, Boston, 1987, p. 99-111.
28. Mainord, W.A., Rath, B. and Barnett, F . Anesthesia and suggestion. Paper presented at the American Psychological Association Annual Convention. Los Angeles, California, 1983,
29. Sebel, P.S. and Bovill, J.G. Br J Anaesth. 54:1149-1150, 1982.
30. Wilson, S.L., Vaughan, R.W. and Stephen, C.R. Anesth. Analg. 54::609, 1975.
31. Saucier, N., Walts, L.F. and Moreland, J.R. Anesth. Analg. 62:239, 1983.
32. Mark, J.B. and Greenberg, L.M. Anesth. Analg. 62:698, 1983.
33. Hilgenberg, J.C. Anesthesiology. 54:341, 1981.
34. Mummanemi, N., Rao, T. and Montoya, A. Anesth. Analg. 59:943, 1980.
35. Crawford, J.S., James, F.M., Davies, P. and Crawley, M. Br J Anaesthesia. 48:661-666,, 1976.
36. Utting, J.E. In: Lunn, J.N. and Rosen, M. (eds.). Consciousness, awareness and pain in general anesthesia. Butterworth, Boston, 1987, p. 171-180.
37. Ghoneim, M.M., Dhanaraj, J. and W.W., Choi. Anesth. Analg. 63:405-412, 1984.
38. Stanley, T.H. and Lathrop, G.D. Anesthesiology. 46:166, 1977.
39. Stanley, T.H., Philbin, D.M. and Coggins, C.H. Can Anaesth. Soc J. 26:168, 1979.
40. Bailey, P.L., Wilbrink, J., Zwanikken, P. and et al. Anesth. Analg. 64:48, 1985.
41. Stanley, T.H. and de Lange, S. Can Anaesth. Soc. J. 31:368, 1985.
42. Stanley, T.H., Leysen, J., Niemegeers, J.E. and et al. Anesth. Analg. 62:705, 1983.
43. Shafter, A., White, P.F., Schüttler, J. and Rosenthal, M.H. Anesthesiology. 59:245, 1983.
44. Siebert, B.S., Rosow, C.E., Keegan, C.R., et al. Anesth. Analg. 67:717, 1986.
45. Stoelting, R.K. Anesth. Analg. 56:615, 1977.
46. Stanley, T.H., Bennett, G.M., Loeser, E.A. and et al. Anesthesiology. 44:255, 1976.

47. Tomichek, R.C., Rosow, C.E., Philbin, D.M., et al. Anesth. Analg. 62:881-884, 1983.
48. Blacher, R.S. JAMA. 234:67, 1975.
49. Lowenstein, E., Hallowell, P., Levin, F.H. and et al. N. Engl. J. Med. 281:1389, 1969.
50. van de Walle, J., Lauwers, P. and Adriaensen, H. Acta. Anaesthesiol. Belg. 27:129, 1976.
51. Sebel, P.S. and Bovill, J.G. Anesth. Analg. 61:115, 1982.
52. Nauta, J., Stanley, T.H., de Lange, S., et al. Can. Anaesth. Soc. J. 30:53-60, 1983.
53. Moldenhauer, C.C., Griesemer, R.W., Hug, C.C. and Holbrook, G.W. Anesth. Analg. 62:276, 1983.
54. Schmidt, C.F and Livingston, A.E. J. Pharmacol. Exp. Ther. 47:411, 1933.
55. Moffitt, E.A., Sethna, D.H., Bussell, J.A, et al. Anesth. Analg. 61:979-985, 1982.
56. Vasko, J.S ., Henney, R.P., Brawley, R.K and et al. Am. J. Physiol. 210:329:329, 1966.
57. Stanley, T.H., Isern-Amaral, J. and Lathrop, G.D. Can. Anaesth. Soc. J. 22:478, 1975.
58. Stanley, T.H., Isern-Amaral, J. and Lathrop, G.D. Anesth. Analg. 54:509, 1975.
59. Balasariswathi, K., Glisson, S.N., El-Etr, A.A. and et al. Can. Anaesth. Soc. J. 25:198, 1978.
60. Fahmy, N.R., Sinder, N. and Soter, N.A. Clin. Pharmacol. Ther. 33:615-620, 1983.
61. Flacke, J.W., Van Etten, A.P., Bloor, B.C., et al. Anesth. Analg. 66:723-730, 1987.
62. Liu, W.S., Bidwai, A.V., Lunn, J.K. and et al. Can. Anaesth. Soc. 24:371, 1977.
63. Stanley, T.H., Berman, L., Green, O. and et al. Anesthesiology. 53:250, 1980.
64. Hicks, H.C., Mowbray, A.G. and Yhap, E.O. Anesth. Analg. 60:563-568, 1981.
65. Lunn, J.K., Stanley, T.H., Webster, L.R, et al. Anesth. Analg. 58:390, 1979.
66. Kentor, M.L., Schwalb, A.J. and Lieberman, R.W. Anesthesiology. 3:S95, 1980.
67. Rendig, S.V., Amsterdam, E.A., Henderson, G.L. and Mason, D.T. J. Pharmacol. Exp. Ther. 215:259-265, 1980.
68. Hamm, D., Freedman, B., Pellom, G., et al. Anesthesiology. 59:A86, 1983.
69. Freedman, B., Hamm, D., Pellom, G., et al. Anesthesiology. 59:A35, 1983.
70. Drew, J.H., Dripps, R.D. and Comroe, J.H. Anesthesiology. 7:44-61, 1946.
71. Conahan, T.J., Ominsky, A.J., Wollman, H. and Stroth, R. Anesthesiology. 38:528-535, 1973.
72. Lappas, D.G., Geha, D., Fischer, J.E, et al. Anesthesiology. 42:153-159, 1975.

73. Rosow, C.E., Moss, J., Philbin, D.M. and Savarese, J.J. Anesthesiology. 56:93-96, 1982.
74. Moss, J. and Rosow, C.E. Anesthesiology. 59:330-339, 1983.
75. Rosow, C.E., Philbin, D.M., Keegan, C.R. and Moss, J. Anesthesiology. 60:489-491, 1984.
76. Stanley, T.H., Gray, N.J., Staford, W. and Armstrong, R.. Anesthesiology. 38:536, 1973.
77. Lowenstein, E., Whiting, R.B., Bittar, D.A., et al. J. Pharmacol. Exp. Ther. 180:359-367, 1972.
78. Henney, R.P., Vasko, J.S., Brawley, R.K., et al. Heart. J. 72:242-250, 1966.
79. Ward, J.M., McGrath, R.C. and Weil, J.L. Am. J. Cardiol. 29:659-666, 1972.
80. Stanley, T.H., Gray, N.H., Isern-Amaral, J. and Patton, C.P. Anesthesiology. 41:34-38,, 1974.
81. Greene, J.F., Jackman, A.P. and Krohn, K.A. Circ. Res. 42:479-486, 1978.
82. Greene, J.F., Jackman, A.P. and Parsons, G. Circ. Res. 42:474-478, 1978.
83. Hsu, H.O., Hickey, R.F. and Forbes, A.R. Anesthesiology. 50:98-102, 1979.
84. Zelis, R., Mansour, E.J., Capone, R.J. and Mason, D.T. J. Clin. Invest. 54:1247-1258, 1974.
85. Priano, L.L. and Vatner, S.F. Anesthesiology. 55:236-243, 1981.
86. Wong, K.C., Martin, W.E., Hornbein, T.F., et al. Anesthesiology. 38:542-549, 1973.
87. Moores, W.Y., Weiskopf, R.B., Baysinger, M. and Utley, JR. J. Thorac. Cardiovasc. Surg. 81:163-170, 1981.
88. Hoar, P.F., Nelson, N.T., Mangano, D.T., et al. Anesth. Analg. 60:406-411, 1981.
89. Strauer, B.E. Anesthesiology. 37:304-310, 1972.
90. Bennett, G.M. and Stanley, T.H. Anesthesiology. 52:520-522, 1980.
91. King, B.D., Elder, J.D. and Dripps, R.D. Surg. Gynec. Obstet. 94:591-597, 1952.
92. Freye, E. Anesth. Analg. 53:40-47, 1974.
93. Stanley, T.H., Bidwai, A.V., Lunn, J.K. and Hodges, M.R. Anesth. Analg. 56:836-841, 1977.
94. De Castro, J., Van de Water, A., Wouters, L., et al. Acta. Anaesth. Belg. 30:5, 1979.
95. Stanley, T.H. and Liu, W.S. Anesth. Analg. 56:669-673, 1977.
96. Sugioka, K., Boniface, K.J. and Davis, D.A. Anesthesiology. 18:623-633, 1957.
97. Stoelting, R.K., Gibbs, P.S., Creasser, C.W. and Peterson, C. Anesthesiology. 42:319, 1975.
98. Waller, J.L., Hug, C.C., Nagle, D.M. and Craver, J.M. Anesthesiology. 55:212-217, 1981.
99. Wynands, J.E., Wong, P., Whalley, D.G., et al. Anesth. Analg. 62:476-482, 1983.
100. Hamm, D., Freedman, B., Pellom, G., et al. Anesthesiology. 59:A37, 1983.

101. Motomura, S., Kissin, I., Aultman, D. and Reves, J.G. Anesth. Analg. 63:47-50, 1984.
102. Miller, D.R., Wellwood, M., Teasdale, S.J., et al. Can. J. Anaesth. 35:219-233, 1988.
103. Lake, C.I. and DiFazio, C.A. Anesth. Analg. 66:S99, 1987.
104. Liu, W.S., Bidwai, A.V., Stanley, T.H, et al. Canad. Anaesth. Soc. J. 23:395-403, 1976.
105. Hill, A.B., Nahrwold, M.L., de Rosayro, M., et al. Anesthesiology. 55:452-454, 1981.
106. Flacke, J.W., Flacke, W.E., Bloor, B.C. and Olewine, S. Anesth. Analg. 62:305-313, 1983.
107. Flacke, J.W., David, L.J., Flacke, W.E., et al. Anesth. Analg. 64:1053-1059, 1985.
108. Starck, T., Hall, D., Freas, W., et al. Anesth. Analg. 68:S277, 1989.
109. Mathews, H.M.L., Furness, G., Carson, I.W., et al. Br. J. Anaesth. 60:530-535, 1988.
110. Niemegeers, C.J.E. and Janssen, P.A.J. Drug Dev. Res. 1:83-88, 1981.
111. Schauble, J.F., Chen, B.B. and Murray, P.A. Anesthesiology. 59:A85, 1983.
112. de Bruijn, N.D., Christian, C., Fagraeus, L., et al. Anesthesiology. 59:A33, 1983.
113. Takemori, A. Adv. Biochem. Phychopharmacol. 8:335, 1974.
114. Ausems, M.E., Hug, C.C. Jr and de Lange, S. Anesth. Analg. 62:982-986, 1983.
115. Bartkowski, R.R. and McDonnell, T.E. Anesth. Analg. 63:330-334, 1984.
116. Lemmens, H.J.M., Bovill, J.G., Burm, A.G.L. and Hennis, P.J. Anaesthesia. 43:850-856, 1988.
117. Rucquoi, M. and Camu, F. Br. J. Anaesth. 55:223S-230S, 1983.
118. Thomson, I.R., Putnins, C.L. and Friesen, R.M. Anesth. Analg. 65:91-95, 1986.
119. Gaumann, D.M., Yaksh, T.L., Tyce, G.M. and Lucas, D.L. Anesthesiology. 68:743-753, 1988.
120. James, T.N., Isobe, J.H. and Urthaler, F. Circulation. 52:179-192, 1975.
121. Arens, J.F., Benbow, B.P., Ochsner, J.L. and Theard, R. Anesth. Analg. 51:901-909, 1972.
122. Hasbrouck, J.D. Ann. Thorac. Surg. 10:364-369, 1970.
123. Bedford, R.F. and Wollman, H. Anesthesiology. 43:1, 1975.
124. Bailey, D.R., Miller, E.D., Kaplan, J.A. and Rogers, P.W. Anesthesiology. 42:538-544, 1975.
125. Quinton, L., Whalley, D.G., Wynands, J.E., et al. Anesth. Analg. 60:412-416, 1981.
126. Wynands, J.E., Townsend, G.E., Wong, P., et al. Anesth. Analg. 62:661-665, 1983.
127. Edde, R.R. Anesthesiology. 55:444-446, 1981.
128. Sebel, P.S., Bovill, J.G., Boekhorst, R.A.A. and Rog, P. Acta. Anesthesiol. Scand. 26:308, 1982.

129. de Lange, S., Stanley, T.H. and Boscoe, M. Comparison of anesthetic requirements and cardiovascular responses in Salt Lake City and Leiden, Holland. Paper presented at the Seventh World Congress of Anaesthesiology. Amsterdam, Excerpta Medica, 1980, 313.
130. de Lange, S., Stanley, T.H., Boscoe, M.J. and Pace, N.L. Anesthesiology. 56:112-118, 1982.
131. Wynands, J.E., Wong, P., Townsend, G.E., et al. Anesth. Analg. 63:101-105, 1983.
132. Sebel, P.S., Bovill, J.G., Schellekens, A.P.M. and Hawker, C.D. Brit. J. Anaesth. 53:941-947, 1981.
133. Bennett, G.M. and Stanley, T.H. Anesth. Analg. 58:179-182, 1979.
134. Stoelting, R.K., Creasser, C.W., Gibbs, P.S. and Peterson, C. Anesth. Analg. 53:449-455, 1974.
135. Bland, J.H.L., Chir., B. and Lowenstein, E. Anesthesiology. 45:287-293, 1976.
136. Freedman, B., Christian, C., Hamm, D., et al. Anesthesiology. 59:A25, 1983.
137. Howie, M.B., Reitz, J., Reilley, T.E., et al. Anesthesiology. 59:A146, 1983.
138. Hickey, P.R. and Hansen, D.D. Anesth. Analg. 63:117-124, 1984.
139. McDonnell, T.E., Bartkowski, R.R. and Williams, J.J. Anesthesiology. 60:136-140, 1984.
140. Nauta, J., de Lange, S., Koopman, D., et al. Anesth. Analg. 61:267-271, 1982.
141. de Lange, S., Stanley, T.H. and M.J.,.Boscoe. Br. J. Anaesth. 53:1291-1296, 1981.
142. Reitan, J.A., Stengert, K.B., Wymore, M.L. and Martucci, RW. Anesth. Analg. 57:31-36, 1978.
143. Tammisto, T., Takki, S. and Toikka, P. Brit. J. Anaesth. 42:317-324, 1970.
144. Liu, W.S., Bidwai, A.V., Stanley, T.H. and Isern-Amaral, S. Anesth. Analg. 55:168-172, 1976.
145. Prakash, 0., Verdouw, P.D., De Jong, J.W., et al. Can. Anaesth. Soc. J. 27:223-229, 1980.
146. Hornbein, T.F., Martin, W.E., Bonica, J.J., et al. Anesthesiology. 31:250-260, 1969.
147. Smith, N.T., Eger, E.I., Stoelting, R.K., et al. Anesthesiology. 32:410-421, 1970.
148. Meuleman, T., Port, J.D., Stanley, T.H. and Williard, K.F. J. Wildl Mange. 48:258, 1984.
149. Reddy, P., Liu, W.S., Port, D., et al. Can. Anaesth. Soc. J. 27:345-350, 1980.
150. Williard, K.F., Port, J.D. and Stanley, T.H. Anesthesiology. 59:A321, 1983.
151. Port, J.D., Stanley, T.H. and McJames, S. Anesthesiology. 59:A325, 1983.
152. de Lange, S., Boscoe, M.J., Stanley, T.H., et al. Anesth. Analg. 61:434-438, 1982.
153. de Lange, S. and de Bruijn, N. Br. J. Anaesth. 55:S183, 1983.
154. Cohn, A.E. Proc. Soc. Exp. Biol. Med. 10:93-96, 1913.

155. Robbins, B.H., Fitzhugh, O.G. and Baxter, J.H., Jr. J. Pharmacol. Exp. Ther. 66:216-223, 1939.
156. Kennedy, B.L. and West, T.C. J. Pharmacol. Exp. Ther. 157:149-158, 1967.
157. Tomichek, R.C., Rosow, C.E., Schneider, R.C., et al. Anesth. Analg. 61:217-218, 1982.
158. De Silva, R.A., Verrierm, R.L. and Lown, B. Cardiovasc. Res. 12:167-172, 1978.
159. Starr, N.J., Sethna, D.H. and Estafanous, F.G. Anesthesiology. 64:521-523, 1986.
160. Maryniak, J.K. and Bishop, V.A. Br. J. Anaesth. 59:390-391, 1987.
161. Sherman, E.P., Leobwitz, P.W. and Street, W.C. Anesthesiology. 66:106, 1987.
162. Rivard, J.C. and Lebowitz, P.W. Anesth. Analg. 67:907, 1988.
163. Royster, R.L., Keeler, D.K., Haisty, W.K., et al. Anesth. Analg. 67:15-20, 1988.
164. Puerto, B.A., Wong, K.C., Puerto, A.X., et al. Canad. Anaesth. Soc. J. 26:263-268, 1979.
165. Blair, J.R., Pruett, J.K., Crumrine, R.S. and Balser, J.S. Anesthesiology. 67:442-443, 1987.
166. Bennett, G.M. and Stanley, T.H. Anesthesiology. 51:S138, 1979.
167. Cahalan, M.K., Lurz, F.W., Eger, E.I., et al. Anesth. Analg. 66:166-170, 1987.
168. Ebert, T.J., Kotrly, K.J., Madsen, K.E., et al. Anesth. Analg. 67:548-554, 1988.
169. Kotrly, K.J., Ebert, T.J., Vucins, E., et al. Anesthesiology. 60:173-179, 1984.
170. Kotrly, K.J., Ebert, T.J., Vucins, E.J., et al. Anesthesiology. 61:558-563, 1984.
171. Zimpfer, M., Kotal, E., Mayer, N., et al. Anaesthetist. 32:259-264, 1983.
172. Murat, J.M., Levron, J.C., Berg, A. and Saint-Maurice, C. Anesthesiology. 68:717-722, 1988.
173. MacLeod, B.A., Augereau, P. and Walker, M.J.A. Anesthesiology. 58:44-52, 1983.
174. Frank, L.P. and Davis, R.F. Anesth. Analg. 65:S50, 1986.
175. Sonntag, H., Larsen, R., Hilfiker, O., et al. Anesthesiology. 56:417-422, 1982.
176. Litak, C., Ansley, D., Wynands, J.E., et al. Canad. Anaesth. Soc. J. 33:S97-S98, 1986.
177. Moffitt, E.A., McIntyre, A.J., Barker, R.A., et al. Anesth. Analg. 65:46-52, 1986.
178. Heikkilä, H., Jalonen, J., Arola, M. and Laaksonen, V. Acta. Anaesthesiol. Scand. 29:457-464, 1985.
179. Goehner, P., Hollenberg, M., Leung, J., et al. Anesthesiology. 69:A32, 1988.
180. Skourtis, C.T., Nissen, M., McGinnis, L.A., et al. Anesthesiology. 61:A6, 1984.
181. Kleinman, B., Henkin, R.E., Glisson, S.N., et al. Anesthesiology. 64:157-164, 1986.

182. Slogoff, S. and Keats, A.S. Anesthesiology. 70:179-188, 1989.
183. Tuman, K.J., Keane, D.M., Silins, A.I., et al. Anesth. Analg. 67:S236, 1988.
184. Blaise, G., Sill, J.C., Nugent, M. and Vanhoutte, P.M. Can. Anaesth. Soc. J. 33:S104-S105, 1986.
185. Beland, A., Blaise, G.A., Lenis, S.G., et al. Can. Anaesth. Soc. J. 34:S72-S73, 1987.
186. Craythorne, N.W.B. and Darby, T.D. Br. J. Anaesthesia. 37:560-565, 1965.
187. Eisele, J.H. and Smith, N.T. Anesth. Analg. 51:956-962, 1972.
188. McDermott, R.W. and Stanley, T.H. Anesthesiology. 41:89-91, 1974.
189. Stoelting, R.K. and Gibbs, P.S. Anesthesiology. 38:45, 1973.
190. Mayer, D.J., Wolfle, T.L., Akil, H., et al. Science. 174:1351-1354, 1971.
191. Bennett, G.M., Ready, P., Liu, W.S., et al. Anesthesiology. 51:S102, 1979.
192. Moffitt, E.A., Scovil, J.E.., Barker, R.A., et al. Anesthesiology. 59:A31, 1983.
193. Michaels, I. and Barash, P.G. Anesth. Analg. 62:275, 1983.
194. Philbin, D.M., Foëx, P., Drummond, G., et al. Anesthesiology. 62:166-174, 1985.
195. Crean, P., Koren, G., Goresky, G., et al. Can. Anaesth. Soc. J. 33:36-40, 1986.
196. Moffitt, E.A., McIntyre, A.J., Glenn, J.J., et al. Can. Anaes. Soc. J. 32:S86-S87, 1985.
197. Hillel, Z., Thys, D., Goldman, M.E., et al. Anesth. Analg. 65:S71, 1986.
198. Heikkilä, H., Jalonen, J., Arola, M., et al. Anesth. Analg. 66:111-116, 1987.
199. O'Young, J., Mastrocostopoulas, G., Hilgenberg, A., et al. Anesthesiology. 66:653-658, 1987.
200. O'Brien, D.J., Moffitt, E.A., McIntyre, A.J., et al. Can. Anaesth. Soc. J. 33:S101-S102, 1986.
201. Mastrocostopoulos, G., Athanasiadis, C., Skourtis, C., et al. Anesth. Analg. 65:S93, 1986.
202. Rydvall, A., Häggmark, S., Nyhman, H. and Reiz, S. Acta. Anaesth. Scand. 28:690-695, 1984.
203. Dauchot, P.J., van Heeckeren, D.W., Bastulli, J. and Anton, A.H. Anesth. Analg. 67:S45, 1988.
204. Heikkilä, H., Jalonen, J., Laaksonen, V., et al. Acta. Anaesth. Scand. 28:357-361, 1984.
205. Benson, K.T., Tomlinson, D.L., Goto, H. and Arakawa, K. Anesth. Analg. 67:996-998, 1988.
206. Streisand, J.B., Clark, N.J., Stanley, T.H., et al. Anesth. Analg. 65:S156, 1986.
207. Butterworth, J.F., Bean, V.E. and Royster, R.L. Anesthesiology. 69:A65, 1988.
208. Thomson, I.R., Bergstrom, R.G., Rosenbloom, M. and Meatherall, R.C. Anesthesiology. 68:194-200, 1988.
209. West, J.M., Estrada, S. and Heerdt, M. Anesth. Analg. 66:693, 1987.

210. Spiess, B.D., Sathoff, R.H., El-Ganzouri, A.R.S. and Ivankovich, A.D. Anesth. Analg. 65:703-705, 1986.
211. Marty, J., Gauzit, R., Lefevre, P., et al. Anesth. Analg. 65:113-119, 1986.
212. Reves, J.G., Kissin, I., Fournier, S.E. and Smith, L.R. Anesth. Analg. 63:97-100, 1984.
213. Komatsu, T., Shibutani, K., Okamoto, K., et al. Anesth. Analg. 65:S82, 1986.
214. Stanley, T.H., de Lange, S., Boscoe, M.J. and de Bruijn, N. Can. Anaesth. Soc. J. 29:319-324, 1982.
215. Zahl, K. and Ellison, N. Anesthesiology. 65:A519, 1986.
216. Harrison, L., Ralley, F., Wynands, J.E., et al. Anesthesiology. 66:413-418, 1987.
217. Newsome, L.R., Roth, J.V., Hug, C.C., Jr and Nagle, D. Anesth. Analg. 65:451-456, 1986.
218. Hamilton, W.K. Anesthesiology. 69:811-812, 1988.
219. Ghignone, M., Quinton, L., Duke, P.C., et al. Anesthesiology. 64:36-42, 1986.
220. Flacke, J.W., Bloor, B.C., Flacke, W.E., et al. Anesthesiology. 67:11-19, 1987.
221. Drasner, K., Bernards, C. and Ozanne, G.M. 67:S42, 1988.
222. Bernard, J.M., Bourréli, B.., Pinaud, M., et al. Anesthesiology. 69:A147, 1988.
223. Hill, D.C., Chelly, J.E., Dlewati, A., et al. Anesthesiology. 68:874-879, 1988.
224. Ramsay, J.G., Arvieux, C.C., Foëx, P., et al. Can. Anaesth. Soc. J. 33:S100-S101, 1986.
225. Kapur, P.A., Norel, E.J., Dajee, H. and Flacke, W. Can. Anaesth. Soc. J. 33:138-144, 1986.
226. Bernard, J.M., Pinaud, M., Carteau, S., et al. Can. Anaesth. Soc. J. 33:308-314, 1986.
227. Thomson, I.R., Mutch, A.C. and Culligan, J.D. Anesthesiology. 61:385-393, 1984.
228. Coriat, P., Daloz, M., Bousseau, D., et al. Anesthesiology. 61:193-196, 1984.

IS ISOFLURANE CONTRAINDICATED IN PATIENTS WITH CORONARY ARTERY DISEASE?

R. MERIN

INTRODUCTION

Data from animal studies show that isoflurane causes direct coronary dilation and can cause steal (1,2). Data from studies in humans indicate direct dilation, but whether or not isoflurane causes steal in humans, and whether or not steal is of clinical importance to the outcome of anesthesia is not yet clear, and will determine whether isoflurane is dangerous for the patient with coronary artery disease.

It is important to understand the basic anatomy required for intracoronary steal, since not all patients with coronary artery disease are at risk. "Steal-prone anatomy" includes three elements: 1) a complete occlusion of one or more coronary arteries, 2) collateral blood flow into the zone previously supplied by the occluded vessel, and 3) hemodynamically significant stenosis of the artery supplying the collaterals (3).

It is also important to understand the mechanism by which arteriolar dilation causes steal. Agents such as dipyridamole, adenosine, nitroprusside, and isoflurane dilate intramyocardial coronary arterioles preferentially over large epicardial coronary arteries. Arteriolar dilation in the zone supplied by the stenosed artery leads to an increase in flow through the stenosis and a greater pressure drop across the stenosis. If aortic pressure stays constant, then the pressure distal to the stenosis decreases and flow through the "pressure-dependent" collateral vessels may decrease as well. While a stenosis of the supplying artery is not absolutely necessary for steal to occur, the stenosis magnifies the

T. H. Stanley and R. J. Sperry (eds.), Anesthesiology and the Heart, 231–237.

effect (4). These elements occur in 19-23% of patients with coronary artery disease severe enough to warrant coronary angiography (5).

Although the proposed and demonstrated deleterious effects of coronary vasodilation on the ischemic heart and the spectre of "silent" or more properly for the anesthetized patient, "non-hemodynamically related myocardial ischemia" have complicated the anesthetic management of patients with ischemic heart disease enormously, it still appears prudent to attempt to control the indices of myocardial oxygen supply and demand during the peri-operative period (6,7). Many anesthesiologists choose to maintain that control using volatile anesthetics. Obviously, this debate is pertinent to that practice.

THE EVIDENCE FROM ANIMAL STUDIES

1. In fact, isoflurane is only a mild coronary vasdodilator especially when compared with the prototype coronary vasodilators which have been been used to demonstrate coronary steal, adenosine and dipyridamole. Even in the classic study of Buffington et al (1), isoflurane did not produce nearly as much coronary vasodilation as an admittedly low dose of adenosine. In addition, Hickey et al showed in a chronically instrumented closed-chest dog preparation that isoflurane produced appreciably less coronary vasodilation than dipyridamole (2). Zimpfer and co-workers, in a direct comparison of dipyridamole and isoflurane, showed very different effects in a chronically instrumented closed chest animal (8). Part of this difference may relate to the well recognized negative inotropic effect of isoflurane as compared to adenosine. Gewirtz and colleagues noted a substantial difference between the effect of adenosine and nifedipine on coronary flow distribution and metabolism distal to a severe stenosis (9). They hypothesized that a major reason for the difference was the negative inotropic effect of nifedipine which decreased myocardial oxygen demand, thus negating the effect of coronary vasodilation.

2. A major criticism of Buffington's study has been the invasive nature of the preparation. Utilizing a similar

chronically instrumented animal with ameroid constriction of a coronary artery to stimulate collateral development, Cason et al were unable to show any coronary steal with either halothane or isoflurane (10). In addition, in another chronically instrumented preparation with constriction producing collateralization, Hartman and colleagues could show no difference between the effect of halothane and isoflurane on myocardial blood flow distribution and ischemia (11).

3. Although the anatomy for the classic coronary steal demands an occluded collateralized area of the myocardium with the collateral supplied by a partially stenosed coronary artery (3), steal may also be transmural with the coronary vasodilator redistributing blood from the more susceptible endocardium to the epicardium. Tatekawa et al showed in an open chest dog model that although isoflurane produced a redistribution of blood flow from the subendocardium to the epicardium distal to a critical stenosis, there was no evidence of ischemia in either area (12). This substantiates the suggestion in a previous section that perhaps the negative inotropic effect of isoflurane mitigates the deleterious effects of the coronary blood flow redistribution. The same group in a further study was able to demonstrate not only redistribution of myocardial blood flow from epi- to endocardium distal to a coronary stenosis but ischemia as well. However, only with higher doses of isoflurane producing both tachycardia and hypotension was the ischemia demonstrated (13).

4. Two studies in chronically instrumented animals have failed to show evidence of ischemia with isoflurane. Zimpfer and Meyer, utilizing a chronically applied critical stenosis, were unable to demonstrate ischemia even with hypotension (14), and Warltier et al showed that both isoflurane and halothane improved the return to function of "stunned" myocardium with no difference demonstrated between the two anesthetics (15).

THE EVIDENCE FROM CLINICAL STUDIES

1. In spite of the fact that isoflurane can produce coronary vasodilation in patients with coronary artery disease, several

studies have shown a beneficial effect of isoflurane. Hess and co-workers demonstrated that either isoflurane or halothane could be used to treat hypertension during coronary artery bypass grafting but that the mechanism was different. Isoflurane predominantly reduced systemic vascular resistance whereas halothane depressed cardiac output (16). In an ingenious study, Tarnow and co-workers showed that patients anesthetized with isoflurane for coronary bypass grafting tolerated a higher paced heart rate before evidence of ischemia than the same patients had demonstrated the previous day awake without anesthesia (17). O'Young et al showed that when hypertension developed during sufentanil anesthesia in another group of patients during coronary artery bypass isoflurane rapidly and efficiently controlled the hypertension, not only without producing further ischemia but in some cases treating ischemia presumably produced by the hypertension (18).

2. The ischemia demonstrated during anesthesia and surgery with isoflurane by Reiz' group (19), Moffitt's group (20), and Sonntag's group (21) was usually related to unfavorable alterations in myocardial oxygen supply-demand (tachycardia and either hypo-hypertension). In fact, to date, with the exception of the original paper by Reiz (where the patients were already ischemic from hypotension and tachycardia), no clinical study has shown ischemia associated with isoflurane unless there was hypotension and/or by tachycardia.

3. a) Control of the indices of myocardial oxygen balance still appears to be important in anesthetizing the patient with ischemic heart disease. Two presentations at the 1988 American Society of Anesthesiologists Annual Meeting demonstrated this. Stanley et al randomized patients for coronary artery bypass grafting to receive increasing doses of either sufentanil, halothane or isoflurane, and monitored ischemia by the transesophageal echocardiogram (TEE), the current gold standard for clinical ischemia monitoring (22). As might be expected, the two inhalation anesthetics produced dose-related decreases in regional wall motion, but there was no difference between the two anesthetics and

the effect appeared to be related to the negative inotropic properties of the anesthetics rather than ischemia. In addition, from preoperative coronary angiography, regions at risk for ischemia were defined and there was no difference in the effect of the anesthetics on regional wall motion in these "risk areas." Goehner and colleagues specifically attempted to control myocardial oxygen balance very tightly during isoflurane or sufentanil for coronary artery bypass grafting. They showed that this tight control resulted in a significantly lower incidence of intra-operative ischemia than had been reported previously by their group and, furthermore, that there was no difference in incidence of peri-operative ischemia when isoflurane and sufentanil were compared.

b) One high risk group for myocardial ischemia during surgery are patients with carotid artery stenosis, for the most common cause of postoperative death in these patients is myocardial infarction (23). Two clinical studies have shown that isoflurane is not associated with a higher incidence of intra-operative ischemia (24) or postoperative myocardial infarction (25) in patients being operated for carotid endarterectomy.

c) Two large scale outcome studies on patients undergoing coronary artery bypass grafting with relative randomization of anesthesia have shown no difference between isoflurane and other anesthetics. Tuman et al (26,27) studied more than a thousand patients receiving either narcotics, ketamine-benzodiazepine, halothane or narcotics supplemented with halothane, enflurane or isoflurane. No difference in any cardiovascular outcome characteristics could be related to the anesthetic. Slogoff and Keats compared sufentanil, halothane, enflurane and isoflurane again in a study of more than a thousand patients for coronary artery bypass grafting (28). Likewise, when a reasonable attempt to control myocardial oxygen balance indices was made, there was no difference in the incidence of ischemia or cardiovascular outcome that could be related to the anesthetic employed.

d) Although perhaps 20% of patients with coronary artery disease may have "steal-prone" anatomy (5), the fact that isoflurane can also cause transmural steal distal to a coronary artery stenosis (13) suggests that the incidence of anatomy conducive to steal is at least 50% in the patient population. Consequently, even though the actual coronary pathophysiology may not be known in the outcome studies, it is likely that should steal be important from ioflurane in patients with coronary artery disease, differences in the incidence of ischemia would be apparent.

CONCLUSIONS

1. It is certainly possible to produce new or worsened ischemia with isoflurane in patients with coronary artery disease. Hypotension and tachycardia probably play a major role in the production of ischemia.
2. Thus far, there has been no completely convincing documentation of "excess risk" associated with isoflurane as compared to other anesthetic techniques in humans, although the ability of isoflurane to cause intercoronary steal in an animal model has been demonstrated.
3. Several studies have documented a beneficial effect of isoflurane and other inhaled agents in patients with coronary artery disease when the drugs are used to treat hyperdynamic cardiovascular states, or supplement narcotic anesthesia.
4. Careful use of isoflurane is probably not dangerous in patients with coronary artery disease; however, the emphasis must be on careful with attention directed towards avoiding hypotension and tachycardia.

REFERENCES

1. Buffington CW, Romson JL, Levine A, Duttlinger NC, Huang AH. Anesthesiology 66:280-292, 1987.
2. Hickey RF, Sybert PE, Verrier ED, Cason BA. Anesthesiology 68:21-30, 1988.
3. Becker LC. Circulation 57:1103-1110, 1978.
4. Patterson RE, Kirk ES. Circulation 67:1009-1015, 1983.
5. Buffington CW, Davis KB. Anesthesiology 69:721-727, 1988.
6. Rao TK, Jacobs KH, El-Etr AA. Anesthesiology 59:499-505, 1983.

7. Goehner P, Hollenberg M, Leung J, et al. Anesthesiology 69:A332, 1988.
8. Zimpfer M. Meyer N, Steinbereithner K. Anesthesiology 67:A587, 1987.
9. Gewirtz H, Gross SL, Williams DO, Most AS. Circulation 69:1048-1057, 1984.
10. Cason BA, Verrier ED, London MJ, Mangano DT, Hickey RF. Anesthesiology 67:665-675, 1987.
11. Hartman JC, Al-Wathiqui MH, Kampine JP, et al. Anesthesiology 69:A26, 1988.
12. Tatekawa S, Traber K, Hantler CB, Tait AR, Gallagher KP, Knight PR. Anesth Analg 66:1073-1082.
13. Wilton NCT, Knight P, Martin B, Ullrich K, Gallagher K: Anesthesiology 69:A25, 1988.
14. Zimpfer M, Meyer N. Appl Cardiopulm Pathophysiol 119-31, 1987.
15. Warltier DC, Al-Wathiqui MH, Kampine JR, Schmeling WT: Anesthesiology 69:552-565, 1988.
16. Hess W, Arnold B, Schulte-Sasse U, Tarnow J: Anesth Analg 62:15-22, 1983.
17. Tarnow J, Markschies-Hornung A, Schulte-Sasse U. Anesthesiology 64:147-156, 1986.
18. O'Young J, Mastrocostopoulos G, Hilgenberg A, et al. Anesthesiology 66:653-658, 1987.
19. Reiz S, Balfors E, Sorensen MB, Ariola Jr S, Friedman A, Truedsson H. Anesthesiology 59:91-97, 1983.
20. Moffitt EA, Barker RA, Glenn JJ, Imrie DD, DelCampo C, Landymore RW, Kinley CE, Murphy DA. Anesth Analg 65:53-61, 1986.
21. Larsen R, Hilfiker O, Philbin DM, Sonntag H. Anaesthesist 35:284-290, 1986.
22. Stanley TE, Clements F, Smith LR, et al. Anesthesiology 69:A8, 1988.
23. O'Donnell TF, Callow AD, Willet C, et al. Ann Surg 198:705-712, 1983.
24. Smith JS, Roizen MF, Cahalan MK, et al. Anesthesiology 69:846-857, 1988.
25. Cucchiara RF, Sundt TM, Michenfelder JD. Anesthesiology 69:783-784, 1988.
26. Tuman KJ, McCarthy RJ, Spiess BD, Ivankovich AD. Anesthesiology 69:A89, 1988.
27. Tuman KH, McCarthy RJ, Spiess BD, et al. Anesthesiology 70:189-198, 1989.
28. Slogoff S, Keats AS. Anesthesiology 70:179-188, 1989.

CARDIOVASCULAR EFFECTS OF LOCAL ANESTHETICS

Benjamin G. Covino, Ph.D., M.D.

It is well known that local anesthetic agents are capable of depressing the cardiovascular system. Since these agents are generalized membrane stabilizers, it is not surprising that excitable cardiac membranes can be markedly effected. This cardiac membrane stabilizing activity is the basis for the clinical use of lidocaine as an antiarrhythmic agent. The antiarrhythmic use of lidocaine was responsible for the performance of a number of studies to evaluate the cardiac electrophysiological and contractile effects of this agent.

The cardiac alterations produced by lidocaine and other local anesthetics were not considered to be clinically revelant when these agents were employed for regional anesthesia. The blood concentrations of local anesthetics associated with profound cardiac depression were believed to be considerably higher than those observed during the performance of regional anesthetic techniques such as epidural blockade. Central nervous system toxicity, i.e., convulsions, were more common manifestations of local anesthetic toxicity and tended to be of greater concern during the clinical performance of various regional anesthetic techniques.

In 1979, two cases reports appeared which described the occurrence of sudden cardiovascular collapse in two patients. (1,2) In one patient an accidental intravenous injection of bupivacaine was presumably made during an attempted interscalene brachial plexus block. In the second case, etidocaine was also presumed to have been injected intravenously during an attempted caudal anesthetic procedure.

Subsequently, an editorial was written based on these two published reports and several other unpublished cases of sudden cardiovascular collapse associated with the use of bupivacaine. (3) As a result, it was hypothesized that the more potent local anesthetic agents such as bupivacaine were relevantly more cardiotoxic than the less potent agents like lidocaine. The enhanced

T. H. Stanley and R. J. Sperry (eds.), Anesthesiology and the Heart, 239–249.

cardiotoxicity was believed related to the greater lipid solubility and protein binding of the more potent local anesthetics.

At the time of these initial reports, the available experimental data suggested that the cardiac depressant effects of local anesthetic agents were directly related to their relative potency in terms of conduction blockade in peripheral nerves. For example, studies on isolated atria from guinea pigs demonstrated that all local anesthetics exerted a dose dependent negative inotropic action. (4) The negative inotropic action of local anesthetic agents was correlated with their ability to suppress conduction in peripheral nerves. Thus, the more potent local anesthetic agents tended to depress cardiac contractility at lower concentrations then the less potent local anesthetic agents. In general, the local anesthetics studied could be divided into three groups in terms of their cardio-depressant effects. The more potent agents, bupivacaine, tetracaine and etidocaine, depressed cardiac contractility at the lowest concentration. The agents of moderate anesthetic potency, i.e., lidocaine, mepivacaine, prilocaine, chloroprocaine and cocaine formed an intermediate group of compounds in terms of their cardiodepressant effects. Finally, procaine, which is the least potent of the local anesthetics, was also the least depressant in terms of decreasing contractility of atrial tissue.

Studies on the isolated whole rabbit heart essentially confirmed the results in the isolated atria. (5) Again, the more potent local anesthetics, bupivacaine, tetracaine and etidocaine, depressed ventricular contractility by 25% at concentrations of approximately 1-1.5 ug/ml. On the other hand, lidocaine, mepivacaine and prilocaine, require concentrations of approximately 15 ug/ml to cause a similar decrease of 25% in the maximum height of tension development.

Investigations in open chest dogs in whom a strain-guage arch was sutured to the right ventricle revealed that all local anesthetic agents evaluated were capable of exerting a negative inotropic action. (6) As in the atrial and ventricular muscle studies, a relationship existed between the local anesthetic potency of the various agents and their ability to decrease myocardial contractility in intact animals. For example, tetracaine is approximately 8 to 10 times more potent than procaine as a local anesthetic and similarly tetracaine was found to be approximately 8 times more potent as a depressant of myocardial contractility in intact dogs. (Table 1)

Additional investigations were conducted in closed chest anesthetized dogs in which cardiac output was measured by means of a thermo-dilution technique. The hemodynamic effects of various clinically useful ester and amino-amide local anesthetics were compared. (7,8)

TABLE 1

Relationship between the negative inotropic action of various local anesthetics as determined in the intact dog and their in vivo anesthetic potency

AGENT ANESTHETIC	RELATIVE NEGATIVE INTROPIC POTENCY	RELATIVE IN VIVO POTENCY
Procaine	1	1
Chloroprocaine	2.5	2
Lidocaine	4.5	4
Cocaine	7.0	6.5
Tetracaine	8	9

TABLE 2

Comparative CC/CNS toxicity ratio of lidocaine, etidocaine, and bupivacaine in adult sheep

AGENT	CC/CNS DOSE RATES	CC/CNS BLOOD LEVEL RATIO
Lidocaine	7.1 ± 1.1	3.6 ± 0.3
Etidocaine	4.4 ± 0.9	1.7 ± 0.2
Bupivacaine	3.7 ± 0.5	1.6 ± 0.1

Statistically significant decreases in cardiac output were observed at doses at approximately 20 mg/kg of tetracaine, 40 mg/kg of chloroprocaine and 100 mg/kg of procaine. The more potent amino-amides, bupivacaine and tetracaine, showed a marked decrease in cardiac output at doses of approximately 5-10 mg/kg while the less potent amide local anesthetics mepivacaine, prilocaine and lidocaine, required doses of 10-30 mg/kg to cause a significant depression of cardiac output.

During the past 10 years, numerous laboratory investigations have been conducted to re-evaluate the comparative cardiac effects of various local anesthetic agents. Most of the studies have compared the cardiac actions of lidocaine and bupivacaine. The results of these investigations indicate that differences do exist with regard to the relative cardiotoxicity of the various local anesthetic agents.

The following types of laboratory studies have been conducted to evaluate the relative cardiotoxicity of the various local anesthetic agents: (1) the ratio of the dosage and blood level of local anesthetics required for irreversible cardiovascular collapse and the dosage and blood level which will produce CNS toxicity (convulsions), i.e., the CC/CNS ratio. (2) the arrythmogenic activity of different local anesthetics following rapid intravenous administration. (3) the comparative cardiotoxicity of certain local anesthetics in pregnant and nonpregnant animals. (4) the ability to resuscitate animals following local anesthetic induced cardiovascular collapse. (5) the effect of acidosis and hypoxia on the cardiotoxicity of local anesthetics.

1. CC/CNS ratio: The dosage and blood level of lidocaine, bupivacaine and etidocaine associated with the development of convulsive activity and cardiovascular collapse have been determined in adult sheep in which continuous intravenous infusions of these various local anesthetics were administered. (9) A CC/CNS ratio of 7.1 $\pm$ 1.1 existed for lidocaine indicating that seven times as much drug was required to induce irreversible cardiovacular collapse as was needed for the production of convulsions. (Table 2) In comparison, the CC/CNS ratio for bupivacaine was 3.7 $\pm$ 0.5 and for etidocaine 4.4 $\pm$ 0.9. Thus, although the central nervous system was still more sensitive to the toxic effects of the more potent local anesthetics, a smaller difference did exist between the dose to cause convulsions and that which led to irreversible cardiovascular collapse as compared to the less potent less anesthetic, lidocaine. Studies in dogs also confirmed that the CC/CNS ratio was lower for bupivacaine as compared to lidocaine. (10)

Studies in sheep in which the blood levels of various local anesthetics were determined and related to the onset of CNS and cardiovascular toxicity also revealed a narrower CC/CNS ratio for the more potent local anesthetics. For example, lidocaine was found to possess a CC/CNS blood level ratio of 3.6 ± 0.3 compared to values of 1.6 to 1.7 for bupivacaine and etidocaine. (Table 2) Tissue levels of the various local anesthetics which were determined at the time of cardiovascular collapse indicated a greater uptake of bupivacaine and etidocaine by the myocardium compared to lidocaine. Thus, the enhanced sensitivity by the myocardium to these more potent agents appears to be due to a greater myocardial uptake.

2. Ventricular arrhythmias: The rapidity with which cardiovascular collapse apparently occurred in some of the patients following the accidental intravascular injection of bupivacaine may be indicative of a severe ventricular arrhythmia. Ventricular tachycardia was reported in one patient following the accidental intravascular injection of 250 mg of bupivacaine with epinephrine during an attempted brachial plexus block. (11) However, it is not certain whether the tachycardia was related to the administration of bupivacaine or the epinephrine. Electrical cardioversion proved successful and no serious adverse sequelae were reported in this patient. Unfortunately, electrocardiographic evidence of ventricular dysrhythmias is lacking in the other reported cases of sudden cardiovascular collapse following the administration of bupivacaine. However, a number of investigators have reported the development of ventricular arrhythmias in animals exposed to toxic doses of bupivacaine. (12-15) Studies in awake dogs in which convulsant and supraconvulsant doses of lidocaine, mepivacaine, bupivacaine, etidocaine and tetracaine were administered intravenously showed that ventricular arrhythmias occurred in approximately 50% of dogs following bupivacaine and 20% of the animals receiving etidocaine. Ventricular arrhythmias were not observed in lidocaine, mepivacaine or tetracaine treated dogs. The results suggest that the occurrence of ventricular fibrillation is not related to the basic piperidine ring structure of bupivacaine since mepivacaine which contains the piperidine moeity failed to cause these cardiac abnormalities. In addition, a precise correlation does not appear to exist between the frequency of ventricular arrhythmias and the lipid solubility and protein binding of local anesthetics. Large doses of etidocaine, which is more lipid soluble than bupivacaine and equally protein bound, may cause ventricular arrhythmias and fibrillation but the incidence appears to be lower than that observed with bupivacaine.

The etiology of bupivacaine associated ventricular arrhythmias is believed related to a prolonged inhibition of sodium conductance in the cardiac membrane. Electrophysiological studies on isolated tissues have shown that bupivacaine can markedly depress the rapid phase of depolarization (V max) of the cardiac action potential. (16) Bupivacaine blocked cardiac sodium channels in a time and voltage-dependent fashion. In particular, bupivacaine was shown to block inactivated sodium channels. At concentrations above 0.2 ug/ml bupivacaine blocked a significant fraction of the sodium channels. Recovery of the blocked channels during diastole was extremely slow with a time constant of 1,557 $\pm$ 304 ms. The depressant effect of bupivacaine on V max was enhanced at higher heart rates, i.e., rates of 60-150 beats/min. Thus, bupivacaine was characterized as an agent which blocks sodium channels in a fast in - slow out fashion which effect is more apparent at fast heart rates. By contrast, 5-10 ug/ml of lidocaine were required to block a significant number of sodium channels. Moreover, recovery from block was more rapid with a time constant of 153.8 $\pm$ 51.2 ms. Lidocaine was characterized as a fast in - fast out agent which would not show much enhancement of sodium channel blockade at normal heart rates. Subsequent studies have confirmed that both bupivacaine and etidocaine cause a significantly greater depression of Vmax at fast rates of stimulation of guinea pig papillary muscle, i.e., 2-3 Hz. (17) On the other hand, lidocaine caused only minimal depression of Vmax even at high stimulation rates.

A detailed study of the cardiac electrophysiological effects of bupivacaine and lidocaine was conducted in an isolated rabbit Purkinje fiber-ventricular muscle preparation. (18) Bupivacaine at concentrations of 1-5 ug/ml resulted in a significant decrease in the Purkinje fiber maximum diastolic potential (MDP), action potential amplitude (APA), and Vmax. Exposure to 30 ug/ml of bupivacaine for 2 minutes caused a marked decrease in conduction between Purkinje fibers (PF) and ventricular muscle (VM) and ultimately PF-VM conduction block and PF inexcitability. Recovery from PF-VM conduction block and PF inexcitability following perfusion of the preparation with drug-free solution required approximately 40 and 20 minutes respectively. By contract 5-20 ug/ml of lidocaine caused minimal changes in MDP, APA and Vmax. Exposure to 100ug/ml lidocaine did result in PF-VM conduction slowing. PF-VM conduction block and PF inexcitability did occur in some of the preparations. However, recovery from PF-VM block and PF inexcitability took place within 5 minutes in these lidocaine treated tissues.

One other difference between bupivacaine and lidocaine was noted in these studies. A peculiar notching was observed during the phase 2 plateau phase of the PF action potential following exposure to high concentrations of bupivacaine only. It was suggested that this phenomenon may be due to prolonged sodium inactivation or inhibition of slow calcium channels by bupivacaine. Studies on guinea pig papillary muscle demonstrated that 10^{-4}M concentration of bupivacaine and 5 x 10^{-4} concentration of lidocaine could block completely slow action potentials indicating that local anesthetics can inhibit the slow calcium channels in ventricular muscle. (19) Lynch also reported a significant depression of the slow depolarization phase which is consistant with a possible inhibition of slow calcium channels. (17) However, this effect was only noted with 10mM of bupivacaine and was not seen with lidocaine or etidocaine.

Electrocardiographic studies in intact dogs and pigs have demonstrated significant decreases in cardiac conduction at high serum concentrations of bupivacaine. For example, marked increases in the PR, QRS, QTU and RR intervals were observed in dogs when bupivacaine was infused at a rate sufficient to produce serum concentrations of approximately 8 ug/ml. (20) These serum levels of bupivacaine also caused a significant decrease in the ventricular tachycardia threshold Moreover, bupivacaine treated dogs demonstrated an unusual polymorphic undulating ventricular tachycardia which is believed to be similar to the clinical syndrome of Torsades de Pointes. These studies in isolated cardiac tissue and intact animals indicate that high concentrations of bupivacaine result in unidirectional conduction blockade which ultimately leads to a re-entrant type of ventricular arrthymia.

It has been generally assumed that the arrhythmogenic activity of bupivacaine is related to a direct effect of this agent on cardiac membranes. Ventricular arrhythmias have been reported in isolated whole heart exposed to bupivacaine (21) and following the direct intracoronary injection of this agent in pigs. (22) Other data suggest that the arrhythmogenic action of bupivacaine may be indirectly caused by its effect on the central nervous system. For example, ventricular arrhythmias have been observed following the direct intraventricular injection of small doses of bupivacaine in cats and rats. (23.24) Although the development of ventricular arrhythmias associated with the rapid intravascular administration of bupivacaine is probably due primarily to a direct action on the myocardium, the possibility also exists that an indirect effect subsequent to the CNS toxicity of bupivacaine may also be responsible in part for the arrhythmogenic action of this agent.

3. Enhanced cardiotoxicity in pregnancy. A number of the cardiotoxic reactions reported following the use of bupivacaine have apparently occurred in pregnant patients although few published reports are available. As a result, the 0.75% solution is no longer recommended for use in obstetrical anesthesia in the U.S.A. Studies

in pregnant and non-pregnant sheep have shown that the CC/CNS dosage ratio decreased from 3.7 $\pm$ 0.5 in non-pregnant sheep to 2.7 $\pm$ 0.4 in pregnant animals. (9) However, little difference was observed in the CC/CNS blood level ratio which varied from 1.6 $\pm$ 0.1 in non-pregnant animals to 1.4 $\pm$ 0.1 in pregnant ewes. The blood concentration of bupivacaine associated with the onset of cardiovascular collapse was significantly lower in pregnant animals compared to non-pregnant sheep. These studies suggest that in terms of local anesthetic dosage to produce CNS and cardiovascular toxicity, the myocardium of the pregnant animal may be somewhat more sensitive. Measurements of cardiac tissue levels failed to demonstrate a greater myocardial uptake of bupivacaine in pregnant sheep at the time of cardiovascular collapse which indicates that the possible enhanced vulnerability of the pregnant animal is not related to a greater myocardial uptake of drug.

Similar studies conducted with mepivacaine in pregnant and nonpregnant sheep did not show any change with regard to the CC/CNS dose or blood level ratio. (25) Moreover, the blood concentration of mepivacaine associated with the onset of cardiovascular collapse was similar in both pregnant and nonpregnant animals. These data suggest that the enhanced cardiac toxicity in pregnant animals may be unique to the more potent agents such as bupivacaine. Preliminary studies in isolated Purkinje fiber-ventricular muscle preparations from rabbits injected for several days with high doses of progesterone indicate that the cardiodepressant effects of bupivacaine are enhanced while no changes were observed with regard to the electrophysiological effects of lidocaine. Thus, some interaction between bupivacaine and the hormones associated with pregnancy may account for the greater sensitivity of pregnant animals to the cardiotoxic properties of bupivacaine.

4. Cardiac resuscitation: Cardiopulmonary resuscitation has been reported to be extremely difficult in patients in whom cardiotoxicity has occurred following the administration of a toxic dose of bupivacaine. Studies in sheep have also indicated that cardiac resuscitation following bupivacaine induced toxicity is difficult. Chadwick compared the ability to resuscitate cats in whom cardiovascular collapse was induced with either lidocaine or bupivacaine. (27) Successful resuscitation was accomplished in approximately 5 minutes in both lidocaine and bupivacaine treated animals. However, all lidocaine treated animals were successfully resuscitated while two of 10 cats treated with bupivacaine did not survive. This difference was not statistically significant. Studies in dogs also demonstrated that resuscitation could be achieved following cardiovascular collapse due to a massive intravenous dose of bupivacaine. (28) Bretylium proved

effective in those animals in whom ventricular tachycardia occurred. Dogs which demonstrated electromechanical dissociation were successfully resuscitated with open chest cardiac massage and large doses of epinephrine, atropine and $NaHCO_3$. Kasten and Martin also reported that bretylium could successfully reverse bupivacaine induced ventricular tachycardia while lidocaine was ineffective. (14) Moreover, bretylium consistently raised the ventricular tachycardia threshold (VTT) which was lowered by bupivacaine. On the other hand, lidocaine caused either a further decrease in the VTT or no effect.

The currently available data indicate that resuscitation may be difficult but not impossible following bupivacaine induced cardiovascular collapse. Ventricular tachycardia and fibrillation probably should be treated rapidly by electrocardioversion. If pharmacologic antiarrhythmic therapy is attempted, bretylium would appear to be more effective than lidocaine. In addition, artifical ventilation with 100% oxygen should be rapidly instituted and large doses of epinephrine, atropine, Ca Cl_2 and $NaHCO_3$ administered in conjunction with closed or open chest cardiac massage if necessary.

5. Effect of acidosis and hypoxia: The combination of hypoxia and acidosis markedly potentiates the cardiodepresant effects of bupivacaine in isolated atrial tissue. (29) Hypoxia and acidosis also increased the frequency of cardiac arrhythmias and the mortality rate in sheep following the intravenous administration of bupivacaine. (26) Marked hypercarbia, acidosis and hypoxia occur very rapidly in some patients following seizure activity due to the rapid accidental intravascular injection of local anesthetic agents. (30) Thus, the cardiovascular depression observed with the more potent agents such as bupivacaine may be related in part to the severe acid-base changes that occur following the administration of toxic doses of these agents. The mechanism by which acidosis and/or hypoxia increases local anesthetic induced cardiac toxicity is not clear. Acidosis decreases the plasma protein binding of local anesthetics resulting in a greater fraction of drug in the free form. (31) On the other hand, acidosis favors the formation of the ionized form of local anesthetics which do not diffuse readily through membranes. However, it is obviously important to rapidly reverse or prevent the development of hypoxia and acidosis following the administration of a toxic local anesthetic dose.

Summary: All local anesthetic agents are capable of producing cardiovascular collapse if an excessive dose is administered or an accidental rapid intravascular injection occurs. The studies conducted in recent years indicate that the more potent local anesthetics agents such as bupivacaine and etidocaine are relatively more cardiotoxic than the less potent agents such as lidocaine. In particular, the ratio of the dose required for cardiovascular collapse and CNS toxicity, i.e., CC/CNS ratio, is lower for bupivacaine and etidocaine compared to lidocaine. Pregnant animals also appear more sensitive to the cardiac toxic effects of bupivacaine but not mepivacaine. However, the major differences between bupivacaine and lidocaine appears to be the ventricular arrhythmias which are frequently observed following toxic doses of bupivacaine. Lidocaine overdosage is not associated with arrhythmogenic activity.

The arrhythmogenic action of bupivacaine is related to a rapid and prolonged blockade of cardiac fast sodium channels and possibly slow calcium channels. This results in undirectional conduction blockade in the ventricular conduction pathways leading to a reentrant type of arrhythmia which can be fatal. Acidosis and hypoxia appear to enhance the arrhythmogenic potential of bupivacaine.

Resuscitation may be difficult following local anesthetic induced cardiovascular collapse. However, animal studies indicate that resuscitation is possible if appropriate measures are rapidly instituted. In the past few years no new reports of sudden cardiovascular collapse associated with the use of bupivacaine have been reported. This suggests that anesthesiologists are aware of the potential cardiac toxic effects of these potent agents and are employing greater caution when these local anesthetics are used for various regional anesthetic techniques. For example, it is generally accepted that a fractionated dose technique should be used when large doses of local anesthetics are administered for procedures such as epidural or brachial plexus blockade. The use of appropriate precautions to avoid an accidental intravascular injection or administration of an excessive dose has allowed the safe continued employment of valuable local anesthetic agents such as bupivacaine.

<u>References</u>:

1. Edde R and Deutsch S. Anesth Analg 56:446-7, 1977.
2. Prentiss J.: Anesthesiology 50:51-53, 1979.
3. Albright GA.: Anesthesiology 51:285-87, 1979.
4. Feldman HS, Covino BM, Sage DJ.: Reg Anesth 7:149-156, 1982.
5. Block A and Covino BG.: Reg Anesth 6:55-61, 1982.
6. Stewart DM, Rogers W, Mahaffrey N, Witherspoon S and Woods E.: Anesthesiology 24:621-24, 1963.
7. Liu P, Feldman SH, Covino BM, Giasi R, Covino BG.: Reg Anesth 7:14-19, 1982.
8. Liu P, Feldman HS, Covino BM, Giasi R, Covino BG.: Anesth Analg 61:317-322, 1982.
9. Morishima HO, Pederson H, Finster M, Hiraoka H, Tsuji A, Feldman H, Arthur GA, Covino BG.: Anesthesiology 63:134-139, 1985.
10. Sage D, Feldman H, Arthur G, Doucette A, Norway S and Covino B.: Reg Anesth 10:175-183, 1985.

11. Mallampati SR, Liu PL, Knapp RM.: Anesth Analg 63:856-9, 1984.
12. deJong R, Ronfeld R and DeRosa R.: Anesth Analg 61:3-9, 1982.
13. Kotelko DM, Shnider SM, Dailey PA, Brizgys R, Levinson G, Shapiro A, Koike M, Rosen MA.: Anesthesiology 60:10-18, 1984.
14. Kasten GW, Martin ST.: Anesth Analg 64:911-916, 1985.
15. Reiz S and Nath S.: Br J Anaesth 58:736-746, 1986.
16. Clarkson C and Hondeghem L.: Anesthesiology 62:396-405, 1985.
17. Lynch C.: Anesth Analg 65:551-59, 1986.
18. Moller RA and Covino BG.: Anesth Analg 67:107-14, 1988.
19. Coyle DE and Sperelakis N.: J Phar Exp Ther 242:1001-1005, 1987.
20. Kasten GW.: Reg Anesth 11:20-26, 1986.
21. Tanz R, Heskett T, Loehning R and Fairfax C.: Anesth Analg 63:549-56, 1984.
22. Nath S, Haggmark S, Johansson G and Reiz S.: Anesth Analg 65:1263-1270, 1986.
23. Heavner JE.: Anesth Analg 65:133-138, 1986.
24. Thomas RD, Behbehani MM, Coyle DE, Denson DD.: Anesth Analg 65:444-450, 1986.
25. Santos AC, Pedersen H, Harmon TW, Morishima HO, Finster M, Arthur GR, Covino BG.: Anesthesiology 70:991-995, 1989.
26. Rosen M, Thigpen J, Shnider S, Foutz S, Levinson G, Koike M.: Anesth Analg 64:1089-96, 1985.
27. Chadwick HS.: Anesthesiology 63:385-390, 1985.
28. Kasten GW, martin ST.: Anesth Analg 64:491-7, 1985.
29. Sage D J, Feldman HS, Arthur GR, Datta S, Ferretti AM, Norway SM, Covino BG.: Anesth Analg 63:1-7, 1984.
30. Moore DC, Crawford RD, Scurlock JE.: Anesthesiology 53:259-260, 1980.
31. Burney RG, DiFazio CA, Foster JA.: Anesth Analg 57:478-480, 1978.

PULMONARY EDEMA: IS YOUR FLUID MANAGEMENT BREATHTAKING?

P. BARASH

I. Physiologic Basis

A. Pulmonary Edema:

1. Classic Definition = extravascular water content of lung abnormally increased.
2. Current Definition = change in rate of fluid and protein flow through the interstitium of the lung.

B. Starling Forces

Key to a discussion of pulmonary edema is the Starling equation which describes fluid movement across capillary membranes. Starling hypothesized that the sum of capillary hydrostatic pressure (CHP) and the tissue oncotic pressure (TOP) was exactly balanced by the sum of the tissue hydrostatic pressure (THP) and the plamsma colloid oncotic pressure (PCOP). However, in the lung, unlike other capillary beds, the tissue hydrostatic pressure is negative. Thus, the PCOP is the only force which theoretically moves fluid into the capillary. Subsequently, it has been shown that the capillaries are permeable to various proteins, including albumin. The Starling equation has been modified to account for this observation by the addition of the reflectance coefficient.

T. H. Stanley and R. J. Sperry (eds.), Anesthesiology and the Heart, 251–261.

Abnormalities in these parameters increase the risk of pulmonary edema. Due to the effectiveness of the lymphatic system and other "edema-safety factors" the extravascular water content of the lung can increase by 47% before any abnormalities in pulmonary function are observed.

II. Plasma colloid oncotic pressure (PCOP)

Chief among the Starling forces that effect fluid flow across the pulmonary capillary membrane is PCOP. PCOP can be defined as the pressure exerted by plasma colloids across a semi permeable membrane (capillary endothelial wall) which tends to attract fluid into the intravascular space. PCOP helps regulate the movement of fluid between the intravascular and pulmonary interstitial space. The normal range of PCOP = 22-25 mmHg. Albumin (MWT=69,000) is the prime, contributor to the PCOP. Other blood proteins contribute the remainder.

Protein Contribution to PCOP

	MWT	GM%	ONCOTIC PRESSURE	% OF PCOP
Albumin	69,000	4.0	18.4	68.0
Globulin	200,000	1.2	1.7	6.0
Fibrinogen	333,000	0.3	0.2	0.7
Other		1.5	6.7	25.3
TOTAL		7.0	27.0	100%

The differences between oncotic pressure and osmotic pressure are:

	Plasma Colloid Oncotic Pressure	Plasma Osmotic Pressure
Measurement	Oncotic	Osmotic
Instrument	Oncometer	Osmometer
Units	mmHg	mOsm
Components	Plasma proteins	Electrolytes
Physiologic Site	Capillary membrane Intravascular	Cell membrane Intracellular

III. Fluid Therapy

A. Crystalloid
- Ringer's Lactate
- Normal saline
- Dextrose

B. Colloid
- Albumin
- Dextran
- Mannitol
- Hetastarch
- Whole blood
- Plasma protein

One gram of albumin osmotically attracts 18-20 cc of fluid. In clinical studies, plasma expansion is more rapid with albumin (or colloid) than crystalloids. If speed of restoration of intravascular volume is not critical, than crystalloid will suitably expand the intravascular space, but at a slower rate. On the basis of a decrease in PCOP and potential increase in pulmonary interstitial water (pulmonary edema), advocates of colloid therapy claim that respiratory impairment may result if large volumes of crystalloid are administered. However, numerous studies have shown that PCOP doesn't correlate well with intrapulmonary shunt, and when administered under controlled conditions, there is no difference in respiratory performance between a colloid and crystalloid group of patients.

C. Albumin: guidelines for clinical use

1. Appropriate Use
   Shock, burns, ARDS, cardiopulmonary bypass
2. Occasional Use
   Acute liver failure, RBC suspension media, ascites, with surgery, acute nephrosis, renal dialysis.
3. Additional Data Required
   Detoxification
4. Unjustified Use
   Under nutrition, chronic nephrosis, chronic cirrhosis

IV. Etiology of Pulmonary Edema

A. Increased capillary hydrostatic pressure
   1. Cardiogenic
      1. Left ventricular failure
      2. Valvular heart disease (MS)
   2. Fluid overload
   3. Narcotic reversal

B. Decrease plasma colloid oncotic pressure
   1. Hypoalbuminemia (nutritional)
   2. Overhydration

C. Increased interstitial pressure
   1. Expansion of pneumothorax
   2. Removal pleural diffusion

D. Altered permeability (noncardiac pulmonary edema)

1. Drug	2. Physiochemical	3. Miscellaneous
Antibiotics	Aspiration	Sepsis
Darvon	Oxygen toxicity	ARDS
Librium	Smoke inhalation	Transfusion reaction
Aspirin	Fat emboli	

E. Lymphatic insufficiency

1. Silicosis
2. Lymphangitic carcinoma
3. Chemical agents (Bleomycin)

F. Unknown etiology

Heroin	Eclampsia	Cardiopulmonary Bypass
Neurogenic	Cardioversion	High altitude
Pulmonary Embolism	Pulmonary parenchymal disease	

V. Pulmonary Edema and Emergence from Anesthesia

1. D/C positive pressure ventilation
2. Decreased cardiac output 2° venous return
3. Hypoventilation
   a. decreased $PaCO_2$
   b. increased $PaCO_2$
4. Airway obstruction
5. Increased BP

VI. Treatment Pulmonary Edema

A. General

1. Increase inspired oxygen concentration
2. Endotracheal suction
3. Positive end expiratory pressure (PEEP)
4. Diuretics
5. Digitalis
6. Bronchodilators
7. Morphine

B. Specific Treatment

1. Reduce Capillary Hydrostatic Pressure
   LV Function

a. Preload = Diuretics, venodilators
b. Afterload = Vasodilator
c. Contractility = Inotrope

2. Reduce Capillary Permeability
a. Treat underlying problem
b. Pulmonary capillary wedge pressure
c. Antihistamines, ?Steroids

3. Decreased plasma oncotic pressure
a. Albumin

References:

1. Albert RK, Lakshminarayan S, Charan NB, Kirk W, Butler J: Extra-alveolar vessel contribution to hydrostatic pulmonary edema in situ dog lungs. J Appl Physiol:54:1010-1017, 1983.
2. Baraka A, Moghrabi R, Yazigi A: Unilateral pulmonary oedema/atelectasis in the lateral decubitus position. Anaesthesia, 42:171-174, 1987.
3. Barash P, Chen Y, Kitahata LM, and Kopriva C: The Hemodynamic Tracking System: A method of data management and guide for cardiovascular therapy. Anesth & Analg 59:169-174, 1980.
4. Barin ES, Stevenson IF, Donnelly GL: Pulmonary oedema following acute upper airway obstruction. Anaesth Intens Care 14:54-57, 1986.
5. Braude N, Ludgrove T: Neurogenic pulmonary oedema precipitated by induction of anaesthesia. Br J Anaesth 62:101-103, 1989.
6. Brigham KL, Kariman K, Harris TR, Snapper JR, Bernard GR, Young SL: Correlation of oxygenation with vascular permeability-surface area but not with lung water in humans with acute respiratory failure and pulmonary edema. J Clin Invest 72:339-349, 1983.

7. Brigham KL, Kariman K, Harris TR, et al.: Correlation of oxygenation with vascular permeability-surface area but not with lung water in humans with acute respiratory failure and pulmonary edema. Am Soc Clin Invest 72:339-349,1983.
8. Brigham KL, Woolverton WC, Blake LH, Staub NC: Increased sheep lung vascular permeability caused by pseudomonas bacteremia. J Clin Invest 54:792-804, 1974.
9. Calvin JE, Driedger AA, Sibbald WJ: Positive end-expiratory pressure (PEEP) does not depress left ventricular function in patients with pulmonary edema. Am Rev Resp Dis 124:121-128, 1981.
10. Civetta JM: A new look at the Starling equation. Crit Care Med 7:84-91, 1977.
11. Cooper JD, Maeda M, Lowenstein E: Lung water accumulation with acute hemodilution. J Thorac Cardiovasc Surg 64:957-965, 1975.
12. Cooperman LH, Price HL: Pulmonary edema in the operative and postoperative period: A review of 40 cases. Ann Surg 172:883-891, 1980.
13. Dohi S: Postcardiopulmonary resuscitation pulmonary edema. Crit Care Med 11:434-437, 1983.
14. Flacke JW, Flacke WE, Williams GD: Acute pulmonary edema following naloxone reversal of high-dose morphine anesthesia. Anesthesiology 47:376-378, 1977.
15. Frank LP, Schreiber GC: Pulmonary edema following acute upper airway obstruction. Anesthesiology 65:106, 1986.
16. Gabel JC, Drake RE: Pulmonary capillary pressure and permeability. Crit Care Med 7:92-97, 1977.

17. Gallagher JD, Moore RA, Kerns D, Jose AB, Botros SB, Flicker S, Naidech H, Clark DL: Effects of colloid or crystalloid administration on pulmonary extravascular water in the postoperative period after coronary artery bypass Grafting. Anesth Analg 64:7530758, 1985.

18. Gutupalli KK: Acute pulmonary edema. Card Clin 2:183-200,1984.

19. Helbert C, Paskanik A, Bredenberg CE: Effective of positive end-expiratory pressure on lung water in pulmonary edema caused by increased membrane permeability. Ann Thor Surg 36:42-48, 1983.

20. Klancke KA, Assey ME, Kratz JM, Crawford FA: Postoperative pulmonary edema in postcoronary artery bypass graft patients. Chest 84:529-534, 1983.

21. Klausner JM, Paterson IS, Mannick JA, Valeri CR, Shepro D, Hechtman HB: Reperfusion pulmonary edema. JAMA 261:1030-1035, 1989.

22. Kopman EA, Ferguson TB: Interaction of right and left ventricular filling pressures at the termination of cardiopulmonary bypass. J Thorac Cardiovas Surg 89:706-708, 1985.

23. Krause LM, Langdale LA, Rice CL, Gould SA, Moss GS: Does interstitial pressure oppose lung water formation? J Surg Res 34:510-514, 1983.

24. Lee DS, Kobrine A: Neurogenic pulmonary edema associated with ruptured spinal cord arteriovenous malformation. Neurosurgery 12:691-693, 1983.

25. Lorch DG, Sahn SA: Post-extubation pulmonary edema following anesthesia induced by upper airway obstruction. Chest 90:802-805.

26. Lowe RJ, Moss GS, Jilek J, Levine HD: Crystalloid versus colloid in the etiology of pulmonary failure after trauma: a randomized trial in man. Crit Care Med 7:107-112, 1977.

27. Lydon JC: Furosemide may be detrimental in the treatment of pulmonary edema. (Letter to the Editor) Anesthesiology 64:298-299, 1986.

28. Maggart M, Stewart S: The mechanisms and management of noncardiogenic pulmonary edema following cardiopulmonary bypass. Ann Thorac Surg 43:231-236, 1987.

29. Matthay M: Resolution of pulmonary edema: Mechanisms of liquid, protein, and cellular clearance from the lung. Clin Chest Med 6:521-545, 1985.

30. Matthay MA,: Pathophysiology of Pulmonary Edema. Clin Chest Med 6:301-314, 1985.

31. Milne B, Spence D, Lynn RB, Sleeman D: Unilateral reexpansion pulmonary edema during emergence from general anesthesia. Anesthesiology 59:244-245, 1983.

32. Oswalt CE, Gate GA, Homstrom MG: Pulmonary edema as a complication of acute airway obstruction. JAMA 238:1833-1835, 1977.

33. Pare PD, Warriner B, Baile EM, Hogg JC: Redistribution of pulmonary extravascular water with positive end-expiratory pressure in canine pulmonary edema. Am Rev Resp Dis 127:590-593, 1983.

34. Paterson IS, Klausner JM, Pugatch R, Allen P, Mannick JA, Shepro D, Hechtman HB: Noncardiogenic pulmonary edema after abdominal aortic aneurysm surgery. Ann Surg 209:231-236, 1989.

35. Pavlin DJ, Raghu G, Rogers TR, et al.: Reexpansion Hypotension: A complication of rapid evacuation of prolonged pneumothorax. Chest 89:70-74, 1986.

36. Pavlin DJ: Lung Reexpansion - For better or worse? Chest 89:2-3, 1986.

37. Peterson BT, Ross JC, Brigham KL: Effect of naloxone on the pulmonary vascular responses to anesthetized sheep. Am Rev Respir Dis 128:1024-1029, 1983.

38. Pilato MA, Fleming NW, Katz NM, O'Connell JJ, Krucoff MW, Siegelman RE, Kim YD: Treatment of non-cardiogenic pulmonary edema following cardiopulmonary bypass with veno-venous extracorporeal membrane oxygenation. Anesthesiology 69:609-514, 1988.

39. Popovsky MA, Abel MD, Moore SB: Transfusion-related acute lung injury associated with passive transfer of antileukocyte antibodies. Am Rev Resp Dis 128:185-189, 1983.

40. Prough DS, Roy R, Bumgarner J, Shannon G: Acute pulmonary edema in healthy teenagers following conservative doses of intravenous naloxone. Anesthesiology 60:485-485, 1984.

41. Rafferty T, Ljungquist R, Firestone L, Curtis A, Raven C, Hui S, Barash P: The plasma colloid oncotic pressure - pulmonary artery occlusion pressure gradient - A poor predictor of pulmonary edema in surgical intensive care unit patients. Arch Surg 118:841-843, 1983.

42. Rao CC, McNiece WL, Krishna G: Acute pulmonary edema after removal of an esophageal foreign body in an infant. Crit Care Med 14:988-989, 1986.

43. Rasanen J: Conventional and high frequency controlled mechanical ventilation in patients with left ventricular dysfunction and pulmonary edema. Chest 91:225-229, 1987.

44. Rooke NT, Milne B: Acute pulmonary edema after regional ansthesia with lidocaine and epinephrine in a patient with chronic renal failure. Anesth Analg 63:363-364, 1984.

45. Sgouris JT, Rene A: Proceedings of the Workshop on Albumin. DHEW Publication No (NIH) 76-925, 1975.

46. Shoemaker WC, Hauser CJ: Critique of crystalloid verses colloid therapy in shock and shock lung. Crit Care Med 7:117-124, 1977.

47. Sivak ED, Richmond BJ, O'Donavan PB, Borkowski GP: Value of extravascular lung water measurement vs portable chest x-ray in the management of pulmonary edema. Crit Care Med 11:498-501, 1983.

48. Slutsky RA, Peck WW, Higgins CB: Pulmonary edema formation with myocardial infarction and left atrial hypertension: intravascular and extravascular pulmonary fluid volumes. Circulation 68:164-169, 1983.

49. Snapper JR, Brigham KL: Pulmonary Edema. Hosp Practice 87-101, 1986.

50. Sprung CL, Caralis PV, Marcial EH, et al.: The effects of high-dose corticosteroids in patients with septic shock: A prospective, controlled study. N Engl J Med 311:1137-1143, 1984.

51. Symons NLP, Hobbes AFT, Leaver HK: Analphylactoid reactions to vancomycin during anaesthesia: two clinical reports. Can anaesth Soc J 32:178-181, 1985.

52. Taff Rh: Pulmonary edema following naloxone administration in a patient without heart disease. Anesthesiology 59:576-577, 1983.

53. Tranbaugh RF, Elings VB, Christensen JM, Lewis FR: Effect of inhalation injury on lung water accumulation. J Trauma 23:597-604, 1983.

54. Tranbaugh RF, Lewis FR: Mechanisms and etiologic factors of pulmonary edema. Surg Gynecol Obstet 158:193-206, 1984.

55. Tullis JL: Albumin. 2. Guidelines and Clinical Use. JAMA 237:460-463, 1977.

56. Tullis JL: Albumin. 1. Background and Use. JAMA 237:335-360, 1977.

57. Vandyke WH, Jr, Cure J, Chakko CS, Gheorghiade M: Pulmonary edema after pericardiocentesis for cardiac tamponade. N Engl J Med 309:595-596, 1983.

58. Virgilio RW, Smith DE, Zarins CK: Balanced electrolyte solutions: experimental and clinical studies. Crit Care Med 7:98-106, 1977.

59. Ward HN: Pulmonary infiltrates associates with leukoagglutinin transfusion reactions. Ann Intern Med 73:689-694, 1970.

60. Weil MH, Henning RJ, Puri VK: Colloid oncotic pressure: clinical significance. Crit Care Med 7:113-116, 1977.

61. Willms D, Shure D: Pulmonary edema due to upper airway obstruction in adults. Chest 94:1090-1092, 1988.

Should We All Have a Sympathectomy at Birth? Or at Least Preoperatively? *

Michael F. Roizen, M.D.

The sympathetic nervous system appears useful to wild animals in helping to mobilize energy stores and in facilitating escape from threatening situations. But, as Stone *et al.*[1] suggest, such reactions may not be beneficial in anesthetized humans inasmuch as myocardial oxygen requirement may increase beyond supply. Do the adverse effects of stress now outweigh the benefits an intact sympathetic nervous system conveys? Should we ideally all be sympathectomized at birth, or at least preoperatively? Before answering this not so tongue-in-cheek question, we should first consider the details of the study by Stone *et al.*[1] which has stimulated this question.

Stone *et al.* gave one of a variety of beta-adrenergic blocking drugs or a placebo as preoperative medication to a group of mildly hypertensive patients and, knowing to which group the patients were assigned, the investigators then looked for ischemic episodes. They observed a significantly greater incidence of brief ischemic episodes during induction and emergence in the untreated patients compared with patients receiving a beta-adrenergic blocking drug as premedication. Although, on the surface, the results seem to clearly establish the efficacy of beta blocking drugs in reducing ischemic episodes, there are two limitations to this study which might cause us to temper our enthusiasm. First, there seems to be a problem with the randomization; although characteristics of the groups are not statistically different, they are numerically different. One wonders, therefore, whether bias was introduced by the fact that the control group underwent more vascular operations and had more pre-existing coronary artery disease than did the treatment groups. Second, the observers' awareness of which patients belonged to which treatment group could have resulted in subtle differences in management, such as provision of inadequate anesthesia or looking more closely for myocardial ischemia and

* Permission requested for reprint from Anesthesiology (68:482-484, 1988).

T. H. Stanley and R. J. Sperry (eds.), Anesthesiology and the Heart, 263–266.

sampling electrocardiographic strips for longer periods in the control group. While one wishes one could perform a double-blind study in such a situation, and maybe it is possible to do so, the effect upon heart rate induced by beta-adrenergic blockade may make this difficult. The authors clearly note these limitations of their own study, and should be congratulated for not extrapolating or expanding their conclusions beyond that allowed by their data.

There are those who, upon reading this study, would comment that the tachycardia which was allowed to occur was severe, indicating inadequate anesthesia, and that all the authors have demonstrated is that beta-adrenergic blockade takes the place of a skillful anesthesiologist. I would hesitate to come to that conclusion, because I believe that these investigators really tried to provide the best anesthesia care possible. I doubt whether even the subtle bias of an unblinded study could have caused this degree of inadequate anesthesia, but one nevertheless must consider that possibility. This study, and two recently published papers[2,3] demonstrating that clonidine depressed sympathetic nervous system responses during anesthesia, all imply that modifying the response of the sympathetic nervous system, whether on the alpha-adrenergic side with clonidine, or the beta-adrenergic side with one of the beta-adrenergic blocking drugs used here, may be beneficial perioperatively. I think that is also what Yeager *et al.*[4] showed in their study, and what we have shown in our studies[5]–that perioperative stress is hazardous to those least able to tolerate stress, and that blockade of sympathetic responses ablates the adverse myocardial effects of the perioperative response to stress. I think this may also be what Bland and Lowenstein[6] showed in their classic study on halothane decreasing myocardial ischemia in the non-failing canine heart, and what Klassen *et al.*,[7] Maroko and Braunwald,[8] and Norris *et al.*[9] have shown in other experimental situations. In fact, the whole cult of avoiding Type A behavior is probably based on a similar rationale.

Should we all undergo sympathectomy before operation, or, perhaps, even sympathectomy at birth? Support for such a proposal might derive from the observations that, following sympathectomy, one might experience less myocardial ischemia, less hemodynamic alteration, and less arthritis; there are even implications of less inflammatory bowel disease, lower anesthetic requirements, a more stable perioperative course, and improved small vessel flow allowing less arteriolar and arterial thromboses in the extremities.[1-10] What's wrong with being sympathectomized at birth? Why has evolution not eliminated the sympathetic nervous system? Normally, one would expect evolution to continue in the species those functions that are useful, and to foster disappearance of those that are not as useful in humans–in such a way, we've lost our tails. Thus, if the sympathetic nervous system wasn't useful, we should have lost it, but clearly this has not occurred. Although space does not permit me to develop a complete argument for or against survival of the sympathetic nervous system, several points are worth highlighting. The sympathetic nervous system is crucial for avoiding and treating asthma, and is very important for maintaining blood flow and the even distribution of transmural blood flow in the coronary circulation. Feigl[11] and others have shown that adrenergic coronary vasoconstriction, by preventing a "steal" to the outer layer of myocardium, seems useful in preventing inadequate oxygen delivery to the inner layers of myocardium. This same theory means that the vasoconstriction in larger coronary vessels might be precipitated by beta-adrenergic blockade, thus actually making myocardial ischemia worse in some people, although the majority would be less likely to suffer ischemic episodes.

Thus, while the article by Stone *et al.*[1] and others in the anesthesia literature imply that being sympathectomized preoperatively might be useful, other data make this issue less clear. To me, the issue is perhaps best expressed by the thought that, in those least able to tolerate myocardial ischemia, an adequate dose of anesthesia is that which provides the heart with the least stress. This concept does not necessarily mean giving so much of one type of anesthesia so as to get side effects, but, perhaps, implies including drugs (adrenergic blocking drugs) or techniques (regional anesthesia) that induce sympathectomy as part of the overall anesthetic technique. Maybe this is why so many clinicians use combinations of agents to induce and maintain anesthesia (often scientific rationale lags behind clinical practice). Like most good studies, the Stone *et al.* article leaves us with more questions than answers, and certainly leaves us with many issues to investigate.

References

1. Stone JG, Foex P, Sear JW, Johnson LL, Khambatta HJ, Triner L. Anesthesiology 68:495-500, 1988
2. Flacke JW, Bloor BC, Flacke WE, Wong D, Dazza S, Stead SW, Laks H. Anesthesiology 67:909-917, 1987
3. Ghignone M, Calvillo O, Quintin L. Anesthesiology 67:901-908, 1987
4. Yeager MP, Glass DD, Neff RK, Brinck-Johnsen T. Anesthesiology 66:729-736, 1987
5. Roizen MF, Lampe GH, Benefiel DJ, Sohn YJ, Lichtor JL, Smith JS, Stoney RJ, Ehrenfeld WK, Goldstone JS, Reilly LM, Thisted RA, Eger EI, Hamilton WK. Anesthesiology: 67:A1, 1987
6. Bland JHL, Lowenstein E. Anesthesiology 45:287-293, 1976

7. Klassen GA, Bramwell RS, Bromage PR, Zborowska-Sluis DT. Anesthesiology 52:8-15, 1980
8. Maroko DR, Braunwald E. Ann Intern Med 79:720-733, 1973
9. Norris RM, Clarke ED, Sammel NL, Smith WM, Williams B. Lancet 2:907-909, 1978
10. Levine JD, Dardick SJ, Roizen MF, Helms C, Basbaum AI. J Neurosci 6:3423-3429, 1986
11. Feigl EO. Circulation 76:737-745, 1987

Cardiopulmonary Bypass

John H. Tinker, M.D.

Cardiopulmonary bypass is not a particularly physiological state. It has been likened to a "shock like" state, but actually it is a complex set of physiologic circumstances during which the patient is in great jeopardy. Despite this, anesthesiologists have traditionally not been very interested in it,with respect to its physiology. In many countries, including the United States, perfusionists are under the medical supervision of someone, nearly always the surgeon. While this arrangement works very well from the standpoint of coordinating the perfusionist's activities during surgical maneuvers that are occurring, surgeons in general are not particularly interested in the nuances of cardiovascular physiology, cerebral or other organ protection, anticoagulation, complement fixation or consumption, etc. In short, there are many controversies in the field of cardiopulmonary bypass which have not been satisfactorily resolved. In this presentation, we will be trying to emphasize various sides of the controversies and will stay away from relatively routine aspects of cardiopulmonary bypass.

Available Circuits

The anesthetist should understand the kind of circuits that are available. Most commonly, flow is diverted from either the vena cavae or the right atrium to the pump oxygenator and back to the aorta. It is also possible to divert flow from the femoral vein to the aorta. Thirdly, it is possible to divert flow from any of the above venous drainage sites and replace it at the femoral artery instead of the aorta. It is even possible to use the

T. H. Stanley and R. J. Sperry (eds.), Anesthesiology and the Heart, 267–284.

brachial artery as an arterial inflow site, but this is seldom done due to size limitations. The usual circuit in use today is depicted in figure 1.

FIGURE 1

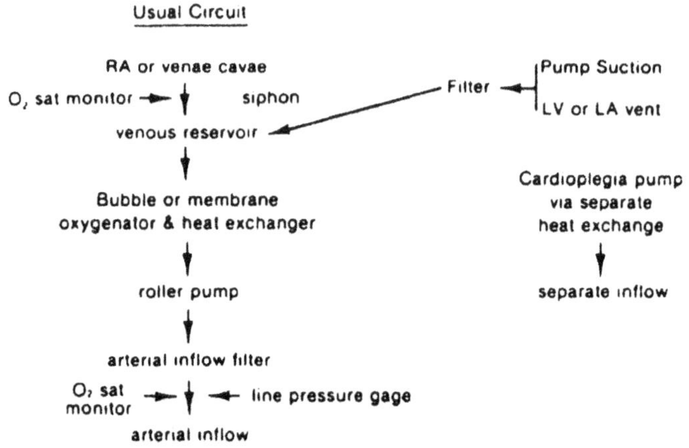

There are several things of special interest about this circuit. First, an oxygen saturation monitor can be placed on the venous outflow and also on the arterial inflow lines. There is also a device which allows the perfusionist to read directly PaO_2, $PaCO_2$, and pH as well as inflowing perfusate temperature, all from the arterial inflow line itself. This device uses fluorescent refractometry and does not actually contact blood.

Next, again referring to figure 1, note that the blood flowing via the venous drainage is in fact a siphon. No pumps are involved in this side of the circuit. It is very possible to have an airlock i.e. a disruption of the siphon by a large air bubble. This is especially likely during complex congenital surgery where the right side of the heart is being operated upon with little room to manuever.

The roller pumps in use today are almost, but not quite, occulsive. The adjustment of tension of these pumps is a critical factor and manufacturer's recommendations must be followed closely. Note also that the roller pump in use today is powered by "constant speed" electric motor. Most electric motors are inherently variable speed devices, when changes in load are placed upon them, speed and therefore output varies greatly. This is obviously an undesirable feature for a bypass pump. The pumps in use today are sophisticated constant speed motors wherein the speed, once set, remains constant even if the pressure load (afterload) changes over a wide range. The pump can be cranked by hand also in cause of failure.

Again referring to figure 1, note that there is an arterial inflow filter in most circuits today. Microemboli, particulate matter from the cardiotomy suction, etc, are removed by filtration, usually at 40 microns. The perfusionist must be able to instantly bypass this filter should it become an obstacle.

The other roller pumps on the machine are used for the following purposes: 1) cardioplegia infusion should be done by the perfusionist today because large volumes of very cold solution need to be pumped rapidly and at a known and controlled pressure; 2) there is almost uniform use today, if surgically possible, of a left ventricular venting device so as to not permit excessive distention of the left ventricle. Today, this suction is usually placed through the right superior pulmonary vein, into the left atrium, through the mitral valve into the left ventricle. 3) The cardiotomy suction. The perfusionist must not permit this suction to overly traumatize blood by use of excessive speeds on the pumps heads. On the other hand, when much blood is being shed, this suction may not be able to keep up with the blood loss. Blood suctioned by the cardiotomy suction and by the left ventricular vent is added to the circuit continuously. Inexperienced surgical assistants, in their zeal to obtain as dry a field for the surgeon as possible, often use the "high power" or wall suction. Blood sucked into this device is lost to the bypass circuit and is lost permanently unless a centrifugation type blood washer is in use. I have seen experienced anesthetists caution surgical assistants against the use of the wall suction, making light of it if necessary, but with the clear purpose in mind of saving the patient exogenous transfusion.

Again referring to figure 1, note the location of the arterial inflow line pressure gauge. This is an important component of a safe cardiopulmonary bypass circuit and, unfortunately, is not in universal use throughout the U.S. During bypass, this gauge usually reads 200 to 300 mm Hg, and represents the pressure in the arterial inflow line, not the pressure in the arterial system of the patient. The arterial inflow line is quite small relative to the size of the aorta and is quite long as well. Therefore, a large pressure differential across it is to be expected. It is entirely possible to have arterial inflow line pressures in excess of 250 mm Hg, whilst having radial artery pressures less than 50 mm Hg. Despite the fact that this is not arterial pressure, this arterial line inflow pressure is important monitor for at least two reasons: 1) If pressures exceed 300 to 350 mm Hg, there is danger that one or more of the high pressure fittings on the tubing will disrupt, resulting in disaster; 2) after the aortic inflow line is placed in the aorta and the pump is attached to it, before going on bypass it is important that the arterial line be opened and the perfusionist state clearly that he sees pulsations on the arterial line inflow pressure gauge. Further, the pressure reading on the gauge <u>before</u> the patient is placed on bypass should correlate closely with the pressure transduced from the arterial line placed by the anesthetists. Absence of pulsations at this stage may indicate several things, all bad. The patient might have been attached to the pulmonary bypass circuit backwards! The surgeon might have, inadvertently, placed the tip of the arterial inflow line not into the aorta itself but into a false lumen. This will result in an immediate major dissection upon assumpton of bypass. Despite these important points, there is controversy among perfusionists about the necessity of having an arterial inflow line pressure gauge. I believe strongly in it and have seen patients saved from disasters by it.

Finally, when everything is thought to be ready to go on bypass and the surgeon says "on bypass", the perfusionist starts the pump head turning. At this stage, the presence of the arterial inflow line pressure gauge will tell the perfusionist rapidly whether or not a clamp has been inadvertently left on the arterial line in the surgical field somewhere. If this is the case, the arterial inflow line pressure will rise immediately to dangerous levels and the perfusionist will know to turn off the pump. In the absence of such a pressure gauge, a rather spectacular explosion is possible next!

Blood gas measurement on bypass and the CO_2 question

In my visitations to various centers, I have seen centers in which no blood gases are measured during bypass at all and other centers where 15 or 20 separate samples for blood gases are taken during cardiopulmonary bypass. Every center has its protocol, but there does not seem to be much agreement. Worse, the question of what to do about "temperature correction" of blood gases is controversial. If the patient is at a perfusate temperature of 28°C, and you tell that fact to the blood gas technician, who is, of course, measuring the blood gases with an electrode kept constant at 37° C, then the blood gas technician will "temperature correct" the blood gases back to the patient's temperature. The blood gases you receive, at least if the patient is at equilibrium with the perfusate temperature, will be the absolute actual blood gas partial pressures that were present when the sample was drawn.

Many perfusionists use "corrected" blood gases and try to add sufficient CO_2 so as to produce an actual "corrected" $PaCO_2$ at or near 35 - 40 mm Hg. Using this method, because of the efficiency of elimination of CO_2 by most oxygenators, the perfusionist will be required to add large volumes of CO_2, circa 5% or more, in order to do this. The rationale behind this method of CO_2 management during bypass is as follows. Control of the cerebral circulation is, even at hypothermia, probably still under the influence of CO_2. If this is true, then maintenance of these relatively high PCO_2 values might be important. There is much controversy about this thinking however. In the first place, the addition of this much CO_2 during bypass, at such cold perfusate temperatures, results in very high quantities of dissolved CO_2. Whether this is deleterious or not is not known.

A second school of thought has developed with respect to CO_2. It is known from the work of Dr. Herman Rahn and many others, for many years now, that poikilothermic animals i.e. animals, who tend to assume room temperature, regulate their own CO_2 in a very curious manner. If you take a poikilothermic animal such as a turtle, and measure his (or her) arterial blood gas at a steady state room temperature of 37^0 C, you will obtain a relatively normal $PaCO_2$ in 35 - 40 mm Hg range. If you then cool that animal to 25^0 C achieve steady state again, with the animal still fully conscious, and draw another arterial blood gas, amazingly enough you will find that the PCO_2 is still about 35 - 40 mm Hg, uncorrected. If you correct it for the actual temperature of the animal, (remember that we are using a 37^0 C electrode) you will now find that the absolute PCO_2 is in the low 20 range, and the pH therefore approximately in the 7.6 range. In other words, these animals ventilate themselves, in the apparently perfectly conscious state, at temperatures below 37^0, into what we might consider to be a severely hyperventilated alkalotic state. The animal has decreased ventilation somewhat during the assumption of this new lower temperature, but CO_2 production has decreased further and therefore the animal is "over ventilating" at least by 37^0 standards. Despite this, the animal appears perfectly conscious. Although it requires a bit of a leap of faith on the reader's part, suffice it to say here that there is a body of evidence to indicate that there may be no reason why the pH of 7.4 and the PCO_2 37 - 40 we all know and love so well at temperatures of 37^0 C is necessarily the "correct" pH which will allow body systems to function optimally at other temperatures. There are enzymes whose function at different temperatures is pH dependent. It is possible that these apparently alkalotic pH's and apparently hyperventilated $PaCO_2$'s are more optimal at these lower temperatures. There is a growing group of perfusionists in the U.S. who believe that PCO_2's should be allowed to fall wherever they may during the pump oxygenator run. These perfusionists add no CO_2 at all during cardiopulmonary bypass! Corrected blood gases will show, in many of their patients, PCO_2's in the low 20's, and pH's in 7.6 range. These patients do not apparently do worse with respect to cerebral dysfunction, although specific studies of outcome are lacking. They are said by some at least to do better with respect to post bypass cardiovascular function.

The use of "uncorrected" blood gases is called "alpha-stat" management, because the body's major buffer is the alpha imidazole ring on the histidine moiety of various proteins. The method is based upon the apparent lack of interest in poikilothermic animals in maintenance of pH! These animals (and the same is true for human skin, muscle, etc. at different temperatures) seem to be interested in the maintenance of electrochemical neutrality. The reader is referred to the recent Society of CV Anesthesiologists Monograph for a full discussion of this and other controversial topics regarding bypass (ref. #28).

Therefore, the question about what to do with CO_2 and therefore pH during bypass, especially if patients are to be rendered relatively hypothermic in the circa 25 - 28° C range, is not known with any certainty. Practice varies widely, there may not be major effects of this on outcome, but, perhaps we do not have the sophistication to measure the differences in outcome which are present. Some perfusionists, not knowing which way to go in this controversy, choose to add a little CO_2 and render corrected CO_2's in the high 20's or low 30's during bypass.

Arterial pressure on bypass

When you go on bypass, the patient's arterial pressure nearly always plummets. This is due to the dramatic decrease in viscosity that results from the massive infusion of clear prime. Probably, in addition to that, there is peripheral dilation secondary to the decreased oxygen delivery that occurs in the initial period of extreme hemodilution with the first "wave" of the clear priming solution. Pressures may dip into the 30 - 40 mm Hg range. Many anesthetists are concerned about this and will administer vasoconstrictors. In recent years, however, the clinical practice trend in the U.S. seems to be away from doing this. In many centers now anesthetists are not concerned about this drop in arterial pressure, as long as the patient is being cooled relatively rapidly.

Later, in many but not all patients, for reasons which are still controversial and in doubt, arterial pressure begins to slowly increase. As time goes on, with the patient relatively hypothermic, circa 28° C, arterial pressure may reach alarmingly high levels. During the above hypotensive phase, concern about cerebral protection is paramount. More will be mentioned about this below. During the hypertensive period, although the possibility of cerebral hemorrhage may exist, concern centers more on the myocardium and its protection for the following reasons. During the aortic cross clamped phase of bypass, when the surgeon is working on the stilled heart, kept cold by external applications of ice plus "internal" applications of cold cardio plegia solution, it is entirely possible to see red blood appearing in the coronary arteries. This is so-called non-coronary collateral circulation, and results from pericardial reflections of vessels which arise from the thoracic aorta. The higher the arterial pressure, the greater is the possibility for disturbing amounts of this non-coronary collateral flow. It is important to remember that this flow is at 25 or 28° C, depending on the perfusate temperature and will therefore warm whichever parts of the heart it goes to. Usually, this is the posterior wall of the myocardium. This flow, coupled with the fact that the posterior wall of the myocardium is anatomically near the descending thoracic aorta, both combine to render imperfect the surgeon's ability to keep the posterior wall of the myocardium very cold during the ischemic phase. This is a major reason why, sometimes, there is disturbing posterior papillary muscle dysfunction resulting in mitral regurgitation during emergence from bypass. Thus it is not in the best interest of the patient to ignore the steadily climbing arterial pressure.

What should the arterial pressure be? There is no convincing experimental evidence for any particular pressure range. In this author's experience, and based on travels around to many institutions, it does seem reasonable that arterial pressures above 30 mm Hg during the initial phase of bypass should be tolerated. This author no longer administers vasoconstrictors during the initial hypotensive phase of bypass. During the cold cardioplegic cross clamp phase of bypass, this author does not tolerate arterial pressures greater than 65 mm Hg and is aggressive about treating pressures approaching that level.

There is also controversy about how this hypertension should be treated. In many centers, the relatively vasodilating anesthetic isoflurane is used via a vaporizor placed on the pump. The problems with this are manyfold. First, it is the use of a drug for a side effect because, below 30° C, the need for anesthesia is minimal. Second, these vaporizors are often "in limbo" from an administrative point of view i.e. do they belong to the perfusionist? Do they belong to the anesthesia department? Who calibrates them? Who maintains them? Third, if the anesthetist forgets to turn the vaporizor off during the rewarming phase after removal of the aortic cross clamp, hypotension may result which may in turn result in the otherwise unnecessary administration of vasoconstrictors. Also, emergence from bypass with a negative inotrope in high concentrations on board can be problematic. This author, for the above reasons, has removed the anesthetic vaporizers from all pumps. This author prefers uses nitroprusside to control arterial pressure during bypass. Nitroglycerin can be tried, but does not seem to work very well, probably because of its absorption to various plastic surfaces inside the oxygenators and its volatility in high gas flow situations plus the fact that it is largely a venodilator. Thorazine is mentioned to <u>condemn its use during cardiopulmonary bypass</u>. This author has been in a major medical center where the perfusionist administered 5 mg boli of thorazine at various points during cardiopulmonary bypass without medical direction from anyone. Thorazine is a cumulative drug and certainly deserves its European and Canadian name namely, "largactil". It is also not a drug which is particularly reliable since, again, this is use of a drug for a side effect, namely alpha adrenergic blockade. Finally, alpha adrenergic blockade will not necessarily reduce arterial pressure in these patients since the hypertension is not often primarily due to alpha adrenergic stimulation.

To summarize the question of "where should the arterial pressure be during bypass?", it is important to state again that there is no solid body of experimental evidence, in either animals or man, with respect to either cerebral or cardiac or any other vital organ outcome, that would strongly dictate any arterial pressure at any time during bypass. There is evidence that cerebral autoregulation lower limits are extended downward during cardiopulmonary bypass and that cerebral blood flow is reasonably well maintained at arterial pressures greater than 30 mm Hg.

Pump flow during bypass

In the late 1950's, largely at Mayo Clinic, flow rates of 2.4 l/m^2/min were established for performance of bypass. Many institutions still use recipes with flows of 2.0 - 2.4 l/m^2/min. In a parallel direction, at Stanford, flows of approximately half these levels, namely 1.0 - 1.2 l/m^2/min have been utilized. Neurologic results are not obviously different between institutions using these quite different flow rates. On the other hand, well controlled neurologic testing has not been done when flows were at the low rates mentioned above. There are many centers in which different surgeons use different flows and perfusionists must keep track of each individual surgeon's preferences! Clearly definitive studies need to be done, but the problem is that neurologic outcome is probably the most important outcome criterion. Since that is true, the performance of these kinds of studies in animals will probably not give us the answers we need. It is clear that "low flow" bypass does result in less blood trauma, less non- coronary collateral flow, and might therefore be expected to result in better myocardial protection. The Stanford group's most powerful argument, may be that it is after all the heart on which we are operating, the organ which the most disease, and therefore we should be very concerned about that organ. Nonetheless, neurologic and neuropsychiatric damage following cardiopulmonary bypass (see below) is a major ongoing and continuing problem associated with these procedures. It has been thought for many years that some of this neuropsychiatric and neurologic damage is related to flow and pressure, although many surgeons believe that most damage is related to emboli of various sorts. The purpose of this discussion is to make the reader aware of this controversy. In the future, many centers may come to a compromise between the "high" and the "low" flow recipes, and use flow rates circa 1.6 l/m^2/min.

Cerebral protection during cardiopulmonary bypass

As mentioned above, inadequate flow, particulate and gaseous emboli have been considered causative of the various kinds of cerebral damage which have been reported over the years following bypass. It is increasingly obvious that some of the damage is quite subtle and is of a psychologic or neuropsychiatric nature rather than a more gross or "neurologic" nature. Individual skills, tested pre versus post bypass may show dramatic declines in a patient who seems to have overall excellent function. This problem remains one of the most significant continuing problems of cardiopulmonary bypass.

Barbiturates have been discussed as possible cerebral protectants for many years now. They have the theoretical advantage of being able to dramatically (circa 50%) lower $CMRO_2$ without disturbing basal cerebral integrity. In other words, they seem to be able to disassociate cerebral functional activity, which requires approximately 50% of the $CMRO_2$, from basal cerebral cellular integrity, which seems to require approximately the other half. Because of this theoretical advantage, many experiments have been done, mostly in animals, to try to ascertain whether in fact barbiturates might be clinically protective. As far back as 1982, it was considered that the human model which might be best controlled for a study of barbiturate cerebral protection might be the human cardiopulmonary bypass. In 1982, Slogoff et al studied a large number of patients who underwent aortocoronary bypass grafting with vs. without barbiturates injected before cardiopulmonary bypass. No statistically or clinically significant cerebral protection was found, but the level of neurologic dysfunction was relatively low in these patients who, of course, underwent superficial cardiac operations rather than open heart operations. In 1986, Nussmeier et al performed a similar study at the same institution, namely Texas Heart Institute, using patients who underwent open heart surgery. The endpoint for the administration of the barbiturates was an isolectric EEG, a point at which numerous previous studies have shown that the barbiturate-related depression of $CMRO_2$ is maximal. Thiopental was used, and sufficient dosage was administered before and during bypass to keep the EEG nearly isolectric. It is important to note, at the Texas Heart Institute, that normothermic bypass was utilized. These patients required very large doses of barbiturates to maintain EEG isolectricity. They reported statistically and clinically significant neurologic and neuropsychologic "protection" in the group of patients given barbiturates. It is also important to note, at the Texas Heart Institute at the time of this study, arterial inflow line filters were not utilized. The performance of normothermic bypass, and lack of utilization of arterial inflow line filtration, are probably important in the interpretation of the results of the study. During hypothermic bypass, far smaller doses of barbiturate are required to flatten the EEG. Since most centers in the U.S. use hypothermic, not normothermic, bypass, administration of barbiturates in high dosages, without EEG control, to patients undergoing hypothermic bypass, does not seem justified to this author. If the clinician does wish to use barbiturates because of the results reported in the Nussmeier study, this author would strongly suggest use of EEG control and titration of the barbiturate dosage based on the observation of that EEG. In the Texas Heart Institute study, there was indeed a "price" to be paid for use of such large doses of barbiturates, namely an extra 5 hours of intubation, and a statistically significant increased requirement for inotropic agents during emergence from bypass. Studies from other centers which use hypothermic filtered bypass which show barbiturate cerebral protection have not been forthcoming.

The presence of the hypothermia itself might be as "protective" as the barbiturates were in the Texas Heart Institute study. If this is true, addition of barbiturates to hypothermic bypass, even with EEG control, may not provide additional protection. It is nonetheless true that the Nussmeier et al study, represents a major attempt at ameliorating the difficult problem of neuropsychiatric damage following cardiopulmonary bypass, and will certainly stimulate continued research effort. Anesthesiologists must read studies like this carefully and not apply them to their practices without careful thought and detailed study.

Awareness during bypass

The point at which awareness is most likely is during rewarming. Cerebral structures are rewarmed rapidly because of relatively high blood flows. Volatile agents have probably been discontinued by this time. Large doses of narcotics have likely been given previously, but are not total anesthetics in many patients and the blood levels of them may have declined by this time. There are many anecdotal reports of awareness during this period. There is no reliable monitor of whether or not the patient is aware. Therefore, we believe that early during the rewarming period is the time to administer some sort of hypnotic or amnesic agent. Lorazepam, 2 - 4 mg, diazepam, 5 -10 mg, or scopolamine, 0.5 mg, can be given to accomplish this task. We do not see harm in routinely doing this, because it is so difficult to decide whether or not awareness is occurring. Some anesthetists believe that pupillary signs are valuable at this stage, this author is not in agreement. During rewarming, profuse sweating is the rule rather than the exception. This says nothing about awareness one way or the other. It means that the hypothalamic perfusate temperature has risen above a level wherein the patient sweats. Many trainees are tempted to treat this sweating with thiopental. This results in the administration of relatively large doses of a negative inotropic agent just at the time before emergence from bypass. This makes no sense at all to this author.

Cardioplegia and myocardial preservation

Virtually all cardioplegia solutions contain a high concentration, circa 25 - 30 meq/liter of potassium. They contain numerous other ingredients, the recipes for which vary from institution to institution. The purpose of the potassium is to stop the heart in diastole rapidly, thus reducing oxygen demand. Subsequent doses of cardioplegia certainly do not need the potassium, but it is usually administered anyway. The only point that this writer wishes to make here, is that myocardial preservation beyond the initial cooling, mandates frequent, circa 20 minutes, re-administration of the cardioplegia. There is extensive literature support for the statement that the re- administration of cardioplegia is crucial to myocardial protection during this phase of bypass. Surgeons who ignore the repeated warnings of the perfusionist and/or anesthetist that too much time has elapsed, are placing their patients in jeopardy. The purposes of the re-administration of the cardioplegia solution are at least twofold, namely reestablishment of the cold state and washout of lactate. As lactate builds up from anaerobic glycolosis, further anaerobic glycolosis can be shut off and, as is obvious, the heart cannot continue to utilize anaerobic glycolosis. Therefore, anesthetists and perfusionists should pay attention to the time periods that are elapsing between re- administration of cardioplegia.

Emergence from bypass

This critical period is, in fact, the replacement of the cardiac workload on the heart. Many surgeons apply this workload at far to rapid a pace, resulting in a period of time during which the heart is distended, beating rapidly, with poor subendocardial oxygen delivery, and poor output. It makes sense to replace the cardiac workload gradually, never allowing the heart to distend, and adding pharmacologic inotropic support early.

The anesthetist must understand that new a "disease" may now be present, namely post ischemic global myocardial dysfunction. This new disease process is added to whatever difficulties were present before bypass. Many anesthetists get bogged down in their thinking about this in in the following way. The usual reason for doing the bypass in the first place was coronary artery disease, and was therefore a myocardial oxygen supply or potential supply problem. In the emergence phase their attention gets focused on delivery of myocardial oxygen supplies. This may not be the problem at all. After all, hopefully, the major coronary stenoses have been bypassed. Many anesthetists concentrate on the application of an adequate arterial pressure "head" in order to provide enough coronary driving pressure to assure oxygen delivery to the myocardium. To be sure, this sometimes can be accomplished with peripheral vasoconstriction with neosynephrine. The question is whether this is indeed the whole answer to the problem. If indeed the heart is suffering from post ischemic global myocardial dysfunction, there may be reasonably adequate supplies of oxygen and nutrients being delivered to this damaged myocardium. The nature of the above mentioned new disease process is that the heart is unable to adequately utilize the oxygen delivered to it. This, in essence, is acute heart "failure" and, in this author's strong opinion, needs to be treated with inotropic support. It is invalid to allow a heart to sit for 15 minutes or so post bypass at high filling pressures, namely left atrial pressures of 15 - 20 mm Hg, and low arterial pressures, namely systolic arterial pressures of less than 85 mm Hg or so, at relatively high heart rates, while the momentous decision about whether or not to use an inotrope is debated between surgeon and anesthetist. To be sure, most patients come off bypass without the necessity for an inotrope i.e. they come off bypass with very adequate arterial pressures, cardiac outputs, at relatively low filling pressures and at reasonable rates (circa 90 beats per minute). (Incidentally, part of the reason this is so, is because endogenous catecholamine levels are usually high at this stage.) The percentage of patients who have the above mentioned post ischemic global myocardial dysfunction syndrome varies among institutions and depends on the length of cross clamp, quality of myocardial preservation during cross clamp, and the population of patients being operated upon. The diagnosis of such global post ischemic myocardial dysfunction must be made and made early, and inotropic support must be provided with dispatch.

The anesthetist should have reliable methods of estimating in advance which patient will need this kind of support. A long cross clamp time, a surgeon who delays the re- administration of cardioplegia, a surgeon who lifts the heart out into the hot lights very frequently, a patient with severe pre-bypass dysfunction, or poor coronary run off, or major ventricular hypertrophy, may be such a candidate. If so, it is reasonable and prudent to mix the appropriate inotrope, figure out what the dosage at least initially should be, and have it ready in a calibrated drug pump (not a gravity flow device) for emergence from bypass.

What should that inotrope be? Nature evolved epinephrine to have a good combination of qualities which are useful at this point. Strong inotropic action, little tachyphylaxis, without massive increases in peripheral vascular resistance are all strong attributes of "nature's remedy", namely epinephrine. An obvious disadvantage to epinephrine is the fact that nature has also evolved it to be a venous squeezer in order to provide increased preload in situation of of "fight or flight". With epinephrine there will, often, be the necessity to overcome this with a peripheral venous dilator, either nitroprusside or nitroglycerin. Many people say that epinephrine is "too strong" an inotrope to start with and that they would prefer to use one of the "less dangerous" drugs such as dobutamine or dopamine. This makes little sense to this writer because this is a resuscitation situation. Obviously, epinephrine is not the world's greatest drug with respect to renal blood flow, but after we get the heart started, we can worry about renal blood flow over the next few minutes or hours. Our first job, however, is clearly to get the heart started and it is wishful thinking, in this writer's opinion, to start with one of the "weaker" drugs. If the patients really has severe post ischemic global myocardial dysfunction, dobutamine and dopamine will not be sufficient. Epinephrine may not be either, and a balloon may be necessary, but long periods of time should not be spent debating about which inotrope to use in the presence of a poorly functioning heart with high filling pressures, low outputs, acidosis, dysrhythmias, etc. Why not start with epinephrine and, if successful, taper the epinephrine and switch to one of the less renally problematic drugs? Some centers use Levarteranol (levophed) plus regitine. This is more complex, but at least Levarteranol is also a naturally evolved "major league" substance for fight or flight.

Finally, if post ischemic global myocardial dysfunction, coupled with patient disease, appears to be defeating all our efforts, the balloon should be used if possible. The balloon is the only way to really separate myocardial oxygen supply from demand. To be sure, the balloon has major complications associated with its use sometimes, but in this situation it can be lifesaving.

The future

The future of cardiopulmonary bypass holds many promising and exciting challenges. The advent of the membrane oxygenator allows prolonged bypass, although bleeding and depletion of clotting factors are still major problems. Ventricular assist devices are also being used in increasing numbers. The armamentarium of the cardiac surgeon in the future may include a whole "shelf" full of devices designed to tide the patient's own myocardium over until it can "heal", though at this stage it is not known whether such healing will necessarily take place if the myocardium is severely damaged. Also, these devices may tide the patient over until cardiac transplantation can be undertaken, though again donor supply will severely limit this treatment modality. Nonetheless, this writer believes that it is nearly certain that cardiopulmonary bypass will not stay in the confines of the operating room in the future. Whether or not pulsatile bypass will "catch on" is more debatable, because although it seems to offer some hormonal and mechanical advantages, it is not obvious that it results in significant outcome benefits and does add some complexity. Clearly we need to make much more progress in our understanding of pressures, flow, cerebral dysfunction, and acid/base balance during cardiopulmonary bypass. Although the success of cardiopulmonary bypass has lulled many physicians into a state of complacency, the truth is that this field of endeavor is ripe for advancement now and, hopefully, will be targeted for considerable research effort in the near future.

References

1. Tinker JH, Roberts SL. In: Cardiac Anesthesia, 2nd edition, vol. 2. J A Kaplan, Ed. Grune & Stratton, Orlando, FL. pp. 895- 926, 1987.
2. Debakey ME. New Orleans Med Surg J 87:386-389, 1934.
3. Ehrenhaft JL, Claman JA. J Thor Cardiovasc Surg 41:503-508, 1961.
4. Rahn H. Pneumonologie 151:87, 1974.
5. White FN, Weinstein Y. Chapter 5. In Utley, JR, Ed. Pathophysiology and techniques of cardiopulmonary bypass. Vol. II, Baltimore, Williams and Wilkins, 1983. pp. 40-48.
6. Severinghaus JW, Stupfel N, Bradley AF. J Appl Physiol 9:197, 1956.
7. Severinghaus JW, Stupfel N, Bradley AF. J Appl Physiol 9:189, 1956.
8. McConnel DH, White FN, Nelson RL, et al. Surg Forum 26:263, 1975.
9. Becker H, Vinten-Johansen J, Buckberg GD, et al. J Thoracic Cardiovasc Surg 82:810, 1982.
10. Swain JA, White FN, Peters RM, et al. Proc Samson Thor Surg Soc, 1982.
11. Halasz NA, Collins GM, White FN. In Pegg D, Ed. Organ Preservation III. London, Churchill-Livingstone, p. 259, 1979.
12. Carter JN, White FN, Collins GM, et al. Transplantation 30:409, 1980.
13. Romolo JL, Aoiyan S, Halasz NA. Cryo Biology 8:407, 1971.
14. Blayo MC, Lecompte Y, Pocidalo JJ. Respir Physiol 42:287, 1980.
15. Swan H. J Extra-Corp Tech 17:65-73, 1985.
16. Follettee DM, Fey K, Livsey J, et al. Surgery 32:149-155, 1977.
17. Govier AV, Reves JG, McKay, et al. Anesthesiology 59:A70, 1983.
18. Govier AV, Reves JG, McKay RD et al. Ann Thor Surg 38:592, 1984.
19. Fox LS, Blackstone EH, Kirklin JW, et al. J Thorac Cardiovasc Surg 83:239-248, 1982.
20. Kirklin JW, Dushane JW, Patrick RT, Donald DD, Hetzel PS, Harshbarger HG, Wood EH. Proc Mayo Clin 30:201, 1955.
21. Kolkka R, Hilberman M. J Thorac Cardiovasc Surg 79:432, 1980.
22. Slogoff S, Girgis KV, Keats AS. Anesth Analg 61:903-911, 1982.
23. Stockard JJ, Bickford RG, Myers RR, et al. Stroke 5:730, 1974.
24. Ellis RJ, Wisniewski A, Potts R, et al. J Thorac Cardiovasc Surg 79:173, 1980.
25. Sotaniemi KA. J Neurol Neurosurg Psych 43:127, 1980.
26. Hickey RF, Hoar PF. J Thorac Cardiovasc Surg 86:903-906, 1983.
27. Nussmeier NA, Arlund C, Slogoff S. 64:165-170, 1986
28. Tinker JH, Ed. Cardiopulmonary Bypass: Current Concepts and Controversies. Saunders, Philadelphia, 1989.

ANESTHESIA FOR CAROTID ARTERY SURGERY

J. KATZ

INTRODUCTION

The only real indication for cartoid endarterectomy (CE) is to reduce the risk of future cerebral infarction. If the stroke rate from surgery approaches the incidence of stroke in the natural history of the disease, there is no benefit to the patient. Whereas it is widely held that the majority of ischemic events associated with CE are thromboembolic in origin, the preponderance of literature is aimed at diminishing the risk of stroke from low flow induced by carotid clamping during surgery. Despite this paradox, countless clinical studies exist which are contradictory as to necessity and best means of affecting cerebral protection by the use of intraoperative monitoring and internal shunts.

Recently Winslow, et al (1) tackled the issue of "appropriateness" of carotid endarterectomy. They concluded that 35% had CE for appropriate reasons, 32% for equivocal reasons and 32% for inappropriate reasons. Between 100,000 and 120,000 CEs are performed annually in the U.S.A. This raises the possibility that near 60,000 CEs are performed annually that have doubtful indications. In this study, 48% of patients undergoing CE had less than 50% stenosis of the carotid artery operated on. Yet, most surgeons require a minimum of 70% stenosis before surgery is considered. It has been claimed that carotid occlusive disease needs to reduce the lumen to 2 mm in diameter before blood flow is decreased. (2)

One area which has received consistent criticism is the

T. H. Stanley and R. J. Sperry (eds.), Anesthesiology and the Heart, 285–293.

performance of CE on patients with asymptomatic bruits. An estimated 35-50% of CEs fall into this group. The evidence that CE is beneficial in preventing strokes in this group is unconvincing. Indeed the perioperative stroke-death (combined) rate in asymptomatic patients is 5.3% which is double the 1-2% annual stroke rate in asymptomatic patients not coming to surgery. (3) The performance of "proplylactic" CE in asymptomatic patients seems ill-advised in view of the current experience.

Although stroke appears to be decreasing, it is still amongst the four leading causes of death in the U.S.A. It is estimated that 160 new strokes occur for every 100,000 population per annum. Although there are many other causes of stroke, 90% are based on atherosclerotic cerebrovascular disease.

Atherosclerotic disease is most frequently located at the carotid bifurcation, but it also occurs at the carotid siphon, and just proximal to the origin of the ophthalmic artery. Clinically, carotid occlusive disease presents in a number of ways; transient ischemic attaches (TIA), are transient focal, neurological deficits following ischemia less than 24 hours in duration; amaurosis fugax is temporary blindness resulting from transient obstruction and ischemia of the retina; a reversible neurological deficit (RIND) is a neurological deficit that persists for longer than 24 hours; a progressing stroke is a stepwise or gradual progressing neurological deficit; a slow stroke presents with weakness which changes to a deficit if the area is used or exercised, usually associated with severe stenosis, not occlusion; generalized cerebral ischemia is a general non-focal cerebral hypotension related to the erect position in patients with multiple occlusions of major extracranial vessels; and cerebral infarction (stroke) refers to an area of neuronal death which may be silent or present with deficits.

COMPLICATIONS

Complications associated with CE can be broadly divided into 2 groups: 1) Neurological 2) Non-neurological

1) Neurological. These deficits can be transient or

or permanent, and minor or major. In a previously neurologically intact patient, a permanent major deficit is devastating, hence the persistent efforts to detect and prevent ischemic events intraoperatively. Patients can also be left with various forms of migraine and a variety of seizure abnormalities. Any of the above neurological complications can occur because of ischemic stroke or intracerebral hemorrhage. Intraoperative embolization of plaque, fibrin, or air account for 1/3 of post-operative deficits. Post-operative internal artery occulusion also is a major cause of ischemic complication. Embolizations are related to soft thrombi in the internal carotid artery, and frequently occur prior to carotid clamping. Strokes in the distribution of the non-operative carotid could be associated with low flow or embolic phenomena. Low flow at the time of carotid clamping accounts for a small number of transient deficits. Most of the minor deficits and transient deficits are thought to reflect microembolization.

Hyperfusion in patients who have large increases in flow and perfusion following the procedure account for the epileptiform and migraine variant complications.

2) Non-neurological. In many studies myocardial infarction is a primary cause of mortality, followed by stroke. Myocardial infarction also can be responsible for low perfusion states which give rise to neurological deficits. The high rate of myocardial infarction is related to the type of patient rather than the procedure itself.

When the surgery involves a significantly larger segment of the internal carotid artery, mechanical injury to adjacent structures can occur. In one study from the Cleveland Clinic, (4) injuries to the recurrent laryngeal, hypoglossal, marginal mandibular, and superior laryngeal nerves were reported. Cricothyroid and thyroarytenoid dysfunction has also been reported. Facial nerve injury can occur when there is a high dissection and the trunk of the facial nerve is exposed. Hemorrhage from the carotid repair has occurred and carries with it the danger of airway compromise from pharyngeal swelling and difficulty with intubation. These are highly emergent cases when they occur.

Although rare, infections at the wound site can arise. These are more likely to occur if prophylactic antibiotics have not been used. Occasionally patients bleed into the wound while still in the recovery room and develop wound hematomas. These are commonly associated with aspirin. They respond well to platelet administration after surgical removal. Overall mortality from CE is in the region of 1-7% resulting mostly from new strokes or myocardial infarctions. In a recent series of articles appearing in Stroke (15:6, 1984) several neurologists raise concern over the results of the surgery compared to the risk of stroke without operation. They also point out a difference in outcome between CE done in large communities versus those done in major centers with an interest in carotid artery stenosis. This underscores the risk of this surgery and emphasizes the need for careful judgement and meticulous surgical technique. One study estimated a 10% nation wide morbidity-mortality rate from this operation. (5)

CONTROVERSIAL ISSUES

Surgery in the High Risk Patient

Some argument still persists over whether to operate on patients who are at high risk for complications or not. It stands to reason that those patients at high risk for neurological deficits also have the most to gain from CE. Dramatic improvements can be achieved in patients with crescendo TIA not controlled by anticoagulants, which are in direct contrast to prophylactic surgery in asymptomatic patients. There seems to be a generalized move towards more careful patient selection, and tighter control of the indications for surgery. Surgery for asymptomatic patients should decrease.

Monitor or No Monitor

A major neurological deficit in a previously intact patient is such a painful event that it seems logical to go to any lengths to prevent this complication. Current monitoring techniques include: surgery under local anesthesia, measuring carotid back (stump) pressures, intraoperative electroencephalography, and intraoperative cerebral blood flow measurements. Careful monitoring by experienced experts seems to be able to reduce the need for shunting which can change certain technical aspects of the surgery.

However, skeptics over monitoring abound. In 1984, Morawetz et al (6) found that complications were related more to preoperative risk category than to intraoperative EEG changes or low flow during clamping. In an editorial in Stroke in 1982, (7) Ferguson reviews the literature and concludes that "internal shunts are necessary to avoid intraoperative stroke in carotid endarterectomy, as the usual cause for such stroke is an embolus." Perhaps a policy of "selective monitoring" might add an element of rationality to an already emotional issue.

Shunt or No Shunt

Vast numbers of papers logically support either side of this argument. Skilled surgeons have reported excellent results both with or without shunts. There is no doubt that the presence of a shunt can in certain circumstances interfere with surgical access and technique. Also, shunts do not favorably affect the incidence of embolic complications. They do prevent low flow during carotid clamping. Since the majority of ischemic complications originate from embolic events, it is easy to decide against shunts. Ferguson (7) has claimed that "the best results have been reported by those who avoid shunts." Several surgeons, under the supposition that very few patients require shunting if the surgery is performed expediently under the added protection of general anesthetia, have elected to adopt a policy of selective shunting when they believe the risks are too great. Several reports have now emerged with a combined stroke morbidity mortality rate of around 1.5% using selective shunting.

Cerebral Protection

It is understood that because general anesthetics decrease brain activity, metabolism, and therefore oxygen demand, they afford the patient a certain measure of protection. However, the only agents which reliably provide additional focal protection from ischemia are the barbiturates. When used in doses large enough to impart protection, barbiturates also prolong anesthesia and severely depress the cardiovascular system, both of which are undesirable effects in CE. Furthermore, when effective barbiturates depress the electroencephalogram (EEG) to the level of burst suppression, EEG monitoring becomes worthless.

THE PATIENT

By far the majority of patients coming to surgery for CE, are in the older age group. Patients over 70 years old are considered to be at higher risk.

It is rare to find patients who have isolated cerebrovascular disease. Most frequently patients will have coexisting arterial disease such as ischemic heart disease, renal artery stenosis or generalized peripheral vascular disease. Thirty to fifty percent of patients will have had previous myocardial infarctions or established ischemic heart disease. It is not uncommon for patients to need a coronary artery bypass before CE is undertaken, or for bypass to be done during the same anesthetic as CE.

Fifty to seventy-five percent of patients needing CE have previous hypertension. These patients are reported to have increased morbidity after CE. A varying percentage of them will be on some antihypertensive medication which may or may not adequately control their blood pressure.

In addition to the above cardiovascular problems, 20% of patients will have diabetes and be on insulin or oral hypoglycemia agents.

Although it is thought that over 50% of patients needing CE smoke, only a half of these will also have some form of chronic obstructive lung disease.

It should be clear that these patients frequently present complex medical problems to the practicing anesthesiologist. Anesthetic technique should be carefully weighed, taking into account all the medical aspects and balancing the requirements for major vascular surgery. In major centers, anesthesiologists frequently give these patients a "cardiac anesthetic". Patients that have had a cerebral ischemic event in under 6 weeks prior to CE have a 20-fold increase in stroke rate following CE and every effort should be made to postpone surgery until CNS stability has been restored.

ANESTHETIC MANAGEMENT

Whatever the technique, it is essential to have the patient fully awake at the end of the procedure so that the surgeon can conduct a full neurological examination and detect deficits that require immediate re-operation. Anesthetic technique should also provide maximum cerebral protection, safe induction for cardiac patients, and a stable hemodynamic profile to ensure optimum cerebral blood flow. Also, anesthetic technique should be compatible with the technique of "selective shunting" which utilizes some measure of EEG to detect ischemia during cross-clamping and enables the surgeon to shunt only those that need it.

Since this is a relatively short procedure, harm could be caused by time consuming monitor placement. Although some patients may require a pulmonary artery catheter, the majority probably don't. Several studies have recently found no difference in outcome in coronary artery bypass performed with or without pulmonary artery catheters. (8)

Monitoring should include an ECG configuration which indicates left ventricular ischemia such as a V5 precordial lead. Blood pressure should be monitored with an indwelling arterial catheter to detect rapid changes. If appropriate, a central venous catheter provides a good indication of blood volume and is a good route for administration of vasoactive drugs. If selective shunting is performed a reliable monitor of EEG, stump pressure, or cerebral blood flow is necessary.

Although local anesthesia does provide the ultimate monitor of cerebral function, there is no reduction in cerebral oxygen demand and patients can develop profound anxiety, feelings of suffocation under the drapes, and have problems clearing airway secretions because of local anesthetic spread to the laryngeal nerve supply. This is especially difficult in patients with chronic obstructive lung disease. Most centers have opted for a well conducted general anesthetic with thorough monitoring.

The actual agents utilized are of considerably less importance than the maintenance of normal to slightly hypertensive blood pressure levels, adequate oxygen saturation, and normocarbia. The technique should provide good operating conditions, and allow rapid emergence and extubation.

In the post-operative period every effort should be made to control frequently labile blood pressures. Patients should be monitored intensively for the first 24 hours so that the onset of reversible neurological injuries can be readily detected and treated.

CONCLUSION

Carotid endarterectomy is probably an overdone operation according to current statistics. In experienced and expert hands with appropriate monitoring and selective shunting, the neurological deficit rate has been reduced to about 1.5%. This is considerably lower than the stroke rate in older patients with stenosis of greater than 70%. However, it is unlikely that patients with asymptomatic bruits really benefit from this procedure.

Anesthetic complications are rare, largely because these are sick patients and the level of vigilance and care is high. Future research will most likely be in the area of safe non-invasive monitoring for the detection and treatment of intra and post-operative ischemic events. It is tempting to speculate on whether the laser will ultimately offer a less invasive, but satisfactory method of reducing the degree of carotid stenosis without sending emboli towards the cerebral microvasculature.

REFERENCES

1. Winslow, C.M., Solomon, D.H., Chassin, M.R., et al. New England Journal of Medicine. 318:721-727, 1988.
2. Brice, J.G., Dowsett, D.J., Lowe, R.D. Lancet. 1:84-85, 1964.
3. Brott, T.G., Labutta, R.J. JAMA. 255:2609-2612, 1986.
4. Hertzer, N.R., Feldman, B.J., Beven, E.G., et al. Surgery, Gynecology, Obstetrics. 151:781-784, 1980.
5. Barrett, H.J.M., Plum, F., Walton, J.N. Stroke. 15:941-943, 1984.
6. Morawetz, R.B., Zeiger, H.E., McDowell, H.A., et al. Surgery. 96:184-189, 1984.
7. Ferguson, G.G. Stroke. 13:287-289, 1982.
8. Tuman, K.J., McCarthy, R.J., Spiess, B.D., et al. Anesthesiology. 70:199-206, 1989.

REGIONAL ANESTHESIA FOR PATIENTS WITH CARDIAC DISEASE

Benjamin G. Covino, Ph.D., M.D.

The choice of anesthesia for cardiac patients scheduled for non-cardiac surgery remains controversial. The frequency of perioperative complications is increased in surgical patients with cardiac disease. For example, approximately 6% of patients with a previous history of a myocardial infarction or significant coronary artery disease developed signs of myocardial injury during or following surgery and anesthesia. (1,2) The frequency of myocardial reinfarction during the perioperative period is related to the time interval between the previous infarct and exposure to surgery and anesthesia. The rate of reinfarction is reported to decrease from 27-37% in patients in whom myocardial infarction occurred within three months of surgery to 6% in patients who had an infarct six months or longer prior to surgery. (1,3) However, these studies provide little information concerning the relationship between various types of anesthesia, e.g., general or regional anesthesia, and the complications rate in patients with coronary artery disease.

<u>Hemodynamic Considerations in Patients with Ischemic Heart Disease</u>: The main concern in surgical patients with ischemic heart disease is the maintenance of adequate myocardial oxygen balance in order to prevent myocardial damage. Myocardial oxygen balance is the resultant of myocardial oxygen supply and utilization. (Fig. 1) Myocardial oxygen supply is determined by (1) the arterial oxygen content which, in turn, is a function of hemoglobin concentration, oxygen saturation, and hemoglobin dissociation curve (2) coronary blood flow (CBF). The determinants of CBF are coronary perfusion pressure (diastolic pressure-left ventricular end diastolic pressure), diastolic duration and coronary vascular resistance. Myocardial oxygen utilization is related to heart rate, myocardial contractility and systolic wall tension which, in turn, is a function of aortic pressure (afterload) and ventricular volume (preload).

T. H. Stanley and R. J. Sperry (eds.), Anesthesiology and the Heart, 295–304.

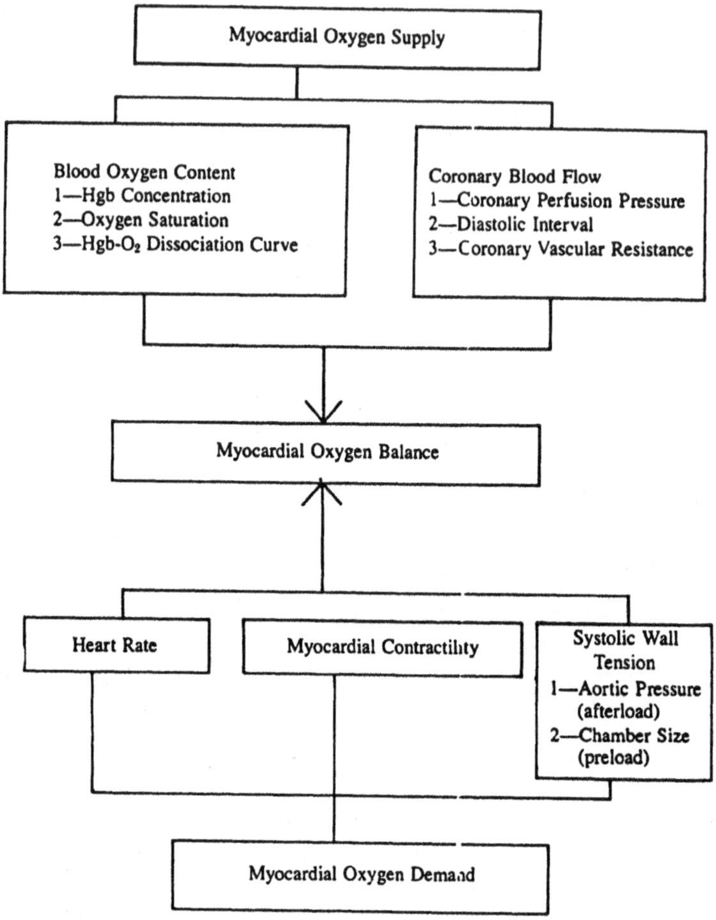

Fig. 1. **Determinants of Myocardial Oxygen Balance.**

Arterial oxygen content is usually well maintained during either general or regional anesthesia provided that the patient is not anemic, has no significant ventilation-perfusion abnormality and no factors exist which may adversely effect the hemoglobin dissociation curve. On the other hand, general and regional anesthesia can alter coronary blood flow, heart rate, myocardial contractility, afterload and preload. Decreases in coronary blood flow and increases in heart rate, contractility, afterload or preload may adversely effect myocardial oxygen balance in patients with ischemic heart disease.

Hemodynamic Effects of Regional Anesthesia: Epidural and spinal anesthesia are the regional anesthetic procedures that are most apt to cause significant hemodynamic alterations. Peripheral nerve blocks such as brachial plexus blockade are rarely associated with changes in cardiovascular function. Spinal anesthesia can profoundly effect the cardiovascular system. Sympathetic nerve fiber blockade is unavoidable during spinal anesthesia. The preganglionic sympathetic nerve fibers originate in the lateral horn of the spinal cord and exit via the ventral roots. Because of the distribution of local anesthetic solution during the conduct of spinal anesthesia, these fibers are blocked along with the other fibers in the ventral roots. The degree of sympathetic efferent denervation is often unpredictable and may be quite extensive during spinal anesthesia . It is generally assumed that the level of sympathetic blockade during spinal anesthesia exceeds the level of sensory anesthesia by two dermatomes. However, thermographic studies during spinal anesthesia have shown that elevated skin temperature (assumed to represent sympathetic blockade) occurred as much as six dermatomal levels higher than the somatic sensory block. These findings may explain the profound hypotension sometimes associated with relatively low spinal anesthesia.

The cardiovascular effects of spinal anesthesia are basically related to the extent of sympathetic blockade. (4) Levels of spinal anesthesia to T_5 cause minimal changes in pulse rate. Spinal anesthesia extending to the upper thoracic dermatomes can cause a decrease in heart rate. Bradycardia is due to blockade of the cardio-accelerator fibers and to diminished venous return. The cardio-accelerator fibers arise from the T_1-T_4 dermatomes. Levels of spinal anesthesia which include these dermatomes not only inhibit the cardiac accelerator nerves but also result in total preganglionic sympathetic blockade which produces venodilation and decreased venous return. The decrease venous return activates great vein and right atrial cardiac receptors which reflexly slow the heart.

Spinal anesthesia to the T_5 level was reported to decrease mean arterial blood pressure by 21.3 percent, while the decline in total peripheral resistance was only 5.0%. The hypotension seen with spinal anesthesia is clearly the result of a decrease in cardiac output (17.7%). The decline in cardiac output results from venodilation and decreased stroke volume (25.4%). It should be appreciated that all of these cardiovascular effects associated with spinal anesthesia are the direct result of preganglionic sympathetic blockade.

Sympathetic blockade also occurs following the establishment of epidural anesthesia. In most patients, cardiovascular changes are not very marked. On the other hand, profound hypotension may be observed in some patients following the onset of epidural anesthesia. The changes in blood pressure, heart rate and cardiac output are related to the level of blockade, the amount of drug administered, the specific local anesthetic agent employed, the inclusion of a vasoconstrictor in the anesthetic solution and the cardiovascular status of the patient. (5-7)

The dermatomal level of sympathetic blockade will determine the degree of hypotension following the epidural administration of local anesthetics. Blocks below T_5 are seldom associated with marked hypotension due to compensatory vasoconstriction in unblocked segments. Higher blocks will not only prevent compensatory vasoconstriction but also effect the cardiac sympathetic nerves which arise in the T_{1-4} segments. At these dermatomal levels of block, a fall in heart rate and cardiac output may occur. The blockade of sympathetic fibers to the heart and the failure to block the vagus nerves can cause vasovagal attacks which are associated with profound bradycardia and, in some patients, with transient cardiac arrest. This may represent the most common cause of profound hypotension following high levels of epidural anesthesia. The venous capacitance vessels will also be effected by the sympathetic block. Pooling can occur if the venous return is obstructed by gravity or a pregnant uterus. Thus, patients are very susceptible to the head-up posture, which causes expansion of the capacitance vessels and can lead to a marked decrease in venous return and cardiac output.

Relatively large amounts of local anesthetic drugs are required to achieve a satisfactory degree of epidural blockade. Local anesthetic agents are absorbed rather rapidly from the epidural space and may produce systemic effects involving the cardiovascular system. For example, it has been shown that blood levels of lidocaine greater than 4 $ug.ml^{-1}$ caused hypotension owing in part to the negative inotropic action of lidocaine and the peripheral vasodilator effect of this agent.

Differences in the onset of epidural anesthesia occur as a function of the specific agent employed. The more rapidly acting agents such as chloroprocaine and etidocaine tend to produce a more profound degree of hypotension due to the more rapid blockade of sympathetic fibers. In addition, certain agents such as etidocaine can penetrate myelinated fibers more readily and again may be associated with a more profound degree of sympathetic blockade and hypotension.

A more profound degree of hypotension may occur following the use of epinephrine-containing local anesthetics for epidural blockade. The absorbed epinephrine is believed to stimulate B_2-adrenergic receptors in peripheral vascular beds, leading to an enhanced state of vasodilation and a fall in diastolic pressure. The B_1 adrenergic receptor stimulating effect of epinephrine results in an increase in heart rate and cardiac output which will counteract the peripheral vasodilator state to some extent. Although absorbed epinephrine may be responsible for the early cardiovascular changes observed following epidural block, the more prolonged hypotension seen with local anaesthetics containing epinephrine is probably related to the achievement of a more profound degree of sympathetic blockade.

Cardiovascular depression is more severe and more dangerous following the production of epidural anesthesia in hypovolemic subjects. Epidural anesthesia in mildly hypovolemic volunteers was associated with profound hypotension and bradycardia. Hypovolemia is usually accompanied by compensatory vasoconstriction which will be abolished by the block and cardiovascular collapse may ensue. The addition of epinephrine to the anaesthetic solution may result in a less profound degree of hypotension in hypovolemic subjects. However, even the positive inotropic and chronotropic action of absorbed epinephrine cannot completely counteract the hypotensive effect of epidural blockade owing to the reduced circulating blood volume in these patients.

Since the sympathetic nervous system plays an important part in regulating regional blood flow, blockade of sympathetic nerve fibers during spinal or epidural anesthesia will alter the distribution of cardiac output. With regard to the coronary circulation, investigations in monkeys have shown that a T_{10} dermatomal level of anesthesia did not result in a significant change in coronary blood flow. High levels of epidural block (T_1) caused a 55% decrease in coronary blood flow. This decrease in coronary blood flow occurred concomitantly with a 47% decrease in mean arterial blood pressure. The decrease in myocardial work was greater than the decrease in coronary flow. The low coronary flows may be related in part to extensive

sympathetic block or to the peripheral vasodilator effect of lidocaine, both of which will cause systemic hypotension and decreased coronary perfusion.
Hemodynamic Effects of Central Neural Blockade in Cardiac Patients: The effect of lumbar epidural anesthesia extending to a T_6 - T_{10} dermatomal level on global and regional left ventricular function was evaluated in normal subjects and patients with stable effort-related angina. (8) (Table 1) Mean arterial pressure was significantly reduced to a similar extent in both groups without a concomitant change in heart rate. Cardiac index and stroke index also decreased to a similar degree in both groups. Left ventricular ejection fraction increased slightly but significantly in the angina patients. Studies of left ventricular wall motion revealed a lower number of hypokinetic sectors following epidural anesthesia in the angina patients as compared to the control state.

The effect of volume loading with 500ml of lactated Ringer's solution administered over 15 minutes was also evaluated following the establishment of the epidural block. After the increase in preload, mean arterial pressure and cardiac index returned toward the control baseline values in both groups. No change in heart rate occurred. In the angina patients, left ventricular ejection fraction decreased after volume expansion to the pre-anesthetic control level. The number of hypokinetic sectors also returned towards the baseline control level. The results suggest that lumbar epidural anesthesia which is confined to the mid thoracic area can result in an improvement in left ventricular global and regional function in patients with a history of stable mild angina provided that preload is not increased.

The effect of general and regional anesthesia on coronary hemodynamics in patients with ischemic heart disease has also been evaluated. (9) (Table 2) A comparison of neuroleptic anesthesia and thoracic epidural anesthesia combined with light general anesthesia in patients with a recent history of myocardial infarction scheduled for major abdominal surgery revealed significant differences in the two groups with regard to various hemodynamic parameters. A mean pulmonary artery occlusion pressure of greater than 18 mm Hg was observed in 73% of the neuroleptic anesthesia patients compared to 17% in the epidural group. A decrease in coronary vascular resistance of greater than 25% occurred in 59% of the neuroleptic anesthesia patients compared to 13% of the epidural patients. All of the neuroleptic anesthesia patients demonstrated an increase in myocardial oxygen consumption of greater than 25% compared to only one patient in the epidural group. Fifty percent of the neuroleptic anesthesia patients showed ST-T segment depression of

Table 1

Hemodynamic effect of epidural anesthesia before and after volume loading in normal and anginal patients

	H.R.	MAP	CARDIAC INDEX	LVEF	HYPOKINETIC SECTORS
A. Normal Patients					
Control	71 ± 3	101 ± 3	3.6 ± 0.2	64 ± 2	
Pre-Loading	72 ± 3	82 ± 4*	2.8 ± 0.2*	65 ± 3	
Post-Loading	73 ± 4	96 ± 3	3.2 ± 0.2	64 ± 3	
B. Anginal Patients					
Control	76 ± 4	101 ± 3	3.5 ± 0.2	54 ± 2	19
Pre-Loading	77 ± 4	79 ± 4*	2.8 ± 0.2*	59 ± 3*	5*
Post-Loading	75 ± 4	93 ± 3	3.2 ± 0.2	54 ± 2	11

*Significant
From Baron et al. Anesthesiology 66:621, 1987

Table 2

Percent of Patients with various cardiac changes during neuroleptic anesthesia (n=22) and epidural anesthesia (n=22)

Parameter	Neuroleptic Anesthetic	Epidural Anesthesia
Mean Pulmonary Wedge Pressure >18 torr	75	20
Decrease Coronary Vascular Resistance >25%	60	15
Increase Myocardial O_2 Consumption >25%	100	5
ST-T depression > 1mm	50	15
Ventricular Arrhythmias	35	10

From Reiz, S et al. Reg Anesth 7:58:S18, 1982

greater than 1 mm compared to 13% in the epidural group. Finally, ventricular arrhythmias developed intraoperatively in 36% of the neuroleptic anesthesia patients while only 8% of the epidural patients showed signs of ventricular arrhythmias. No difference in the frequency of perioperative myocardial infarction or one month postoperative mortality existed between the two groups. Two patients in the neuroleptic anesthesia group and one patient in the epidural group suffered an intraoperative myocardial infarct. In addition, three patients in the neuroleptic anesthesia group developed a myocardial infarction during the first postoperative week. Two patients in the neuroleptic anesthesia group and one patient in the epidural group died within the first postoperative month. The results of this study suggest that patients with diagnosed cardiac disease who undergo major non-cardiac surgery may develop more serious alterations in coronary hemodynamics and may be at greater risk in terms of myocardial ischemia and ventricular arrhythmias when a genral anesthetic rather than a regional anesthetic technique is employed.

Effect of Regional Anesthesia on Perioperative Morbidity in Cardiac Patients: Little difference in perioperative morbidity exists between various anesthetic techniques in relatively healthy patients scheduled for elective surgery. A number of morbidity and mortality studies have been carried out in geriatric patients who presumably have a certain degree of ischemic heart disease and who have undergone emergency surgery for repair of hip fractures. The comparative influence of general inhalational anesthesia and spinal anesthesia on post-operative survival rates has been controversial. In several studies, a lower mortality rate within the one month post-operative period was observed in patients in whom surgery was performed under spinal anesthesia compared to general anesthesia. Other studies have failed to report any difference in the early postoperative mortality figures between patients in whom either general or spinal anesthesia was employed. In addition, no difference has been observed in the number of deaths during a 1-2 year postoperative period in geriatric patients in whom emergency repair of a hip fracture was performed under general or spinal anesthesia.

Although regional anesthesia may not be associated with a significant decrease in long term post-operative mortality, post-surgical morbidity may be reduced in high risk patients in whom central neural blockade is employed. The influence of surgical epidural anesthesia and postoperative epidural analgesia on morbidity has been evaluated in a group of high risk surgical patients, many of whom presumably had ischemic heart disease. (10)

(Table 3) The rate of postoperative complications was significantly lower in those patients in whom epidural anesthesia and analgesia was employed compared to a similar group of high-risk surgical patients subjected to general anesthesia. The incidence of post-operative cardiac failure was also significantly lower in the epidural group. Perioperative myocardial infarction was diagnosed in three patients all of whom were in the general anesthesia group. In addition, four deaths occurred postoperatively, all of whom were in the general anesthesia group.

Table 3

Percent of patients with postoperative complications following general anesthesia (n=25) or epidural anesthesia (n=28)

Parameter	General Anesthesia	Epidural Anesthesia
Postoperative Mortality	16	0
Cardiovascular Failure	52	14
Major Infections	40	7
Total Complication rate	76	32

From Yeager MP et al. Anesthesiology 66:729-736, 1987

SUMMARY

The choice of anesthesia for non-cardiac surgical patients with ischemic heart disease requires a knowledge of the determinants of myocardial oxygen balance and the anesthetic factors which may alter these determinants. Regional anesthetic procedures such as spinal or epidural blockade can cause profound hemodynamic alterations due primarily to an inhibition of sympathetic nerve fibers. Epidural or spinal anesthesia which extends only to the mid-thoracic level is usually not associated with significant cardiovascular depression and may, in fact, improve cardiovascular function in patients with ischemic heart disease. In addition, epidural anesthesia may be less hazardous than general anesthesia in terms of coronary heart disease. Finally, postoperative morbidity may be lessened in high-risk surgical patients in whom epidural anesthesia and analgesia are employed.

REFERENCES

1. Topkins MJ, Artusio JF.: Anesth Analg 43:716-720, 1964.
2. Steen PH, Tinker JH, Tarhan S.: JAMA 239:2566-2570, 1978.
3. Tarhan S, Moffitt EA, Taylor WF, et al.: JAMA 220:1451-1454, 1972.
4. Ward RJ, Bonica JJ, Freund FG, et al.: JAMA 191:275-278, 1965.
5. Bonica JJ, Berges PV, Morikawa K.: Anesthesiology 33:619-620, 1970.
6. Bonica JJ, Akamatsu TJ, Berges PV, et al.: Anesthesiology 34:514-522, 1971.
7. Bonica JJ, Kennedy WF, Akamatsu TJ, et al.: Anesthesiology 36:219-227, 1972.
8. Baron JF, Coriat P, Mundler O et al.: Anesthesiology 66:621-627, 1987.
9. Reiz S, Balfors F, Bredgaard M, et al.: Reg Anesth 7:S8-S18, 1982.
10. Yeager MP, Glass DD, Noff RK, Brinck-Johnson T.: Anesthesiology 66:729-736, 1987.

ANESTHESIA FOR VASCULAR SURGERY*

Michael F. Roizen, M.D.

Goals of Anesthesia for Vascular Surgery

As in any surgical endeavor, the obvious goal in anesthesia for vascular surgical procedures is to minimize patient morbidity and maximize the surgical benefit. The anesthesiologist may, however, have a greater influence in reducing morbidity in vascular surgery, and perhaps in no other area has morbidity decreased so quickly, from a 6-day mortality rate of more than 25% for major aortic reconstruction in the mid-1960s to 1-2% today.

Despite the fact that the blood flow to many different organs is interrupted, that the stress of clamping and unclamping vessels is different in different operations, and that comorbid conditions of patients are dissimilar in different operations, the data presented here suggest that the heart should be the major focus of the anesthesiologist's attention, as myocardial dysfunction is the greatest cause of morbidity following surgery for cerebrovascular, visceral, or peripheral vascular insufficiency, or following aortic reconstruction for aneurysm.

Causes of Morbidity after Operations for Cerebrovascular Insufficiency

There are two types of operations for correction of cerebrovascular insufficiency: carotid endarterectomy and cerebral bypass. However, the extracranial-to-intracranial (EC-IC) bypass is not performed with even 1/100th the frequency of carotid endarterectomy. The results, morbidity, and mortality

---

* Much of this is taken from Roizen MF: Anesthesia for vascular surgery. Clinical Anesthesia. Barash PG, Cullen BF, Stoelting RK, eds. Philadelphia: Lippincott, 1989, with permission of the author.

T. H. Stanley and R. J. Sperry (eds.), Anesthesiology and the Heart, 305–346.

following carotid endarterectomy vary directly with the preoperative neurologic and cardiac status of patients. In a Mayo Clinic series,[1] those patients with "strokes in progress" or unstable neurologic status had a 2.5% rate of death from postoperative neurologic deficits, and 1% died of cardiovascular complications. Those patients with a history of coronary artery disease (CAD) had a 1.9% rate of deaths from myocardial ischemia. Since more patients in this large Mayo Clinic series had CAD than had unstable neurologic status, the greatest cause of morbidity and mortality following carotid endarterectomy was myocardial.

Table 1. Mortality after Carotid Endarterectomy

Senior Author	Year of Publication	No. of Patients Studied	% Patients with Serious Morbidity or Mortality from Cardiac Causes	Central Nervous System Causes
Sundt[1]	1981	1145	50	31
Hertzer[2]	1981	355	60	17
Ennix[3]	1979	1546	60	30
Burke[10]	1982	1141	67	33
Graham[11]	1986	105	100	0
Smith[12]	1988	60	0	100

In two other surgical series in which routine neurologic and cardiologic examinations were performed, Hertzer and Lees[2] found 60% of the deaths within 60 days of carotid endarterectomy to be due to myocardial dysfunction. Ennix and colleagues[3] reported an 0.8% rate of myocardial infarctions and a 1.1% rate of severe strokes in those patients without CAD symptoms, a 12.9% myocardial infarction rate and a 2.4% severe stroke rate in those patients with symptomatic CAD, and a 2.6% rate of myocardial infarctions and a 1.3% rate of severe strokes in patients with a history of CAD with prior or simultaneous coronary artery bypass grafting (CABG).

Age undoubtedly also plays a role in morbidity. Glaser[4] has shown a strong correlation between age and both myocardial and central nervous system (CNS) morbidity after carotid endarterectomy. Whereas Ennix *et al* [3] and others[5] have stressed the potential benefits of CABG prior to carotid endarterectomy or other surgical procedures, these studies to date show no significant reduction in mortality when the mortality due to the CABG is included in the overall mortality rate. Perhaps the reason for the reduced morbidity and mortality after carotid endarterectomy in patients who have undergone CABGs is that those patients at greatest risk experience myocardial and CNS morbidity and mortality during the first (the CABG) procedure. It may be that identification of high-risk patients by noninvasive tests, or better intraoperative monitoring and management of myocardial ischemia, will alter these results.

Patients with symptomatic carotid artery disease appear to be at as much as 17 times higher risk of stroke during coronary artery bypass grafting than are patients without carotid artery disease.[6] Such statistics have led to simultaneous carotid and coronary vascular procedures, with mortality and serious morbidity in the best series at about 10%.[7,8] However, patients with asymptomatic carotid stenosis do not have a higher stroke rate following coronary artery surgery than do those without carotid stenosis, but they do have a higher mortality after coronary artery surgery, mostly resulting from myocardial infarction.[9]

Thus, the morbidity and mortality statistics from virtually all series but our own surprisingly show that, even when a vessel to the brain is occluded, the major cause of morbidity and mortality after carotid endarterectomy is myocardial (Table 1).[1-4,9-12] Even in our own series, 34% of the patients evidenced myocardial ischemia intraoperatively, but none went on to suffer myocardial infarcts or death from myocardial events during their hospital stay.[12] Perhaps the reason for the difference between our results and the outcome in other published series is that we focus so much on the goal of decreasing myocardial insults, and on maintaining myocardial well-being perioperatively.

Causes of Morbidity after Operations for Visceral Ischemia, Thoracoabdominal Aneurysms, and Aortic Reconstruction for Aneurysm or Atherosclerotic Disease

The major cause of morbidity and mortality following these different procedures relates to the heart (Table 2).[13,14] Despite this common cause, distinct pathologic and physiologic patterns exist for the different diseases.

There are three distinct patterns of occlusive peripheral vascular disease:

Type I is isolated aortoiliac disease. This pattern of atherosclerosis is characterized by disease localized to the bifurcation of the aorta and the common iliac vessels. Despite the association of this disease with smoking, the atherosclerosis tends to be absent in coronary vessels, and to exhibit symptoms only of thigh and hip claudication. Type I disease is associated with a five-year survival rate of 90% following surgery.

Type II aortoiliac disease has a diffuse atherosclerotic pattern, often involving the coronary and cerebral circulation. As with Types I and III, smoking is common in this group of patients. Diabetes and hypertension are more common than in patients with Type I disease. The five-year survival rate following surgery is about 80%.

Type III, atherosclerotic peripheral vascular disease, involves femoral-popliteal and tibial atherosclerosis as well as small-vessel disease. The patients have a 60-65% five-year survival rate following surgery.[15,16]

Although the associated conditions and prognoses for these three types of occlusive peripheral vascular diseases differ, the mortality in most cases and the limiting factor in patient prognosis are the same and are related to the heart (Table 2).[17-32]

Table 2. Percentages of Perioperative Mortality Related to Cardiac Events

Aortic Reconstruction Series	Deaths/Total No. of Patients	% Mortality Caused by Cardiac Dysfunction
Szilagyi *et al*[17] (1966)	59/401	48
Young *et al*[18] (1977)	7/144	100
Hicks *et al*[19] (1975)	19/225	53
Thompson *et al*[20] (1975)	6/108	83
Mulcare *et al*[21] (1978)	14/140	79
Whittemore *et al*[22] (1980)	1/110	100
Crawford *et al*[23] (1981)	41/860	54
Hertzer[24] (1983)	22/523	64
Yeager *et al*[25] (1986)	4/97	100
Benefiel *et al*[26] (1986)	3/96	67

Adapted with permission from Roizen MF, Sohn YJ, Stoney RJ: Intraoperative management of the patient undergoing supraceliac aortic occlusion. Vascular Surgery. Wilson SE, Veith FJ, Hobson RW *et al*, eds. New York: McGraw Hill, 1986

Patients undergoing surgery for aneurysmal disease have higher perioperative morbidity and mortality by a factor of 2 and a lower median survival rate (5.8 years vs. 10.7 years) than do patients undergoing aortic reconstruction for occlusive disease.[33,34] Should patients, then, be exposed to surgery for asymptomatic aneurysms? This question was answered by Szilagyi *et al*[17] in 1966 for aneurysms more than 6 cm in diameter, when he showed that such surgery approximately doubled a patient's life expectancy. Since then, perioperative mortality rates have declined from 18 to 25% in the mid-1960s to 8 to 12% in the early 1970s, to 2 to 4% today. Consequently, even patients with abdominal aortic aneurysms less than 6 cm in diameter are considered candidates for aortic reconstructive surgery. This change is due to three factors: 1) the lessened morbidity of elective repair now versus that in the 1960s; 2) the higher mortality (45-90%) associated with emergency aortic reconstruction versus elective reconstruction; and 3) the lack of predictability as to which patients' aneurysms will enlarge and rupture (19% of aneurysms less than 6 cm in Szilagyi's series[17] resulted in death from rupture).[35-38]

Other causes of morbidity following vascular surgery include pulmonary infections, graft infections, renal insufficiency and failure, hepatic failure, and spinal cord ischemia resulting in paraplegia. The incidence rates of these other causes of morbidity has declined substantially over the last 20 years, with death from renal failure declining from 25% to less than 1% at present.[17,22,26,39] Much of the improvement toward elimination of renal failure has resulted from better perioperative fluid management.[40-44]

Thus, in patients undergoing vascular surgery, the major cause of morbidity, and the factor limiting both perioperative and long-term survival in almost every series, relates to the heart. For this reason, the anesthetist should concentrate on factors that prevent myocardial damage perioperatively in patients undergoing major vascular surgery, whether on the aorta or on the carotid, femoral, popliteal, or other vessels. This concentration on the heart should be kept in mind when decisions are made as to how to manage the patient's comorbid conditions such as hypertension, chronic obstructive lung disease, renal insufficiency, and/or diabetes.

The Patient and the Patient's Disorders

Many disorders are associated with vascular disease; however, diabetes, smoking and its sequelae, chronic pulmonary disease, hypertension, and ischemic heart disease are the most common. Perhaps the most important factor in planning the perioperative management of these comorbid conditions is to understand and to search for the end-organ effects of these diseases and to understand the appropriate drug therapy. Although it would be unusual to administer anesthesia to patients with uncontrolled hypertension, uncontrolled metabolic disease, or untreated pulmonary infections, or to patients within 3 to 6 months following a myocardial infarction when other portions of the myocardium are still at risk of infarct,[45,46] an expanding aneurysm, crescendo transient ischemic attacks (TIAs), or threatened limb loss can force one's hand. Attempts at rapid control of blood pressure or electrolytes may be more hazardous than leaving the condition untreated and trying to control the abnormality slowly. For example, rapid reduction of blood pressure in a patient with TIAs may precipitate cerebral ischemia and should be postponed to the postoperative period (assuming that surgery cannot be delayed to permit gradual preoperative control of blood pressure). Similarly, stopping a drug may be more hazardous than continuing drug therapy and being cognizant of its effects.

Specific attempts have been made to identify, prior to surgical operations, patients at risk of myocardial insult[5,46]; but until these procedures gain widespread acceptance, and until extensive trials are shown to reduce the overall mortality, the goal of optimizing care, with the specific focus on doing what is best to minimize myocardial morbidity, seems logical. This goal is based both on the preoperative likelihood, in patients with vascular disorders, of CAD and on the fact that the major cause of morbidity and mortality after vascular surgery is related to the heart.

Anesthetic Goals and Monitoring Techniques

For minimal morbidity and mortality, the anesthetic goals must be 1) to protect the heart from ischemia and 2) to protect the brain from ischemia. Other prominent anesthesiologists believe that the order of priority for these goals should be reversed.[47,48] However, the major cause of morbidity and the major effect that we as anesthesiologists can have strongly argue for protection of the heart to receive a higher priority than does brain protection in this operation. Unfortunately, the two goals are often in conflict.

To decrease myocardial oxygen requirements, one tries to decrease the heart rate and blood pressure and the contractility of the myocardium.[49] To maintain oxygen delivery to the brain, one tries to increase the cerebral perfusion pressure and to decrease the cerebral metabolic requirements. For increased cerebral perfusion pressure, an attempt is made to increase the arterial blood pressure at least to levels above which the normal brain autoregulates.[12,50,51] This usually also means trying to avoid severe bradycardia, or to decrease central venous pressure.

Not only the blood pressure reduction and augmentation but also the heart rate changes lead to conflicts in priority management between the well-being of the heart and that of the head. However, I believe that there are compromise solutions that allow both goals to be met. To decrease the myocardial work, one tries to decrease the heart rate; but sudden bradycardia can occur when the surgeon stretches the baroreceptor nerve endings directly (because of atherosclerosis, these nerve endings are supersensitive, since they usually have not been stretched easily by blood pressure changes over many years). This sudden bradycardia can result in substantial decreases in arterial pressure which could compromise collateral cerebral perfusion. Injection of the area of the bifurcation with 1% lidocaine 10 to 15 minutes before the carotid is to be occluded unites the two goals by allowing or facilitating a stable heart rate of approximately 70 beats $\cdot$ min^{-1}. In addition, the goals of decreasing myocardial contractility and decreasing the cerebral metabolic rate are consonant, regardless of whether thiopental or isoflurane is used as the major anesthetic.

To maintain blood pressure, we usually employ light anesthesia (without paralysis, so that inadequate anesthesia can be detected), allowing native vasopressor substances to maintain blood pressure. This light-anesthesia technique has been associated with a substantially lower incidence of myocardial ischemia than was possible with deeper anesthesia and administration of phenylephrine.[12] In fact, one of the major benefits of EEG or processed-EEG monitoring is that when the EEG is normal or unchanged from pre- to postclamping of the carotid, one can decrease the blood pressure to facilitate protection of the heart.

The hemodynamic and metabolic means for facilitating the goals of protecting the heart and brain from ischemia as previously described in theory should work in practice. It would be reassuring, however, to have monitors to make certain that these goals are actually being met. Unfortunately, the detection of both myocardial and cerebral ischemia by monitors during general or regional anesthesia is imperfect at present, with both false-negative and false-positive results confusing the technicians who do the monitoring.

Myocardial Ischemia

ST-T Segments of the EKG. Lead V_5 is usually selected. However, in a study that we performed, ST segments of even 7 leads of the electrocardiogram (ECG) did not enable us to detect 75% of the instances of myocardial ischemia detected by changes in regional wall motion and by wall-thickening defects on two-dimensional echocardiograms (2D-TEE).[52] In other vascular surgery, the ECG had a 40 to 60% sensitivity if systolic wall motion abnormalities (SWMA) and wall thickening abnormalities were considered the ultimate standard.[53] In addition, lead V_5 was insensitive compared to other leads (notably II) in detecting ischemia during carotid endarterectomy.

EKG Monitoring with ST-Segment Trend Analysis (2 or 3 Leads). Although devices are purported to facilitate easier detection of myocardial ischemia than can be obtained with simple oscilloscopic ECG traces, and although they might meet this stated goal,[53,54] they should not be expected to be as sensitive as an ECG printout, or 2D-TEE. In our preliminary study, they were approximately 70 to 90% as sensitive as a hard-copy ECG.[53]

Changes in Pulmonary Capillary Wedge Pressure (PCWP) or Appearance of V Waves on PCWP. Although changes in PCWP in the absence of systemic pressure changes or fluid administration may be a sensitive indicator of myocardial ischemia, such changes are not specific. The appearance of V waves on the PCWP may be specific (detection of ischemia where it is present), but V waves are not sensitive (normal where ischemia is not present) detectors of myocardial ischemia.[55] In addition, with the 2% carotid arterial puncture rate during cannulation of the internal jugular vein that has been reported in large series, it is difficult to justify that route during this operation. Most surgeons would postpone the operation to another day after disturbing the contralateral carotid. The risks of pulmonary artery (PA) catheter insertion from subclavian, external jugular, arm, or femoral sites do not justify the benefit. A PA catheter is not justified except in rare cases in which the patient is to undergo general anesthesia and the patient's only documented evidence of myocardial ischemia is that of PCWP changes without ST-segment changes, or in operations in which a 2D-TEE is unavailable or satisfactory echograms cannot be obtained.

Angina in Patients Undergoing Regional Anesthesia. No reports on the usefulness of this symptom are available, and the incidence of myocardial ischemia and death from myocardial mechanisms after carotid endarterectomy performed during regional anesthesia is similar to that following general anesthesia.[56]

Cerebral Ischemia

Repeated Neurologic Evaluation of the Conscious Patient. This evaluation is cited as a major reason for choosing regional anesthesia. If the patient is to cooperate, he or she cannot be heavily sedated. Regional anesthesia thus requires a completely successful blockade and a surgeon who is accustomed to operating under this condition. Usually, the carotid artery is occluded for a 1- to 4-minute trial period; if no deficit is detected by neurologic examination, the surgeon proceeds with the endarterectomy. If a new neurologic deficit occurs, the surgeon releases the clamp. After reperfusion with return of neurologic function, some surgeons immediately proceed to reocclude the vessels and try rapidly to insert a shunt and complete the surgical procedure. However, in my experience, most surgeons prefer to cancel surgery at this point and return on another day to do the procedure under general anesthesia with a shunt. Still other surgeons apparently consider the lack of tolerance for carotid occlusion to be a contraindication for any futher carotid surgery on such patients.[57] The disadvantages of the technique include the need for patient cooperation; the possible loss of patient cooperation with the onset of a neurologic deficit because of confusion, panic, or seizures; the possibility that an unexpected delayed deficit will develop at some time after the test period; the inability to administer drugs such as thiopental which might protect the brain; and the inability to secure the airway if panic, seizure, or oversedation occurs. Those surgeons who revert to general anesthesia in the event of a deficit in response to test occlusion seem to perceive general anesthesia as best for the worst cases; if this is so, as Dr. Michenfelder states, "it should be best for most cases."[57]

The techniques for assaying of neurologic function during general anesthesia include the following:

Electroencephalogram. The scalp-recorded EEG reflects the electrical activity of the underlying cortical tissue. Conventional recording methods provide vast amounts of information, including a voltage value at each instant in time for each pair (16 or more) of electrodes. However, the interpretation of this type of information is unwieldy in the operating room. Data reduction methods have been developed with which the EEG is described in terms of several calculated variables, and the changes in these variables are charted over time.

Various physiologic and anesthetic manipulations have effects on the EEG. Reductions in cerebral blood flow, temperature changes, hypotension, and the administration of anesthetic agents have been shown to have characteristic effects on the EEG. The proper interpretation of EEG changes at surgery depends on familiarity with the effects of the commonly used anesthetic agents and of temperature on the EEG. It should be remembered, however, that the blood flow threshold for electrical failure (approximately 18 ml $\cdot$ 100 $g^{-1} \cdot min^{-1}$) is higher than the blood flow threshold for metabolic failure (approximately 10 to 12 ml $\cdot$ 100 $g^{-1} \cdot min^{-1}$).[58]

The EEG can be viewed in a raw form, or it can be subjected to various transformations. For example, with the development of rapid computer transformation of the EEG by Fourier transform into spectral arrays of power and frequency, on-line assessment of the brain's electrical activity is made simpler.

Generally, if focal ischemia occurs, the usual change is a localized decrease in frequency or amplitude, or both.

How well does the EEG do as an early-warning signal of ischemia? How well does it do in improving the outcome after carotid endarterectomy? These are quite different questions. The EEG is a sensitive early-warning device, but it is not very specific (too many false-positive results), and we have no idea whether outcome is improved by its use. However, myocardial well-being may be improved more than cerebral well-being.

In the Mayo Clinic series of 1145 carotid endarterectomies that were monitored with EEG and xenon blood flow measurements, no patient awoke from anesthesia with a new deficit that had not been predicted by the EEG. An analysis of the results of a series of 111 carotid endarterectomies monitored with a single channel of the EEG that was analyzed in real time to produce a density spectral array[59] revealed that, among patients with no preoperative neurologic deficit, new postoperative deficits appeared in only the 5 patients who had ischemic EEG events of 5 or more minutes' duration. However, the EEG was not as predictive of outcome in patients who had an existing preoperative neurologic deficit. One such patient without intraoperative EEG changes developed a new postoperative deficit, and one patient with EEG changes lasting 13 minutes had no demonstrable new deficit postoperatively.

The need for caution when patients with pre-existing neurologic deficits are monitored was emphasized in a report of 125 patients who had had strokes or reversible ischemic neurologic deficits (RIND) and who underwent carotid endarterectomy.[60] Four patients in that study awoke with new deficits, despite unchanged EEGs.

In a study of a series of 172 carotid endarterectomies,[61] EEG monitoring was undertaken only in the last 93 cases. The use of EEG monitoring was associated with a reduction in the use of indwelling shunts (from 49% to 12%) and a reduction of the combined major neurologic morbidity and mortality (from 2.3% to 1.1%). However, this study suffers from the use of historic controls and non-randomization.

Other investigators have shown that EEG monitoring may be of limited use, because 65 to 95% of neurologic deficits following carotid endarterectomy are due to thromboembolic and not to flow-related events. Although both can easily be detected with the EEG, no major benefit will be achieved from any therapeutic maneuver to the 65 to 95% of patients in whom neurologic problems are detected.

In fact, if more shunts or a higher afterload result, more emboli or worsening of myocardial oxygen balance could ensue. For example, one group[62] reviewed its experience with 176 consecutive patients undergoing carotid endarterectomy without shunt, but with EEG monitoring. The authors concluded that, although the majority of clamp-associated EEG changes were related to lowered regional cerebral blood flow (CBF), postoperative deficits in their series were usually caused by embolism. Other studies have yielded similar results.[63,64]

Other issues which have been raised in the evaluation of the appropriateness of EEG monitoring for carotid endarterectomy include the false-positive and false-negative results and the cost-effectiveness of EEG monitoring. Intraoperative false-positive results, that is, changes in the EEG without accompanying demonstrable deficits, may be related to several factors. First, the brain can tolerate relatively brief periods of ischemia without infarction. Thus, temporary, reversible EEG changes should not be expected in association with postoperative deficits. Second, the EEG must be viewed as a sensitive, but non-specific measure of ischemia. The EEG can be affected by factors such as anesthesia or alterations in temperature and blood pressure in addition to cerebral ischemia. Third, as stated previously, the flow threshold for electrical failure is higher than the flow threshold for metabolic failure. This means that, whereas the EEG may be viewed as an "early-warning system" for cerebral ischemia, not all EEG changes indicate that ischemia is taking place. Fourth, focal embolic events may not be detected by EEG. Except as noted previously, i.e., in patients with pre-existing neurologic deficits, strokes in evolution, or recent RINDs, there are relatively few reports of false-negative results.

In general, patients who do not show intraoperative EEG changes do not awaken with new neurologic deficits. Since most neurologic deficits after carotid endarterectomy are not the result of flow-related ischemia, detection of EEG changes does not guarantee reversibility upon shunt placement. In fact, shunt placement is associated with a low, but definite risk of causing emboli.

The evaluation of the cost-effectiveness of EEG monitoring can be thought of as a comparison of the cost of monitoring with the cost of the deficits that monitoring may prevent. Let us assume that 100,000 carotid endarterectomies are performed each year, with a deficit rate of 3% (3000 new deficits each year), and that use of monitoring devices might prevent one-sixth of these deficits (i.e., 500 deficits per year). One might assume that an additional 15% of patients would receive temporary shunting of their carotid flow because of EEG monitoring and that 0.7%

would experience "shunt insertion-associated" neurologic deficits. This would result in an additional 106 deficits related to the monitoring, or a net 394 deficits preventable by the monitoring. If each deficit costs $100,000, on average, in medical care and loss of wages and productivity, then the deficits preventable by monitoring cost $39,400,000 per year. The break-even point for monitoring costs would be $394 per patient; at that price, the cost of monitoring would equal the cost of the deficits that monitoring would prevent. If monitoring could be provided for less than $394, it would be cost-effective. This analysis neglects the benefit that EEG monitoring may have in preserving myocardial function. It also neglects factors to which no dollar amount can be assigned, such as human suffering. If different values are assumed for the cost per deficit, for the percentage of deficits preventable by monitoring, and for the deficit rate, or for the shunt insertion-caused deficit rate, the break-even point will be higher or lower. But, as long as the percentage of deficits preventable by EEG monitoring is not zero, the break-even point will also not be zero; this implies that there is some cost below which monitoring is cost-effective for large-scale application, assuming that EEG monitoring is better at prevention than are other strategies of monitoring, such as somatosensory evoked potentials (SSEP) or stump pressure.

However, it is entirely possible that EEG monitoring would allow the anesthesiologist to maintain a lower blood pressure during the period of temporary carotid occlusion than would be feasible if only stump pressure were used. Thus, perhaps EEG monitoring provides a benefit in allowing one to decrease the afterload in the patient who is at risk for myocardial ischemic events, as well as permitting an unhurried and technically superior endarterectomy, identifying delayed ischemia, and aiding in the detection of other problems such as shunt malfunction.

Unfortunately, there are no data showing that this method of detection of neurologic dysfunction during carotid endarterectomy results in a better patient outcome than does any other method.

Somatosensory Evoked Potential. Evoked potentials offer a method of processing the neural activity after a stimulus in which activity that is stimulus-related (signal) is separated from activity that is not related to the stimulus (noise). The primary problem with evoked potentials is an unfavorable signal-to-noise ratio. The neural potentials evoked by any sensory stimulus are small compared with the spontaneous activity that is recorded at the same time. When recorded noninvasively from the scalp, evoked cerebral electrical activity (the signal) from electrical stimulation of a peripheral nerve amounts to a few microvolts in amplitude, whereas the spontaneous electrical activity (noise) of the cerebrum can be of the order of 100 or more microvolts. The assumption made for separation of the signal from the noise is that the signal is always found after a certain latency period following the stimulation, whereas the noise bears no temporal relationship to the stimulus. By giving repeated stimuli and summing (or averaging) the resulting responses, one can "average out" the noise.

The most frequently used evoked potential during vascular procedures is the somatosensory evoked potential (SSEP). This evoked potential is usually elicited by electrical stimulation of a selected peripheral nerve at an intensity sufficient to cause a twitch of the muscles supplied by that nerve. The resulting afferent activity may be recorded from rostral portions of the nerve, the spinal cord and brainstem, and thalamocortical projections. The variables that describe evoked potentials are the latency (related to the conduction velocity characteristics of the pathway) and the amplitude (related to the number and synchrony of conducting fibers in the pathway) of the afferent volley recorded at successively higher levels of the nervous system. It has been observed that damage to the pathways mediating these responses is manifested as alterations in these two variables.[64]

Recently, investigators have started to examine the SSEP as a monitor of neurologic function during carotid endarterectomy. A case report on a 69-year-old woman undergoing carotid endarterectomy under general anesthesia without a shunt of the carotid flow is an example.[65] The median nerve was stimulated, and the resulting afferent activity was recorded from a cervical spinous process and from the scalp over the cortical somatosensory receiving area in the parietal cortex. The cortical evoked potential disappeared immediately after carotid cross-clamping, but the potential recorded from the nape of the neck was preserved. Immediately after awakening from anesthesia, the patient was noted to have a paresis and hypesthesia of the contralateral arm, but this effect cleared over the next 24 hours.

A series of 25 carotid endarterectomies was performed under general anesthesia without the use of an intraluminal shunt and with SSEP monitoring.[66] Two patients had no electrical response, one bilaterally and the other unilaterally, following carotid cross-clamping. The patient with the unilateral changes developed a perioperative stroke, the only one that occurred in that series.

Authors who have monitored the SSEP during carotid endarterectomy with both cervical-plexus block and general anesthesia reported, without providing critical evidence, that the SSEP is a sensitive measure of cerebral ischemia and of the need for a shunt.[67,68] The rate of shunt placement based on SSEP was roughly the same as that when selective shunting was based on the EEG, i.e., about 10%. However, the fact that the patients in this series had no complications upon awakening limits the conclusions that can be drawn concerning the predictive value of the SSEP in patients undergoing carotid endarterectomy.

Thus, the benefit of SSEP in monitoring of neurologic function during carotid endarterectomy is even more conjectural than is the role of EEG monitoring.

Regional Cerebral Blood Flow. Measurement of regional CBF usually involves washout of a radioisotope such as xenon-133 after its injection into a surgically occluded carotid artery.[1] Flows above 24 ml $\cdot$ min^{-1} $\cdot$ 100 g^{-1} brain are regarded as satisfactory, and those below 18 ml $\cdot$ min^{-1} $\cdot$ 100 g^{-1} brain are considered to indicate the potential for cerebral ischemia. These measurements require expensive and highly technical equipment in the operating room. Of the few centers that have such equipment, one has reported an excellent correlation between cerebral blood flow and outcome, but flow differences representing ischemia were dependent on the anesthetic agents used.[1,69] Questions about this method of monitoring involve both its sensitivity and its specificity. As with all of the other monitors of neurologic function during carotid endarterectomy, no benefit has yet been shown for it.

Carotid Stump Pressure. Stump pressure (mean blood pressure distal to the carotid clamp, also sometimes called back pressure) is widely used for evaluation of the adequacy of cerebral perfusion during carotid surgery. Cerebral ischemia will rarely occur at stump pressures above 60 mmHg during halothane anesthesia, presumably because of the excellent collateral circulation required for maintaining that pressure,[57,70] and presumably due to the autoregulation that is present at this level. If the stump pressure decreases below that value, the likelihood of ischemia increases. However, since pressure is not identical to flow, it is possible for stump pressures to be below 60 mmHg and for the flow to be perfectly adequate.

The major criticism of the use of stump pressure concerns the large number of false-positive results–that is, a stump pressure of less than 60 mmHg and a regional CBF of more than 24 ml $\cdot$ min^{-1} $\cdot$ 100 g^{-1} brain. Such results occur in about 30% of patients.[70] Thus, a shunt may be placed when none is needed. However, the simplicity of the measurement and its validity when the pressure exceeds 60 mmHg during anesthesia with volatile anesthetics still render it the most useful clinical method for ensuring adequate perfusion during carotid endarterectomy. The stump pressure must be higher during an opioid-based anesthesia for blood flow to be adequate.[70]

As with all other measures, no benefit has been proved for the use of stump pressure, but logic dictates that monitors that ensure adequate cerebral function at the lowest myocardial work have a role during carotid endarterectomy.

Anesthesia for Surgery for Cerebrovascular Insufficiency

Many surgeons have requested general anesthesia in surgery for patients with cerebrovascular insufficiency. If the patient has no medical problem that requires optimization before surgery, the preoperative interview focuses on reducing anxiety, obtaining informed consent, and searching for the status of end-organs likely to be affected by atherosclerosis, hypertension, or other diseases. In addition, multiple blood pressure and heart rate readings are obtained while the patient is in various positions, and the nurses are asked to obtain at least four additional such readings (one every 2 hours while the patient is awake, and one during the night) before surgery.

The preoperative values become important in defining a window of acceptable intraoperative values. To elaborate, such preoperative data are used to determine the individualized range of values considered tolerable for a particular patient during and after surgery; that is, if the blood pressure is 180/100 mmHg and the heart rate 96 beats · min^{-1} on admission, with no signs or symptoms of myocardial ischemia, the patient can probably tolerate these levels during surgery. If the blood pressure decreases during the night to 80/50 mmHg and the heart rate decreases to 48 beats · min^{-1} and the patient does not awaken with signs of a new cerebral deficit, he or she can probably safely tolerate such levels during anesthesia. Thus, from preoperative data, an individualized set of values is derived for each patient. The cardiovascular variables are then kept within that range and, prior to induction of anesthesia, one should decide which therapies to use to accomplish that goal (e.g., administration of more or less anesthesia, nitroglycerin, or nitroprusside/dopamine, dobutamine, phenylephrine, or propranolol/esmolol/isoproterenol, atropine)

This type of planning is especially important for the patient who has suspected cardiovascular disease, such as is usual in the patient undergoing carotid endarterectomy. It is relatively unimportant for the totally healthy patient. It is unknown whether keeping cardiovascular variables within an individualized range of acceptable values improves the surgical outcome, but logic implies that using such a plan would reduce morbidity. For example, in several studies, major intraoperative deviations of the blood pressure from the preoperative level have been correlated with the occurrence of myocardial ischemia.[12,14,71]

These acceptable values are listed at the top of the anesthesia record prior to induction of anesthesia. Prior to working with surgeons who routinely use the EEG, I worked with surgeons who wanted the patient's blood pressure to be at the upper end of his ward pressure. This desire on the part of the surgeons was based on data indicating better collateral CBF distal to a carotid occlusion if the systemic blood pressure was higher.[51] On the other hand, such an increase in blood pressure increases the work the heart has to perform; thus it increases the likelihood of myocardial ischemia.[12,48] If the surgeon requires an increase in the patient's blood pressure above his or her ward upper limits of normal, as is sometimes required for a patient whose carotid flow cannot be shunted because of the anatomy of his lesion, we do so in a test period preoperatively, asking questions about angina and examining seven ECG leads for evidence of ischemia. Only rarely (2 of the approximately 1500 patients to whom I have administered anesthesia for carotid artery surgery) in patients in whom myocardial ischemia is evidenced by PCWP changes without ECG changes will we use a PA catheter during carotid surgery. I have tried to avoid inserting PA catheters during carotid artery surgery for two reasons: 1) There is little fluid shift during these operations, and 2) the rate of complications associated with PA catheters is reported to exceed that from carotid artery surgery at our institution.

Other data obtained during the preoperative visit and assessment are which ECG lead is most likely to reveal ischemia (often found on an exercise ECG study or from evaluation of a thallium redistribution study) and what is the patient's normal $PaCO_2$ level. Usually, the latter can be assumed to be normal if the patient's bicarbonate level on an electrolyte panel is normal, or if the patient does not have a history suggestive of chronic obstructive pulmonary disease.

There is controversy concerning the optimum intraoperative carbon dioxide level in patients undergoing carotid endarterectomy.[51] Most practitioners now opt for slight hypocarbia or normocarbia.[47,51] The maintenance of slight hypocarbia has the possible advantage of preferentially diverting CBF to potentially ischemic areas of the brain by constricting the non-ischemic, normally reactive vessel.[47]

Historically, we have not given any premedication to patients about to undergo carotid artery surgery, because this might delay awakening and might confuse the results of tests of mental function prior to induction of anesthesia. Although we worried about the possibility of increasing anxiety[72] and causing myocardial ischemia because of this lack of premedication, only one patient among the 1500 whom we "premedicated" with only an interview for this operation has arrived in the preoperative holding area or operating room with angina or ECG evidence of myocardial ischemia. Either the preoperative interview is very effective[72] or there is a substantial difference between our patients and those of Slogoff and Keats.[71]

Thus, local custom as well as logical considerations have biased us in our treatment of such patients to seek the following goals with the techniques indicated:

1. Avoid myocardial ischemia by maintaining normal hemodynamics (especially normal heart rates). For this purpose, we usually monitor lead V_5 and lead II of the ECG for ST-T and heart rate changes and the transesophageal echocardiogram for wall-motion and systolic wall-thickening abnormalities.

2. Avoid cerebral ischemia by maintaining normal or high-normal blood pressure, and by shunting carotid flow if an abnormal EEG develops; maintain slight hypocarbia.

3. Use general anesthesia, but have the patient awake at the end of the operation. To accomplish this, we avoid drug premedication and "premedicate" only by interview, and we use light levels of volatile agents for general anesthesia.

4. Delay operations when there is uncontrolled hypertension, untreated pulmonary disease, myocardial infarction less than 3 months old with areas of myocardium still at risk, and uncontrolled metabolic diseases, unless crescendo TIAs are present.

Obviously, some goals are in conflict and have been modified by study results. For example, we could provide deeper anesthesia and maintain blood pressure with an alpha $_1$-adrenergic drug such as phenylephrine. However, we found that "light" general anesthesia and the maintenance of the same systolic pressure is associated with one-third the incidence of myocardial ischemia compared with that of "deep" anesthesia and the use of vasopressors to attain that blood pressure.[12] The usual procedure is as follows:

After the preoperative interview, the patient is made NPO after midnight, and an IV infusion is begun through an 18-gauge plastic cannula, (D_5 0.45 NS) at a maintenance rate of $100\ ml \cdot hr^{-1} \cdot 70\ kg^{-1}$. This fluid administration is intended to ensure that the patient is not hypovolemic and thus subject to a large decrease in blood pressure during induction of anesthesia. When the patient arrives in the preoperative holding area, the IV solution is changed to normal saline and an 18-gauge arterial catheter is placed (after iodine prep and lidocaine skin wheal) in the radial artery contralateral to the planned carotid surgery. This arterial catheter is 18-rather than 20-gauge because no greater morbidity ensues[73] and because the 20-gauge catheter tends to have a 5 to 10% incidence of kinking when surgeons "push" on the arm (with their bellies) during carotid dissection. Normal saline, rather than dextrose or lactated Ringer's solution, is used because lactate is metabolized to dextrose and because recent animal studies indicated that increasing blood glucose may increase neurologic damage after global ischemia.[74] Although some different results have been found for focal CNS ischemia in at least one laboratory (Pearl *et al*, as presented at the meeting of the Association of University Anesthesiologists, Portland, Oregon, May 1987), and some investigators may say that survival is better with fructose than with saline,[75] the most prudent approach at this time seems to be to maintain normoglycemia.

The patient is then brought to the operating room and transferred to an operating table with an already warmed heating mattress. Here, EEG, ECG, blood pressure measurement, pulse oximetry, and other standard monitoring methods are applied and the data are examined prior to induction of anesthesia. The heating mattress[76] is important for maintaining normothermia, which probably helps to reduce circulatory instability postoperatively.

Induction of anesthesia is then begun with a barbiturate. Some anesthesiologists titrate the dose at this time and during carotid occlusion to achieve burst suppression on the EEG,[47] because this electrical suppression is associated with a reduction of cerebral metabolism to as little as 40 to 50% of awake levels and, at the same time, decreases the CBF and intracranial pressure. Once burst suppression occurs, barbiturates have no further cerebral metabolic effect, or any effect in protecting the brain from ischemia.[77] We administer 100% oxygen, and 1-2 $mg \cdot kg^{-1}$ of thiopental and 3 mg of curare, followed by thiopental 25 to 50 mg (70 kg patient) intravenously, along with isoflurane at increasing concentrations in oxygen by mask. When the systolic blood pressure has been reduced by 20-30%, we administer 1.5 $mg \cdot kg^{-1}$ succinylcholine (assuming the patient has no muscle or lower motor neuron [LMN] dysfunction), or atracurium or vecuronium or nothing if muscle or LMN dysfunction is present, and either 100 mg of lidocaine or 100 mg of thiopental (each given IV) to blunt the cardiovascular (blood pressure and heart rate) response to laryngoscopy and tracheal intubation. After the routine checks and after verification of endotracheal intubation by end-tidal capnography, a transesophageal echocardiographic probe is inserted to obtain echocardiographic images of a cross section of the left ventricle at the level of the papillary muscles.

Controlled ventilation of the lungs is instituted at this time, often with 50% nitrous oxide in oxygen, and at other times with oxygen alone, titrating the concentration of isoflurane or enflurane, and adjusting the table position, to achieve the desired blood pressure. We avoid administering more than 10 ml · kg^{-1} of crystalloid or other fluid in this 2-hour operation, because increasing the fluid administration to these patients may contribute to postoperative hypertension. This results from the absence of baroreceptor function, which such patients usually exhibit.[78] The lack of baroreceptor function may also account for the stability that we find in these patients' heart rates intraoperatively.[12]

During the operation, "light" anesthesia is usually administered, with patient movement as well as hemodynamic changes signaling that the anesthesia is inadequate. If we cannot ensure that the patient will be anesthetized sufficiently so that he will not move during the period of temporary carotid occlusion, a muscle relaxant is added, the choice of which is dictated by the heart rate response we wish to obtain.

Although the effects of anesthetics on normal CBF are known, the choice of an anesthetic for this operation appears to have no sound scientific basis. Perhaps the only information suggesting that one should choose isoflurane over other inhalational agents or opioids is that from a nonrandomized study at the Mayo Clinic[69]; it was evident that the CBF associated with ischemic changes in the EEG is 10 ml · min^{-1} · 100 g^{-1} during isoflurane anesthesia, as opposed to about 20 ml min^{-1} · 100 g^{-1} with other agents, and that there is a less frequent need to shunt during isoflurane anesthesia than is the case during anesthesia with other agents.

Our preference to avoid opioids in these operations is based on our ability to have patients awaken shortly after the last stitch is placed (although this may now be possible with alfentanil), and on the desire to avoid the hemodynamic effects of naloxone and of muscle relaxant reversal, not on the anecdotal evidence that opioids worsen the neurologic outcome after focal or global cerebral ischemia.[79]

Before beginning carotid occlusion, the surgeon infiltrates the carotid at the bifurcation with 1% lidocaine, with the hope of preventing the sudden onset of bradycardia during stretching of the baroreceptor or of the nerve from the baroreceptor. The anesthetic depth is kept at a minimum, so that the blood pressure increases to the upper ward level. If no EEG evidence of ischemia is found, or if the stump pressure is comfortably above 50 mmHg, the anesthetic depth is increased somewhat and the systemic blood pressure falls slightly. If myocardial ischemia is indicated by one of our monitors, we treat it by reversing the hemodynamic cause, if any, or by administering nitroglycerin when no obvious hemodynamic cause exists. Such myocardial ischemia occurred between 8 and 35% of the time at this point in the operation in our studies[12]; we do not know the cause of this event at this time, because the hemodynamics did not differ substantially from that just prior to cross-clamping.

After the carotid artery repair is completed and the flow in the carotid is restored, the focus again shifts totally to the patient's myocardial well-being. When the muscle layer is repaired, the patient is allowed to resume spontaneous ventilation. Usually, the surgeons identify the recurrent laryngeal nerve, and this enables us to extubate the trachea in as light a plane of anesthesia as possible, but before the gag reflex is restored. Usually within 2-3 minutes after the last stitch, the patient will respond to pain, and, before leaving the operating room (and usually within 4-6 minutes after the last stitch), the patient is able to follow simple commands.

The four problems feared most in the recovery room are hemodynamic instability, respiratory insufficiency (usually as a result of vocal cord paresis), hematoma formation, and onset of new neurologic dysfunction.

Circulatory instability is usually evidenced by hypertension, but it is reported in the literature that hypotension also occurs. Since we began hydrating patients starting the night before surgery, giving antihypertensives, including diuretics on the morning of surgery, using a heating blanket to help maintain temperature, and limiting our intraoperative administration of crystalloid to 10 ml $\cdot$ kg^{-1}, the incidence of postoperative hypotension has dropped to zero, and the incidence of postoperative hypertension has decreased to about 10% (from 35%). Although this change is based on historical controls and is anecdotal, any hypertension needs vigorous treatment so that the myocardial work is decreased. We often titrate combinations of nitroprusside or hydralazine and propranolol or esmolol or labetalol to achieve normotension. Such therapies have been found superior to administration of nitroglycerin or trimethaphan in an elegant study on post-CABG patients by Stinson *et al*.[80] Other causes of hypertension are sought (pain, a full bladder, myocardial ischemia, hypoxia, hypercarbia). However, the association of hypertension and neurologic deficit postoperatively is too strong (assuming that the patient is neurologically normal) to allow one to let the hypertension persist.[81]

Other authors have stated that hypotension following carotid endarterectomy is due to hypersensitivity of the carotid sinus nerve,[82] but we have found that significant hypotension (< 80 mmHg systolic) often is associated with myocardial ischemia. We routinely obtain a 12-lead ECG shortly after the patient's arrival in the recovery room, and we monitor the ECG lead(s) most noted or likely to detect ischemia in these patients, which often proves to be lead II following carotid surgery (not lead V_5).[52]

Ventilatory insufficiency can appear as stridor owing to unilateral or, more often, bilateral vocal cord paresis (in the patient who has undergone bilateral carotid operations, or a thyroidectomy and a carotid operation), to hematoma, or to deficient carotid-body function in patients who are chronic CO_2 retainers. In the case of stridor, immediate securing of the airway is necessary; treatment of hematomas can consist of opening of the suture line and application of external drainage. (This may need to be done even in the recovery room. I have been involved in only one of each of the two previously mentioned procedures in 1500 anesthetics for carotid artery surgery that I have given.) The chemoreceptor function of the carotid body is predictably damaged for up to 10 months following carotid endarterectomy, with complete loss of the ventilatory and circulatory response to hypoxia following bilateral endarterectomy.[78] Such loss results in an increase in the $PaCO_2$ of 6 mmHg at rest, and for this reason the routine use of supplemental oxygen is justified, at least until the patient ambulates.

Wound hematoma from venous oozing usually accumulates slowly, but both it and arterial hemorrhage can threaten the airway. This is probably the most painful part of most carotid operations (pain relief stronger than that provided by acetaminophen is usually not required for most patients). Reexploration in the operating room is occasionally necessary, but rapid opening of the wound in the recovery room can be life-saving in an emergency.

Anesthetic Goals in Surgery for Aortic and Visceral Artery Reconstruction

For minimal morbidity and mortality, the anesthetic goals are to preserve myocardial, renal, pulmonary, CNS, and visceral organ function. To meet these goals, one must ensure an adequate oxygen supply to the myocardium commensurate with need, at the same time reducing, if possible, the myocardial requirement for oxygen, and maintain adequate perfusion to all other organs. This latter objective usually requires preservation of adequate intravascular volume so that cardiac output can be maintained.

Pathophysiologic Events

To better understand the monitors that are used and why they are used, it is helpful to be aware of the pathophysiologic events that occur on application and removal of aortic cross-clamps.

Occlusion of the aorta causes hypertension in the proximal segment and hypotension in the distal segment. During resection of a congenitally coarcted aorta, acute occlusion of the thoracic aorta has very little effect on cardiovascular variables because of the normal development, over the years, of extensive collateral vessels around the coarctation. However, in patients who have an aortic aneurysm or atherosclerosis and who have no extensive collateral circulation, aortic occlusion increases afterload and peripheral vascular resistance in proportion to the level of the occlusion. We have found that myocardial stress varies with the level of occlusion.[14]

Myocardial performance and circulatory variables remain within an acceptable range after the aorta is occluded at infrarenal levels.[14] This result is in agreement with many of the findings in previous work. In 1968, Perry[83] demonstrated that the increase in afterload after temporary infrarenal aortic occlusion had little effect on circulatory variables. The use of newer, more sophisticated techniques has shown that deepening anesthesia or administering vasodilating drugs at the time of infrarenal aortic occlusion maintains indices of myocardial performance within an acceptable range[28-30,84] even in sick patients (in our series, 25% had severe left ventricular dysfunction before aortic surgery). Abnormalities of ventricular wall motion and systolic thickening, as well as changes in the ejection fraction, appear to be early signs of myocardial ischemia.[85] However, we did not detect abnormal motion of myocardial walls in any of the patients with infrarenal occlusion.[14] Thus far, the results of only one study contradicted the view that myocardial well-being is preserved after infrarenal aortic occlusion. Attia *et al* [31] reported a 30% incidence (three of ten patients) of myocardial ischemia following infrarenal occlusion. Investigators from the same institution (Massachusetts General Hospital), however, later described a technique (the vasodilation already described at the time of cross-clamping) that allows infrarenal aortic occlusion without eliciting evidence of myocardial ischemia.[32] Therefore, on the basis of these data, we consider it safe to assume that aortic occlusion at the infrarenal level increases the afterload only slightly and that current techniques prevent much of the stress on the heart that is associated with such occlusion.

There are few data in published reports on myocardial and cardiovascular effects of occluding the aorta at the suprarenal-infraceliac or supraceliac level in humans. After occluding the descending thoracic aorta in eight patients, Kouchoukos *et al* [34] noted increases of 35, 56, 43, and 90% in mean arterial, central venous, mean pulmonary arterial, and PCWPs, respectively, and a decrease of 29% in cardiac index. These hemodynamic effects are greater than those that we found for supraceliac aortic occlusion and may be attributable to the more proximal level of thoracic aortic occlusion. Occlusion at the supraceliac level causes substantially more myocardial stress, as evidenced by abnormal motion of segments of the left ventricular wall, than does occlusion at the suprarenal-infraceliac or infrarenal level (Table 3).[14]

Table 3. Effect of Level of Aortic Occlusion on Changes in Cardiovascular Variables (%)

	Level of Aortic Occlusion		
	Supraceliac	Suprarenal-Infraceliac	Infrarenal
Mean arterial blood pressure	54	5*	2*
Pulmonary capillary wedge pressure	38	10*	0*
End-diastolic area	28	2*	9*
End-systolic area	69	10*	11*
Ejection fraction	-38	-10*	-3*
Abnormal motion of wall (% of patients)	92	33	0
New myocardial infarctions (% of patients)	8	0	0

* Statistically different ($P< 0.05$) from group undergoing supraceliac occlusion.

Adapted with permission from Roizen MF, Sohn YJ, Stoney RJ: Intraoperative management of the patient undergoing supraceliac aortic occlusion. Vascular Surgery. Wilson SE, Veith FJ, Hobson RW *et al*, eds. New York: McGraw Hill, 1986

Although systemic and PCWPs were kept normal at all times in 10 of 12 patients who underwent occlusion at the supraceliac level, 11 patients had abnormal motion of the left ventricular wall, suggesting ischemia. Some of the factors contributing to this increase in resistance to myocardial ejection may be the more than 100%

increase in peripheral vascular resistance, the change in aortic impedance characteristics, the release of vasoactive substances with intestinal ischemia, or the activation of hormonal systems, all of which lead to ventricular dilation. Despite low ejection fractions, these patients were able to maintain cardiac output and stroke volume via stretch (expansion) of the left ventricle muscle fibers. The PCWP frequently did not reflect this increased left-ventricular end-diastolic volume accurately; however, 2D-TEE made possible the identification and treatment of myocardial dysfunction that was not detected by conventional monitoring techniques.[14,52] The most important lesson learned from the use of 2D echocardiograms on patients undergoing vascular surgery is that dilating the heart with the administration of fluid (as often requested by surgeons for stimulation of urine output) is a likely precursor of myocardial ischemia.

These pathophysiologic changes in hemodynamic variables could result from the effect that clamping has on normal patterns of flow to the arteries. For example, 22% of the cardiac output usually goes to renal vessels, and 27% to the superior mesenteric vessels and celiac trunk.[86] Thus, the expected decrease in flow and the increase in afterload and peripheral vascular resistance after supraceliac aortic occlusion could cause left ventricular dilation. Other factors that may contribute to myocardial dysfunction during operative supraceliac occlusion include release of vasoactive substances from ischemic areas and the presence of unmetabolized citrate from transfused blood.[87]

Results of studies on animals support the view that myocardial function is altered after occlusion of the descending thoracic aorta. Longo *et al* [88] studied coronary and systemic hemodynamic changes in dogs during suprarenal and infrarenal aortic clamping and unclamping. On application of the cross-clamp to the suprarenal aorta, peripheral resistance increased two- to threefold, with immediate hypertension in the proximal segment, marked increases in coronary blood flow and pulse pressure, decreases in aortic blood flow and cardiac output, and little change in the pulse rate. These results were similar to ours.[14] In the study of Longo *et al*,[88] the canine left ventricles were dilated on application of the cross-clamp. Mandelbaum and Webb[89] showed that occluding the descending thoracic aorta in dogs decreased left ventricular function. However, occluding the infrarenal aorta was much less stressful, the cardiovascular consequences being only slight (as they are in human patients with diseased hearts).[14,89]

In normal dogs, the renal artery can be occluded for an hour before the kidneys are injured even slightly.[44] Data from a study which we performed on human subjects support this observation.[42] Preoperative and postoperative renal function did not differ among patients who underwent less than 40 minutes of suprarenal cross-clamping and those who underwent infrarenal aortic occlusion.[42]

Despite the negligible cardiovascular effects of temporarily applying an infrarenal aortic cross-clamp, hypotension ("declamping shock") still occurs on restoration of flow in the aorta. This hemodynamic alteration occurs even when blood flow is restored to only one leg. Although the occurrence of severe hypotension in patients is rare,[32,34,39] moderate hypotension (that is, a decrease in systolic blood pressure of 40 mmHg) is not uncommon.

Two hypotheses are advanced to account for this hypotension. The first suggests that myocardial depression is caused by the washout of acid, acid metabolites, and vasoactive substances from ischemic extremities when blood flow is restored. This hypothesis has largely been discredited in recent years.[28,34,84] Our own work with 2D-TEE supports the second hypothesis, that of a relative depletion of volume. Reactive hyperemia in the freshly revascularized area decreases total vascular resistance, venous return, and blood pressure. Thus, hypotension can be ameliorated by expansion of volume without a decrease in cardiac output; in fact, the expansion may increase cardiac output. However, if hypotension persists for more than 4 minutes after removal of the clamp, and if blood deficits have been replaced, we believe that other causes should be sought. A 2D-TEE of the left ventricle often reveals in these patients that venous return is still inadequate, sometimes as a result of hidden persistent bleeding or misjudged replacement of blood deficits, or that a rare allergic reaction to graft material has occurred.[83]

Because of these complications, we stress, in our monitoring practices, preservation of myocardial, pulmonary, and renal function as well as intravascular volume. We almost always insert a catheter in the radial artery of the nondominant hand. We also monitor urinary output and some form of ventricular filling pressure, the latter usually via a pulmonary-artery catheter. This catheter allows monitoring of systemic vascular resistance, cardiac output, and PCWP. For its insertion, we prefer the external jugular route, although many anesthetists use the internal jugular or subclavian route. We use a modified chest lead to monitor the ECG during the operation, except in those patients who have demonstrated myocardial ischemia in areas other than the anterior myocardial wall. In addition, we almost always monitor body temperature and maintain it meticulously by warming all fluids (starting properatively), and by the use of heating mattresses on the operating room table. If necessary, we humidify the anesthetic gases. We have found 2D-TEE to be an invaluable tool for monitoring of the myocardial consequences of cross-clamping and unclamping of the aorta, and we now use it routinely for such procedures as temporary aortic occlusion at the supraceliac level. A short-axis cross-sectional view of the left ventricle provides an excellent qualitative assessment of left ventricular filling volumes, global ventricular contractility, and regional ventricular function.[90] When a discrepancy exists between pulmonary capillary filling pressures and end-diastolic dimension (volume) obtained by 2D-TEE, we have found the latter to be more reliable and useful.[14,91]

To reduce the incidence of organ ischemia and of pulmonary dysfunction, we manage fluids with the aim of preventing intraoperative hypotension and minimizing cardiac dilation. Although there are no supporting data at present, it is strongly believed that prehydration of patients undergoing vascular reconstructive surgery minimizes the hemodynamic fluctuations that occur with induction of anesthesia, by ensuring that perfusion of vital organs is adequate. During the early period of dissection, intravascular volume is maintained at normal levels by noting ventricular filling on the 2D-TEE or by sustaining a normal PCWP. To accomplish this, we replace blood losses of less than 10 ml $\cdot$ kg^{-1} and insensible losses (assumed to be 5 to 7 ml $\cdot$ kg^{-1} during this dissection phase) are replaced with Ringer's lactate or saline solution.

The indicators used for assessing perfusion of the organs before cross-clamping are: 1) for the heart, myocardial contractility as judged by global and regional motion of the wall on the 2D-TEE,[14,52,91] by the ST segments on the modified chest lead V of the ECG, and by cardiac output; 2) for the kidney, urinary output (2 ml per half hour per 70 kg is adequate, although with 20-30 ml per half hour per 70 kg, it may be easier to convince surgeons of adequacy); urinary flow almost always decreases during dissection around the renal vessels; 3) for the central nervous system, eye signs (although the EEG or sensory evoked potentials or both[92] can be used, we have had little experience with these monitors); and 4) for the lung, gas exchange.

Protection of Myocardium. For the half hour immediately before cross-clamping and aortic occlusion, we keep the patient slightly hypovolemic by examining the ventricular volume, using 2D-TEE, or by keeping pulmonary or arterial pressure at 5 to 12 mmHg. At the time of occlusion, we are prepared to give a vasodilating drug through an intravenous catheter available specifically for that purpose, to avoid hypotension that is secondary to an accidental bolus of vasodilator. This infusion site is often the third lumen of the pulmonary-artery catheter. The difference in our management of aortic occlusion at different levels (e.g., supraceliac versus infrarenal) is that we are absolutely meticulous in planning our management and in executing that procedure in all occlusions planned at renal vessels or above.

During the early part of the aortic dissection, the heart is protected by trying to maintain hemodynamic variables within the range of the preoperative values.[45] Without evidence to the contrary, it is assumed that a little hypertension is just as harmful as a little hypotension. For example, in extreme cases, we might let the systolic blood pressure of a patient whose preoperative range was 110 to 170 mmHg fall to a level as low as 90 mmHg, or rise as high as 190 mmHg. If values approach or exceed these limits, we have a contingency treatment plan. If the blood pressure reaches 150 mmHg, the amount of anesthetic is increased; at approximately 160 mmHg, nitroprusside is infused; at 165 or 175 mmHg, the table is tilted. If the systolic blood pressure drops to 110 mmHg, the anesthetic is decreased and the possible causes of hypotension are reviewed. At 105 mmHg, the amount of anesthetic is decreased even more, and the patient is placed in a head-down position. At 100 mmHg, more fluid is infused, the patient is tilted in a more steeply head-down position, the possible causes of hypotension are reviewed again, and, if possible, the cause is corrected. At 90 mmHg, a dilute infusion of phenylephrine (10 mg in 500 ml, infused at a rate that restores systolic blood pressure to approximately 100 mmHg) is added.

For the heart rate, a range of acceptable values is set based on preoperative determinations. If a preoperative range of 60 to 90 beats · min^{-1} is used as an example, once these limits are exceeded, treatment would be initiated. Here, it is assumed that tachycardia is of greater concern than is bradycardia, and it is avoided more aggressively. At 95 beats · min^{-1}, the level of anesthesia might be increased, more opioid may be given, or an intravenous infusion of a beta-adrenergic receptor blocking drug may be added. At 100 beats · min^{-1}, a bolus is given, or an intravenous infusion of a beta-adrenergic receptor blocker is begun, assuming the intravascular fluid volume is acceptable. At 45 beats · min^{-1}, the anesthetic might be decreased or a dilute solution of dopamine (200 mg in 500 ml) might be administered to keep the heart rate within the acceptable range. It is important to reemphasize that bradycardia is tolerated more than is tachycardia during these operations, because minimizing the myocardial oxygen demand should be of primary importance. Use of 2D-TEE gives some latitude in the range of acceptable values before intervention. However, pulmonary-artery pressures are not allowed to remain abnormal, that is, below 5 or above 15 mmHg, during this procedure, assuming that these values correlate with the echocardiographic values. Increases in pulmonary artery pressure are treated aggressively by administering nitroglycerin or nitroprusside, depending on whether the suspected cause is an increase in preload or an increase in afterload.[93,94] For low pressures, more fluid is infused except in the 1 or 2 minute interval immediately before application of the aortic cross-clamp.

The application of a cross-clamp to the supraceliac aorta probably produces the greatest hemodynamic stress ever experienced by a patient. In fact, 92% of the patients whom we studied had ischemia, as evidenced by abnormal motion and thickening of the wall (Table 3).[14] More distal levels of temporary occlusion are less stressful hemodynamically. Stabilizing pulmonary artery pressure and systemic blood pressure by administering vasodilating drugs before and during suprarenal cross-clamping may not be sufficient. When myocardial ischemia was indicated by abnormal global or regional motion of the wall in patients in our study, we gave more vasodilating drugs, to the point of bringing the systolic blood pressure toward the low end of the normal preoperative range. Once the blood pressure is as low as possible (this is achieved by reduction of the afterload with administration of nitroprusside), we often attempt to decrease the preload with nitroglycerin and, if necessary, to decrease the heart rate with intravenous propranolol or, preferably, with esmolol. If, despite these maneuvers, one sees myocardial dysfunction on placement of the cross-clamp, the surgeon is asked (before he has actually incised the aorta or its branches) to unclamp the aorta partially until myocardial function is more stable. In our study, despite myocardial dysfunction in 11 of the 12 patients who underwent supraceliac cross-clamping, only one of the 11 had perioperative myocardial infarction.[14] Therefore, myocardial contractile function seems to be affected most by ventricular size and by maintenance of vital signs within the normal preoperative range.

Administration of exogenous vasoconstrictors is avoided if possible. Although coronary and cerebral vessels are not prominently innervated, $alpha_1$- and $alpha_2$-adrenergic agents can induce cerebral vasoconstriction. In addition, alpha-adrenergic vasoconstriction appears to be important in maintaining an appropriate distribution of flow between the outer and inner myocardium.[95] Perhaps because of this, or perhaps for other reasons, patients who are deeply anesthetized and whose systemic pressure is maintained with an infusion of phenylephrine have more than twice the incidence of myocardial ischemia than do patients whose blood pressure is maintained simply by light anesthesia and endogenous vasoconstrictors.[12] This ischemia appears to be related to the myocardial dilation induced by these agents (the problem of a stretched, dilated myocardium).[12]

During unclamping of the aorta, a different set of maneuvers is performed for reaching the same goals. To ensure adequate volume when the cross-clamp is removed, blood losses are replaced during occlusion by administering warmed blood, milliliter for milliliter. We normally have only four units of packed cells available during this procedure. The packed cells are diluted with normal saline or lactated Ringer's solution. Although we would prefer to administer whole blood (as that is what is lost), we are unable to obtain it routinely at our institution.

When greater blood loss is anticipated (e.g., for patients previously operated on for the same condition), autotransfusion is often available and a second person to operate it. After the sixth unit of blood has been given and if more blood loss is anticipated, or after eight units of blood have been administered, ten units of platelets are requested for the patient (and occasionally two units of fresh frozen plasma). After giving 8 to 10 units of packed cells, we routinely administer a unit of fresh frozen plasma for each unit of packed cells. When no more blood is at hand, and if it is absolutely necessary (that is, when colloid or crystalloid cannot be used), the best available type-specific, washed packed cells are administered. For example, if B-negative blood is needed but not available, we give B-positive blood. Blood filters are changed after every two units when the blood for transfusion is more than 10 days old, and after every four units when it is less than 10 days old.

Because a large part of the vascular tree is excluded from circulation during temporary aortic occlusion, blood loss can be considerable during supraceliac cross-clamping without onset of hypotension or tachycardia.

Since maintenance of volume status is so important, we monitor more than pulmonary artery pressures or PCWP. Observation of the surgical field is of key importance. When any blood vessel is dissected, the anesthesiologist and surgeon must communicate closely; blood loss can occur with astonishing rapidity, and the attention of the anesthesiologist may not be directed at the operative field. Watching the volumes in the suction bottles supplements the data, as does observation of left ventricular cavity size on 2D-TEE.

Blood loss into the pleural or retroperitoneal cavity may not be detected in the amounts that are measured every 5 to 10 minutes. In addition, evisceration of bowel, often necessary for optimal exposure of the thoracoabdominal aorta, further depletes the intravascular volume. Thus, one must be guided closely by pulmonary artery pressures or echocardiographic estimates of left ventricular filling volumes, or both. Just before opening of the aorta, we allow blood pressure, PCWP, and filling volumes to go as high as possible without the occurrence of myocardial ischemia. The surgeon then opens the aorta gradually to ensure that overly severe hypotension does not develop and that there is not too much bleeding from the suture line.

Pathophysiologic events on removal of the aortic cross-clamp (see previous discussion) are associated with inadequate return of volume to the heart (that is, inadequate preload). Thus, immediately before and during removal of the cross-clamp, we stop infusing nitroprusside and start infusing crystalloid or blood; usually, two units of whole blood are pressured into venous access sites. Guided by filling pressures or echocardiographic estimates of volume, or both, we are careful not to dilate the left ventricle to an abnormal size. Another technique for maintaining normal volumes during cross-clamping is controlled volume depletion, that is, the removal of a specific amount of blood from the patient just before or during application of the cross-clamp for a short period. During the minutes remaining just before the cross-clamp is removed, this amount is replaced. Although we have used this technique, we do not advocate its routine use.

A third techique for maintaining normal hemodynamic values involves the use of halothane, enflurane, or isoflurane, rather than nitroglycerin or nitroprusside, as the vasodilating agent. This is an interesting technique that is usually effective,[96] but it requires very close observation of pulmonary-artery pressures, the echocardiogram, or both, to ensure that myocardial dilation and dysfunction do not occur. This technique is not recommended for routine use.

It is not uncommon for moderate hypotension (that is, decreases in systolic presure of 40 to 60 mmHg) to occur on removal of the aortic cross-clamp, regardless of whether the clamp is replaced infrarenally or in such a way that blood flow to only one leg is obstructed. Our anecdotal impressions, gained in work with 2D-TEE, support the view that such hypotension is caused mainly by relative depletion of volume. Reactive hyperemia in the freshly revascularized area decreases vascular resistance, venous return, and systemic blood pressure. If hypotension persists for more than 4 minutes following removal of the clamp and the pressure does not return toward normal levels after blood deficits have been replaced, other causes should be sought. These include myocardial dysfunction caused by inadequate metabolism of the citrate present in replacement blood; such blood has not yet gone to the liver, where citrate is metabolized. This problem can be treated by administration of calcium, which antagonizes the effect of citrate.[87] Other causes include hidden, persistent bleeding or misjudged replacement of blood deficits; on the echocardiogram, the ventricular cavity is devoid of volume, and on the oscilloscope, filling pressures reflecting pulmonary-artery pressures are low. If necessary, the surgeon can reclamp or occlude the aorta, preferably below the renal arteries. Thus, replacement and maintenance of volume are mainstays of therapy before, during, and immediately after removal of the supraceliac cross-clamp. When blood flow is restored to the first extremity, replacement of volume should also be considered. Removal of the clamp from the second leg usually causes few hemodynamic effects, presumably because of collateral blood vessels across the pelvis.

Central Nervous System Protection. Other investigators have used sensory evoked potentials and the EEG to gauge protection of the spinal cord and cerebrum.[92,97] We have found no benefit in examining the EEG and no evidence that stroke is a predictable consequence of aortic reconstruction, even of supraceliac aortic reconstruction. However, in rare instances, spinal cord ischemia is a predictable consequence of this procedure. Spinal cord sensory evoked potentials may prove useful, but there has not been much experience in the use of this technique. Experiments on animals indicate that isoflurane may allow longer periods of temporary occlusion of the blood supply to the spinal cord before development of permanent neurologic injury than are possible with other anesthetic agents. Other halogenated anesthetics and intravenous anesthetics decrease the interval during which the spinal cord can be ischemic before permanent neurologic damage sets in in this animal model.[98]

Renal Protection. Intraoperative urinary output is not predictive of postoperative renal function.[42] In 137 patients undergoing aortic reconstruction (38 at the supraceliac level), we measured the hourly urine output and calculated each patient's lowest and mean urinary outputs. The PCWP was kept within normal limits in each patient. If urinary output was less than $0.125\ ml \cdot kg^{-1} \cdot hr^{-1}$, patients were given either crystalloid (so that the PCWP was raised to a high-normal level) or furosemide, mannitol, or nothing. For each patient, serum creatinine and blood urea nitrogen (BUN) were assayed on the first, third, and seventh postoperative days. There was no significant correlation between intraoperative mean urinary ouput, or lowest hourly urinary output, and changes from preoperative to postoperative levels of creatinine or BUN. Thus, urinary output, which is believed to be an index of perfusion and therefore is monitored routinely during surgery, was not predictive of postoperative renal function in normovolemic patients.

When patients who underwent aortic occlusion at the suprarenal level were compared with those who underwent occlusion at the infrarenal level, there was no difference in postoperative renal function.[42]

Our results for patients who underwent aortic reconstruction conflict with those of other studies. In investigations in which a period of renal ischemia was imposed on patients and animal models, pretreatment with mannitol lessened post-ischemic increases in creatinine.[99-102] Direct infusion of mannitol into the renal artery sustained renal cortical perfusion (as assayed by the xenon washout technique) in mongrel dogs after infrarenal aortic occlusion.[99] In rabbits, pretreatment with mannitol prevented an increase in serum creatinine after 60 minutes of renal artery occlusion.[102] In dogs subjected to aortic clamping and unclamping, adequate replacement of blood with saline prevented a decrease in renal blood flow, an occurrence that is consistent with the findings of Alpert *et al*[42] In addition, furosemide and ethacrynic acid significantly increase both the total and the cortical components of renal blood flow, as demonstrated by studies of xenon-133 washout.[99] The use of mannitol, furosemide, or ethacrynic acid, however, has not been clearly shown to prevent renal failure. The difference between the results of Alpert *et al* and those of others[99-102] may be due to variations among species, the maintenance of normal intravascular volume by Alpert *et al*, the insensitivity of urinary output as a measure of the adequacy of renal perfusion, or a combination of these factors. We believe that preoperative renal function and the maintenance of an appropriate intravascular volume and of normal myocardial function are the most important determinants of postoperative renal function.

It is important to monitor renal function because development of acute renal failure after aortic reconstruction is associated with high morbidity and a mortality rate of more than 30%.[103] This complication is most frequent in patients with ruptured aneurysms who have significant hypotensive episodes, and in those for whom suprarenal aortic clamping is required. Despite our aforementioned data, infusion of mannitol prior to clamping of the renal arteries is believed by some to be beneficial and is commonly used.[104,105] Furosemide, vasodilators, and angiotensin-converting enzyme inhibitors may also have a place before renal artery clamping. If prolonged renal ischemia is anticipated, selective profound hypothermia of the kidneys may decrease the incidence of postoperative renal impairment. Recently, it was suggested that infusion of verapamil into the renal arteries just before reperfusion may also be beneficial,[105] although the question has been raised as to whether anything better than good surgical technique exists.[42] Our management, however, is biased by the results of our own studies. Thus, when intraoperative urinary output is less than $0.125 ml \cdot kg^{-1} \cdot hr^{-1}$, we ensure that no mechanical problems in urine collection are present and that left-sided cardiac filling volumes or pressures are adequate. We then continue to monitor but do not treat. Urinary output usually returns to acceptable levels within 2 hours. If it does not, or if we are uneasy about low urinary output, 2 to 5 mg of furosemide are administered intravenously for stimulation of urine production.[42]

Thus, virtually all investigators have concluded that the maintenance of adequate intravascular volume and myocardial function largely prevents renal insufficiency and insufficiency of other organs from being major clinical problems and that it is the key to intraoperative perfusion of critical organs.

Surgery for Peripheral Vascular Insufficiency

There are three clinical indications for elective surgery for chronic peripheral occlusive disease: 1) claudication, 2) ischemic rest pain or ulceration, and 3) gangrene.[106] Patients with claudication have symptoms on walking that are relieved by rest. Such patients are not at significant risk for imminent limb loss. Patients with rest pain, ulceration, and/or gangrene are at variable risk for imminent limb loss and may have severe progressive ischemia. Thus, reconstruction is semi-urgent or urgent. Vascular reconstruction procedures are generally categorized as either inflow or outflow procedures. Inflow reconstruction involves bypass of the obstruction in the aortoiliac segment, whereas outflow procedures are those performed distal to the inguinal ligament for bypass of femoralpopliteal or distal obstructions.

The most common inflow reconstruction procedure for obstructions in the aortoiliac segment is aortofemoral bypass. The usual vascular reconstruction below the inguinal ligament is a bypass graft which originates in the common femoral artery and extends to the popliteal or tibial artery. Such a bypass may be performed with a reversed saphenous vein, the saphenous vein *in situ*, or a prosthetic graft.[107] For the vascular surgeon, the differences among these procedures involve different technical aspects of vessel dissection and exposure, of anastomosis, and of tunneling.

The complexity of femoralpopliteal and femoraltibial bypass varies widely. The site for distal anastomosis and the quality of the outflow vessels are assessed by preoperative angiography. The best short- and long-term results are achieved when the saphenous vein is used[108,109]; however, this requires longer operative time and greater technical expertise than are needed for prosthetic grafts. The duration and complexity of the operation are usually determined by the quality of the saphenous vein and the quality and size of the distal outflow vessels. Operative arteriography is commonly used for evaluation of the adequacy of the surgical repair. Major blood loss or hemodynamic changes are not usually encountered with distal reconstruction, but the procedure tends to be lengthy, making intraoperative urinary drainage advisable. Since the major morbidity and mortality with this procedure are related to the cardiovascular system, with rates above 8% and 2%, respectively, the noninvasive nature and the absence of hemodynamic alterations should not lull the anesthesiologist into taking a casual attitude.[107-109]

In a reversed saphenous vein bypass, the vein is dissected from its entrance into the common femoral vein to the level of the distal anastomosis. All branches of the saphenous vein are ligated and divided, and the vein is excised and inspected. After exposure of the proximal and distal vessels, the direction of the saphenous vein is reversed to permit blood flow in the direction of the valves, and the vein is tunneled from the femoral artery to the distal vessel. In this process, the surgeon tries to avoid damaging, injuring, or twisting the vein. After the proximal and distal anastomoses are completed, the adequacy of flow is determined from the quality of pulse and ultrasound signals, and from angiographic images obtained on completion.

The use of the vein *in situ* offers significant advantages over the reversed-vein bypass. The large proximal saphenous vein is sutured to the large common femoral vein, and the small distal vein is sutured to the small distal artery. The size match is particularly important for tibial artery bypass, which permits the use of small saphenous veins that were previously judged unsuitable. In addition, since the vein is not removed from its bed, it is subjected to little trauma, and twisting or kinking is unlikely. These advantages have resulted in improved patency rates.[110,111]

For bypass procedures in which the saphenous vein *in situ* is used, the vein in its bed is dissected, and side branches are ligated. The proximal saphenous vein is then sutured end-to-side to the common femoral artery, and arterial flow is introduced into the vein. The valves that obstruct retrograde flow in the saphenous vein are lysed with a valvulotome or valve cutter, which is introduced through side branches. When all valves have been rendered incompetent, blood is seen flowing from the distal end of the vein. This distal end is then anastomosed to the appropriate arterial site. Here, also, the quality of the repair is determined from the pulse quality, doppler ultrasound studies, and completion angiography.

Prosthetic bypasses can be performed more quickly and require less dissection than does saphenous-vein bypass, because it is not necessary to make multiple incisions for vein harvest. Prosthetic bypasses, however, have significantly lower patency rates than do saphenous-vein bypasses, particularly when they extend below the knee.[110] Incisions are made for exposure of the proximal and distal arteries, and a tunneling instrument is used for tunneling of the graft between the incisions. After completion of the proximal and distal anastomoses, the quality of the anastomoses and the blood runoff to the foot are judged by intraoperative angiography. The patient is usually given heparin during the procedure; in most cases, the heparin effect is not antagonized, since bleeding problems are rare.

Emergency surgery for peripheral vascular insufficiency is required when acute arterial occlusion results in severe ischemia and threatens the viability of a limb. Immediate operation and restoration of blood flow are needed if limb loss is to be avoided. Depending on the etiology of the occlusion, the patient may or may not be at very high risk.

Acute arterial occlusion causes the involved extremity to suddenly become cold and pulseless. Patients usually complain of coldness, pain, numbness, and paresthesias, and they may lose motion and sensation. The severity of ischemia and the urgency of immediate operation can be assessed by examination of leg motion and sensation. Abnormal sensation in the toes, feet, and legs in response to light touch and pin prick, as well as abnormal proprioception and loss of motor function in the feet and toes, are hallmarks of acute ischemia and nonviability. If the ischemia is not reversed in a matter of hours, irreversible loss of viability is likely to result.

Acute arterial occlusion may develop in patients who have pre-existing peripheral occlusive or aneurysmal disease caused by thrombosis of a stenotic or ulcerated atherosclerotic artery. Acute arterial occlusion can also occur in patients with normal peripheral arteries that contain emboli. Such embolism is usually of cardiac origin in patients with cardiac dysrhythmias, recent myocardial infarctions, or ventricular aneurysms.[112,113]

The cause is important in planning of operative treatment. If the cause is an arterial embolus, Fogarty embolectomy through a groin incision under local anesthesia may suffice. However, if the cause is thrombosis of severely diseased atherosclerotic arteries, bypass reconstruction will be required. Preoperative angiography may be of help in the differential diagnosis; often the cause is not uncovered until the vessel is opened. Thus, the anesthesiologist must be prepared for either a simple or a complex, extended procedure.

Patients with acute ischemia (arterial insufficiency) may be very ill. Significant fluid losses can be anticipated when the artery is flushed during thrombectomy, and fluid can be sequestered in edematous revascularized tissue. Serum potassium levels can change quickly, since cell death and release of intracellular potassium into the circulation can be anticipated. Myoglobin may also be released into the circulation, and the development of compartment syndrome is a possibility.

An incision in the groin is usually made for exposure of the femoral artery. Attempts to pass Fogarty catheters proximally and distally are made in the effort to establish flow and extract the thrombus. If flow is not restored in this manner, more complex reconstructive procedures such as aortofemoral, axillofemoral, or femoropopliteal bypass may be required. Femoral venous drainage on restoration of flow to the femoral artery can aid in management by wasting the initial venous effluent from an acutely ischemic extremity. This may entail significant blood loss.

Anesthetic Goals and Management

There is perhaps no other disease entity in which the anesthesiologist can be misled so easily. "Oh, it's just a local procedure"; or, "just put a spinal in and let's get on with it; you don't have to read the chart." The latter was a comment used by an experienced vascular surgeon. However, the morbidity and mortality following these distal operations approach those following infraaortic reconstruction and are mainly of cardiac origin. Thus, although I tend to use epidural anesthesia and epidural opioids for pain relief, attention to body temperature, oxygen delivery, and hemodynamic homeostasis should be just as intense here as in aortic procedures that involve much greater hemodynamic fluctuations. The devices and the previously described concerns apply, with special attention to the postoperative period. It is during the postoperative period that most cardiac problems arise, and this is when pain relief and correction of hemodynamic and fluid dysequilibria are most likely to be needed. Care must be taken not to allow overhydration to occur intraoperatively in support of blood pressure, and then to cause congestive heart failure as the epidural sympathectomy wears off. As is done for patients with aortic disease, I routinely tilt the patient's head down (while monitoring gas exchange closely) for the last hour of the planned surgery. Dye loads given for completion angiography also contribute to fluid shifts; I consider monitoring of left ventricular filling volumes to be important for a successful outcome for these patients.

The surgeons' concerns for patients with peripheral vascular insufficiency include not only those involving the cardiovascular system, but also specific problems related to the operative repair. Graft patency is evaluated carefully in the recovery room. Most surgeons believe that the patient's feet should be kept warm and that the patient should be well hydrated so that peripheral vasoconstriction, which may limit outflow from the new graft, is prevented. If graft thrombosis develops in the early postoperative period, the patient is promptly returned to the operating room for graft thrombectomy and for evaluation and correction of the cause of the thrombosis. It can be anticipated that, during graft thrombectomy, significant blood loss will occur with flushing of the graft.

Conclusion

Perhaps in no other subspecialty can anesthesiologists have as great an influence on patient outcome as they do in anesthesia for vascular surgery. Similar considerations for preopertive patient evaluation can be made for patients with cardiac disease undergoing other noncardiac procedures. The patients undergoing vascular reconstruction are generally elderly. Vascular disease is a generalized process; thus, patients having surgery for a specific vascular disorder are likely to have atherosclerotic disease elsewhere in the vascular system. Most of the patients have coronary artery disease. Many have a history of smoking, and chronic obstructive pulmonary disease, renal insufficiency, and lipid abnormalities are frequently present. Data show that, although blood flow to many different organs may be interrupted, the stress of clamping and unclamping of vessels differs in different operations, and comorbid conditions of patients are not similar in different operations; the major morbidity in each of the operations relates to myocardial well-being; therefore, the heart should be the major focus of the anesthesiologist's attention.

Attempts have been made to segregate patients who have significant coronary artery disease by use of dipyridamole-thallium scanning or coronary angiography or other means, and then to have patients at high risk for myocardial events undergo coronary artery bypass surgery before their vascular surgery. However, it has not been proved that such approaches reduce morbidity. Critics claim that such segregation is useful for identification of high-risk patients, but that coronary angiography and surgery are simply a survival test preparatory to vascular surgery.

In cerebrovascular surgery, the goals in anesthesia management of ensuring adequate myocardial and brain perfusion and a rapidly arousable patient may be facilitated with the use of the EEG as a guide to afterload reduction. In aortic reconstruction, the available data imply that ensuring intact myocardial function is probably the best way of making certain that spinal cord, visceral, and renal perfusion will be adequate.

In the case of peripheral occlusive disease, the absence of hemodynamic changes should not lull the anesthesiologist into believing that vigilance about the patient's myocardial well-being will not be rewarded. It is also important to remember that vigilance in ensuring that routines such as prehydration and use of a warming mattress is probably more important for the outcome than is occasional brilliance. If given the opportunity, I would opt for the diligent, compulsive practitioner rather than the occasionally brilliant one, if I needed vascular surgery.

Perhaps in no circumstance is the mettle of an anesthesiologist determined better than in anesthesia for emergency vascular surgery. The conversion in our mind from being a trauma anesthesiologist to caring for the heart is a difficult challenge that should be undertaken as soon as hemodynamic stability occurs.

In this review, I have expressed my biases regarding both monitoring and anesthetic techniques; but it should be clear that many other approaches can be used for avoiding myocardial dysfunction. Perhaps it is most important to remember that the best patient results probably are achieved when the great vigilance shown intraoperatively is also applied preoperatively as well as postoperatively.

REFERENCES

1. Sundt TM, Sharbrough FW, Piepgras DG, et al: Mayo Clin Proc 56:533-543, 1981
2. Hertzer NR, Lees CD: Ann Surg 194:212-218, 1981
3. Ennix CL, Lawrie GM, Morris GC: Stroke 10:122-125, 1979
4. Glaser RB: In Anesthesia for Vascular Surgery. Edited by Roizen MF. New York, Churchill Livingstone, 1989 (in press)
5. Hertzer NR, Bevan EG, Young JR, et al: Ann Surg 199:223-233, 1984
6. Kartchmer MM, McRae LP: Arch Surg 117:1086-1088, 1982
7. Dunn EJ: Surg Clin N Am 66:385-395, 1986
8. Hertzer NR, Loop FD, Taylor PC, et al: J Thorac Cardiovasc Surg 85:577-589, 1983
9. Barnes RW, Marsalek PG: Stroke 12:497-500, 1981
10. Burke PA, Callow AD, O'Donnell TF, Kelly JJ: Arch Surg 117:1222-1227, 1982
11. Graham AM, Gewertz BL, Zarins CK: Arch Surg 121:595-598, 1986
12. Smith JS, Roizen MF, Cahalan MK, Beaupre PN, Sohn YJ, Benefiel DJ, Lurz FW, Byrd BF, Bouchard A, Schiller NB, Stoney RJ, Ehrenfeld WK, Ellis JE, Aronson S: Anesthesiology 69: 846-853, 1988
13. Roizen MF, Ellis JE, Smith JS, Stoney RJ, Gewertz BL: In Anesthesia and the Heart Patient. Edited by Estafanous FG. Butterworth, 1989, pp.183-195
14. Roizen MF, Beaupre PN, Alpert RA, Kremer P, Cahalan MK, Sohn YJ, Schiller NB, Cronnelly R, Lurz FW, Ehrenfeld WK, Stoney RJ: J Vasc Surg 1:300-305, 1984
15. Nevelsteen A, Suy R, Daenen MD, et al: Surgery 88:642-653, 1980
16. Martinez BD, Hertzer NR, Beven EG: Surgery 88:795-805, 1980
17. Szilagyi DE, Smith RF, Derusso FJ, Elliott JP, Sherrin FW: Ann Surg 164:678-699, 1966
18. Young AE, Sandberg GW, Couch NP: Am J Surg 134:585-590, 1977
19. Hicks GL, Eastland MW, Deweese JA, May AG, Rob CG: Ann Surg 181:863-869, 1975
20. Thompson JE, Hollier LH, Patman RD, Persson AV: Ann Surg 181:654-661, 1975
21. Mulcare RJ, Royster TS, Lynn RA, Conners RB: Arch Surg 113:601-604, 1978
22. Whittemore AD, Clowes AW, Hechtman HB, Mannick JA: Ann Surg 192: 414-421, 1980
23. Crawford ES, Saleh SA, Babb JW III, Glaeser DH, Vaccaro PS, Silvers A: Ann Surg 193:699-709, 1981
24. Hertzer NR: Surgery 93:97-101, 1983
25. Yeager RA, Weigel RM, Murphy SS, McConnell DB, Sasaki TM, Vetto M: Arch Surg 121:278-281, 1986
26. Benefiel DJ, Roizen MF, Lampe GH, Sohn YJ, Fong KS, Irwin DH, Drasner K, Smith JS, Stoney RJ, Ehrenfeld WK, Goldstone JS, Reilly LM, Thisted RA, Eger EI II: Anesthesiology 65:A516, 1986
27. Roizen MF: In Clinical Frontiers in Anesthesiology. Edited by Benumof JL. New York, Churchill Livingstone, 1983, pp 93-104
28. Carroll RM, Laravuso RB, Schauble JF: Arch Surg 111:740-743, 1976
29. Lunn JK, Dannemiller FJ, Stanley TH: Anesth Analg 58:372-376, 1979
30. Meloche R, Pottecher T, Audet J, Dufresne O, Lepage C: Can Anaesth Soc J 24:20-34, 1977

31. Attia RR, Murphy JD, Snider M, Lappas DG, Darling RC, Lowenstein E: Circulation 53:961-965, 1976
32. Silverstein PR, Caldera DL, Cullen DJ, Davison JK, Darling RC, Emerson CW: Anesthesiology 50:462-470, 1979
33. Plecha FR, Avellone JC, Beven EG, et al: Surgery 86:826-834, 1979
34. Kouchoukos NT, Lell WA, Karp RB, Samuelson PN: Surgery 85:25-30, 1979
35. DeBakey ME, Creech O Jr, Morris GC Jr: Ann Surg 144:549-573, 1956
36. Burham SJ, Johnson G Jr, Gurri JA: Surgery 92:1072-1076, 1983
37. Denlin A, Ohlsen H, Swedenborg J: Brit J Surg 72:530-532, 1985
38. Darling RC: Am J Surg 119:397-401, 1970
39. Sabawala PB, Strong MJ, Keats AS: Anesthesiology 33:229-259, 1970
40. Barry KG, Mazze RI, Schwartz FD: N Engl J Med 270:1371-1377, 1964
41. Wheeler CG, Thompson JE, Kartchner MM, Austin DJ, Patman RD: N Engl J Med 275:320-322, 1968
42. Alpert RA, Roizen MF, Hamilton WK, Stoney RJ, Ehrenfeld WK, Poler SM, Wylie EJ: Surgery 95:707-711, 1984
43. Bush HL Jr, LoGerfo FW, Weisel RD, Mannick JA, Hechtman HB: Arch Surg 112:1301-1305, 1977
44. Moyer JH, Heider C, Morris GC Jr, Handley C: Ann Surg 145:41-58, 1957
45. Roizen MF: In Anesthesia. 2nd ed., vol. 1. Edited by Miller RD. New York, Churchill Livingstone, 1986, pp 255-357
46. Boucher CA, Brewster DC, Darling RC, Okada RD, Strauss HW, Pohost GM: N Engl J Med 312:389-394, 1985
47. Larson CP: Anesthesia for cerebrovascular insufficiency: How I do it in Palo Alto. In Anesthesia for Vascular Surgery. Edited by Roizen MF. New York, Churchill Livingstone, 1989 (in press)
48. Hamilton WK: Anesthesiology 45:273-274, 1976
49. Boysen G, Engell HC, Henriksen H: Neurology 22:1133-1144, 1972
50. Stundt TM, Houser OW, Sharbrough FW, Messick JM Jr: Adv Neurol 16:97-119, 1977
51. Ehrenfeld WK, Hamilton WK, Larson CP, Hickey RF, Severinghaus JW: Surgery 67:87-96, 1970
52. Smith JS, Cahalan MK, Benefiel DJ, Byrd BF, Lurz FW, Shapiro WA, Roizen MF, Bouchard A, Schiller NB: Circulation 872: 1015-1021, 1985
53. Ellis JE, Roizen MF Aronson S, Feinstein SB, Briller JE: Anesthesiology 67:A002, 1987
54. Kotrly KJ, Kotter GS, Mortara D, Kampine JP: Anesth Analg 63:343-345, 1984
55. Pichard AD, Diaz R, Marchant E, Casanegra P: Clin Cardiol 6:534- ,1983
56. Riles TS, Kopelman I, Imparato AM: Myocardial infarction following carotid endarterectomy: a review of 683 operations. Surgery 85:249-252, 1979
57. Wylie EJ: Is an asymptomatic carotid stenosis a surgical lesion? Presidential Address, Society of Cardiovascular Surgeons, 1982
58. McCaffrey MT: EEG and its transformation and meaning. In Anesthesia for Vascular Surgery. Edited by Roizen MF. New York, Churchill Livingstone, 1989 (in press)
59. Rampil IS, Holzer JA, Quest DO, et al: Anesth Analg 62:186- , 1983
60. Rosenthal D, Stanton PE, Lamis PA: Arch Surg 116:1569- , 1981
61. Cho I, Smullens SN, Streletz LJ, Fariello RG: Ann Neurol 20:508- , 1986
62. Blume WT, Ferguson GG, McNeil DK: Significance of EEG changes at carotid endarterectomy. Stroke 17:891- , 1986
63. Morawetz RB, Zeiger HE, McDowell HA, et al: Surgery 96:184- ,1984

64. McCaffrey MT: Somatosensory and motor evoked potentials, their interpretation and meaning. In Anesthesia for Vascular Surgery. Edited by Roizen MF. New York, Churchill Livingstone, 1989 (in press)
65. Russ W, Fraedrich G: Thorac Cardiovasc Surg 32:124,1984
66. Jacobs JA, Brinkman SD, Morrell RM, et al: Amer Surgeon 49:338- , 1983
67. Markand ON, Dilley RS, Moorthy SS, Warren C: Arch Neurol 41:375- , 1984
68. Moorthy SS, Markand ON, Dilley RS, et al: Anesth Analg 61:879- , 1982
69. Messick JM, Casement B, Sharbrough FW, Milde LN, Michenfelder JD, Sundt TM: Anesthesiology 66:344- , 1987
70. McKay RD, Sundt TM Jr, Michenfelder JD, Gronert GA, Messick JM Jr, Sharbrough FW, Piepgras DG: Anesthesiology 45:390-399, 1976
71. Slogoff S, Keats AS: Anesthesiology 65:539-542, 1986
72. Egbert LD, Battit GE, Turndorf H, Beecher HK: JAMA 185:553-555, 1963
73. Bedford RF: Anesthesiology 47:37-39, 1977
74. Lanier WL, Stangland KJ, Scheithauer BW, Milde JH, Michenfelder JD: Anesthesiology 66:39- , 1987
75. Farias LA, Willis M, Gregory GA: Anesthesiology 65:595-601, 1986
76. Roizen MF, Sohn YJ, L'Hommedieu CS, Wylie EJ, Ota MK: Anesth Analg 59:852-855, 1980
77. Nehls DG, Todd MM, Spetzler RF, Drummond BC, Thompson RA, Johnson PC: Anesthesiology 66:453- , 1987
78. Wade JG, Larson CP, Hiday RF, Ehrenfeld WK, Severinghaus JW: N Engl J Med 282:823- , 1970
79. Hosobuchi Y, Baskin DS, Woo SK: Science 215:69-71
80. Stinson EB, Holloway EL, Derby G, et al.: Circulation 53 (Suppl I), I-26-33, 1974.
81. Assidoa CB, Donegan JH, Whitesell RC, Kalbfleisch JH: Anesth Analg 61:631- , 1982
82. Tarlov E, Schmidek H, Scott RM, Wepsic JG, Ojemann RG: J Neurosurg 39:323-237, 1973
83. Perry MO: Ann Surg 168:193-200, 1968
84. Bush HL Jr, LoGerfo FW, Weisel RD, Mannick JA, Hechtman HB: Arch Surg 112:1301-1305, 1977
85. Pandian NG, Kerber RE: Circulation 66:597-602, 1982
86. Guyton AC: Textbook of Medical Physiology, 6th ed. Philadelphia, WB Saunders, 1981
87. Olinger GN, Hottenrott C, Mulder DG, Maloney JV Jr, Miller J, Patterson RW, Sullivan SF, Buckberg GD: J Thorac Cardiovasc Surg 72:503-511, 1976
88. Longo T, Marchetti G, Vercellio G: J Cardiovasc Surg 10:36-42, 1969
89. Mandelbaum I, Webb MK: JAMA 186:229-231, 1963
90. Schlüter M, Langenstein BA, Polster J, Kremer P, Souquet J, Engel S, Hanrath P: Brit Heart J 48:67-72, 1982
91. Beaupre PN, Cahalan MK, Kremer PF, Roizen MF, Cronnelly R, Robinson S, Lurz FW, Alpert R, Hamilton WK, Schiller NB: Anesthesiology 59:A3, 1983
92. Laschinger JC, Cunningham JN Jr, Catinella FP, Nathan IM, Knopp TA, Spencer FC: Surgery 92:1109-1117, 1982
93. Flaherty JT, Magee PA, Gardner TL, Potter A, MacAllister NP: Circulation 65:1072-1077, 1982
94. Gerson JI, Allen FB, Seltzer JL, Parker FB Jr, Markowitz AH: Anesth Analg 61:256-260, 1982
95. Feigl EO: Circulation 76:737-745, 1987

96. Roizen MF, Hamilton WK, Sohn YJ: Anesthesiology 55:446-450, 1981
97. Rampil IJ, Correll JW, Rosenbaum SH, Quest DO, Holzer JA: Neurosurgery 13:276-279, 1983
98. Koike M, Roizen MF, Zivin JA, Shnider SM, Krusko N, Joyce JT: Anesthesiology 59:A333, 1983
99. Abbott WM, Austen WG: J Surg Res 16:482-489, 1974
100. Barry KG, Cohen A, Knochel JP, Whelan TJ Jr, Beisel WR, Vargas CA, Leblanc PC Jr: N Engl J Med 264:967-971, 1961
101. Flores J, DiBona DR, Beck CH, Leaf A: J Clin Invest 51:118-126, 1972
102. Hanley MJ, Davidson K: Am J Physiol 241:F556-564, 1981
103. Ostri P, Mouritsen L, Jorgensen B, et al: J Cardiovasc Surg 27:714-718, 1986
104. Lusby RJ: In Anesthesia for Vascular Surgery. Edited by Roizen MF. New York, Churchill Livingstone, 1989 (in press)
105. Miller DC, Myers BD: J Vasc Surg 5:518-523, 1987
106. Zarins CZ: In Anesthesia for Vascular Surgery. Edited by Roizen MF. New York, Churchill Livingstone, 1989 (in press)
107. Veith FJ, Gupta SK, Ascer E: In Vascular Surgery: Principles and Practice. Edited by Wilson SE, Veith FJ, Hobson RW, Williams RA. New York, McGraw-Hill, 1987, pp 353-375
108. Mannick JA, Jackson BT, Coffman JD: Surgery 61:17- , 1967
109. Reichle FA, Tyson R: Ann Surg 182:449- , 1975
110. Leather RP, Shah DM, Karmody AM: Surgery 90:1000- , 1981
111. Buchbinder D, Singh JK, Karmody AM, Leather RP, Shah DM: J Surg Res 30:213- , 1981
112. Abbott WM, Maloney RD, McCabe RD, et al: Am J Surg 143:460-464, 1982
113. Connett MC, Murray DH Jr, Denneker WW: Am J Surg 148:14-19, 1984

DEVELOPMENTS IN CRITICAL CARE MEDICINE AND ANESTHESIOLOGY

1. Prakash, O. (ed.): Applied Physiology in Clinical Respiratory Care. 1982. ISBN 90–247–2662–X.
2. McGeown, Mary G.: Clinical Management of Electrolyte Disorders. 1983. ISBN 0–89838–559–8.
3. Stanley, T.H., and Petty, W.C. (eds.): New Anesthetic Agents, Devices and Monitoring Techniques. 1983. ISBN 0–89838–566–0.
4. Scheck, P.A., Sjöstrand, U.H., and Smith, R.B. (eds.): Perspectives in High Frequency Ventilation. 1983. ISBN 0–89838–571–7.
5. Prakash, O. (ed.): Computing in Anesthesia and Intensive Care. 1983. ISBN 0–89838–602–0.
6. Stanley, T.H., and Petty, W.C. (eds.): Anesthesia and the Cardiovascular System. Annual Utah Postgraduate Course in Anesthesilogy. 1984. ISBN 0–89838–626–8.
7. van Kleef, J.W., Burm, A.G.L., and Spierdijk, J. (eds.): Current Concepts in Regional Anaesthesia. 1984. ISBN 0–89838–644–6.
8. Prakash, O. (ed.): Critical Care of the Child. 1984. ISBN 0–89838–661–6.
9. Stanley, T.H., and Petty, W.C. (eds.): Anesthesiology: Today and Tomorrow. Annual Utah Postgraduate Course in Anesthesiology. 1985. ISBN 0–89838–705–1.
10. Rahn, H., and Prakash, O. (eds.): Acid-base Regulation and Body Temperature. 1985. ISBN 0–89838–708–6.
11. Stanley, T.H., and Petty, W.C. (eds.): Anesthesiology. 1986. Annual Utah Postgraduate Course in Anesthesiology. 1986. ISBN 0–89838–779–5.
12. de Lange, S., Hennis, P.J., and Kettler, D. (eds.): Cardiac Anaesthesia: Problems and Innovations. 1986. ISBN 0–89838–794–9.
13. de Bruijn, N.P., and Clements, F.M.: Transesophageal Echocardiography. 1987. ISBN 0–89838–821–X.
14. Graybar, G.B., and Bready, L.L. (eds.): Anesthesia for Renal Transplantation. 1987. ISBN 0–89838–837–6.
15. Stanley, T.H., and Petty, W.C. (eds.): Anesthesia, the Heart and the Vascular System. Annual Utah Postgraduate Course in Anesthesiology. 1987. ISBN 0–89838–851–1.
16. Ronai, A.K.: Autologous Blood Transfusions. 1988. ISBN 0–89838–899–6.
17. Stanley, T.H. (ed.): What's New in Anesthesiology. Annual Utah Postgraduate Course in Anesthesiology. 1988. ISBN 0–89838–367–6.
18. Woerlee, G.M.: Common Perioperative Problems and the Anaesthetist. 1988. ISBN 0–89838–402–8.
19. Stanley, T.H., and Sperry, R.J. (eds.): Anesthesia and the Lung. 1989. ISBN 0–7923–0075–0.
20. De Castro, J., Meynadier, J., and Zenz, M.: Regional Opioid Analgesia. Physiopharmacological Basis, Drugs, Equipment and Clinical Application. 1989. ISBN 0–7923–0162–5.
21. Crul, J.F. (ed.): Legal Aspects of Anaesthesia. 1989. ISBN 0–7923–0393–8.
22. Freye, E. (ed.), Cerebral Monitoring in the Operating Room and the Intensive Care Unit. (In prep.) ISBN 0–7923–0349–X
23. Stanley, T.H., and Sperry, R.J. (eds.): Anesthesiology and the Heart. 1990. ISBN 0–7923–0634–1

GPSR Compliance

The European Union's (EU) General Product Safety Regulation (GPSR) is a set of rules that requires consumer products to be safe and our obligations to ensure this.

If you have any concerns about our products, you can contact us on ProductSafety@springernature.com

In case Publisher is established outside the EU, the EU authorized representative is:

Springer Nature Customer Service Center GmbH
Europaplatz 3
69115 Heidelberg, Germany

Batch number: 10761599

Printed by Printforce, the Netherlands